Coming Too Late

SUNY series, Insinuations: Philosophy, Psychoanalysis, Literature

Charles Shepherdson, editor

Coming Too Late

REFLECTIONS ON FREUD AND BELATEDNESS

ANDREW BARNABY

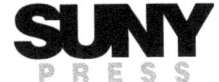

René Magritte, "La Reproduction interdite (Reproduction Forbidden)"
Cover art: © 2017 C. Herscovici / Artists Rights Society (ARS), New York.

Published by State University of New York Press, Albany

© 2017 State University of New York

All rights reserved

Printed in the United States of America

No part of this book may be used or reproduced in any manner whatsoever without written permission. No part of this book may be stored in a retrieval system or transmitted in any form or by any means including electronic, electrostatic, magnetic tape, mechanical, photocopying, recording, or otherwise without the prior permission in writing of the publisher.

For information, contact State University of New York Press, Albany, NY
www.sunypress.edu

Production, Diane Ganeles
Marketing, Michael Campochiaro

Library of Congress Cataloging-in-Publication Data

Name: Barnaby, Andrew Thomas, author.
Title: Coming too late : reflections on Freud and belatedness / Andrew Barnaby.
Description: Albany, NY : State University of New York Press, [2017] | Series: SUNY series, Insinuations: Philosophy, psychoanalysis, literature | Includes bibliographical references and index.
Identifiers: LCCN 2016034117 | ISBN 9781438465777 (hardcover : alk. paper) | ISBN 9781438465760 (pbk. : alk. paper)
Subjects: LCSH: Parent and child. | Childbirth—Psychological aspects. | Pre-existence. | Oedipus complex. | Freud, Sigmund, 1856–1939.
Classification: LCC BF723.P25 B295 2017 | DDC 150.19/52—dc23
LC record available at https://lccn.loc.gov/2016034117

10 9 8 7 6 5 4 3 2 1

*For Emma and Ian,
and in loving memory of Claire (1996–1998)*

Contents

Note on Citations for Major Primary Works   ix

Acknowledgments   xi

Introduction   1

Part I
The Refusal of Being Born:
Psychoanalysis, Belatedness, and Existential Trauma

Introduction to Part I
Why Are We Born? Inversion in Freud's "Theme of the
Three Caskets"   23

Chapter 1
"Awakening is itself the site of a trauma": Rethinking Caruth
on Freud   35

Chapter 2
Owing Life: The Birth Trauma and its Discontents (Rank and Freud)   53

Part II
Tardy Sons: Shakespeare, Freud, and Filial Ambivalence

Chapter 3
"More than his father's death": Mourning at Elsinore and Vienna   77

Chapter 4
The Afterwards of the Uncanny   119

Part III
"Is not He your Father who created you?": Belatedness and the Judeo-Christian Tradition

Introduction to Part III Gazing on God	151
Chapter 5 Satan's Gnostic Fantasy	169
Chapter 6 Choosing the Father in *Moses and Monotheism*	199
Epilogue	231
Notes	245
Works Cited	293
Permissions	299
Index	301

Note on Citations for Major Primary Works

*For full bibliographical entries, see Works Cited.

1. *Freud*

   a) Most of the citations of Freud's writings will be from *The Standard Edition of the Complete Psychological Works of Sigmund Freud*, ed. and trans. James Strachey et al., 24 vols. London, 1953–74. Citations will be given by volume and page number(s) with work identified as necessary.

   b) Citations of some of Freud's earliest writings, including letters, will be from *The Origins of Psycho-Analysis: Letters to Wilhelm Fliess, Drafts and Notes, 1887–1902*, ed. Marie Bonaparte, et al.; trans. Eric Mosbacher and James Strachey, New York, 1954. Citations will be given by page number(s) following *Origins*.

   c) Citations of Freud's "Theme of the Three Caskets" will be from C. J. M. Hubback's translation in *The Collected Papers*, ed. Joan Riviere, 5 vols. New York, 1959, IV, 244–56. Citations will be given by page number(s).

   d) Citations of select letters will be from *Letters of Sigmund Freud*, ed. Ernst L. Freud; trans. Tania and James Stern, New York, 1960. Citations will be given by page number(s) following *Letters*.

   e) Citations of Freud's *Moses and Monotheism* will be from Katherine Jones's translation, New York, 1954. Citations will be given by page number(s).

f) Citations from the original German texts, identified as necessary, will be from *Gesammelte Werke*, 18 vol., ed. Marie Bonaparte, et al., Frankfurt am Main, 1968–78. Citations will be given by volume and page number(s).

2. *Bible*

   a) Unless otherwise noted, citations of the Hebrew Bible, by chapter and verse number(s), will be from *Tanakh: A New Translation of the Holy Scriptures According to the Traditional Hebrew Text*, New York, 1985.

   b) Unless otherwise noted, citations of the New Testament, by chapter and verse number(s), will follow the NRSV.

3. *Shakespeare*

   Unless otherwise noted, all citations from Shakespeare's plays, by act, scene, and line number(s), will be from *The Riverside Shakespeare*, 2nd ed., ed. G. Blakemore Evans, et al., Boston, 1996.

4. *Milton*

   a) Citations of Milton's *Paradise Lost* will be from *The Riverside Milton*, ed. Roy Flannagan, Boston, 1998. Citations will be given by book and line number(s).

   b) Citations of Milton's prose writings will be from *The Complete Prose Works*, ed. Don M. Wolfe et al., 8 vols. New Haven, 1953–82. Citations will be given by volume and page number(s).

5. *Hoffmann*

   a) Citations of E. T. A. Hoffmann's "The Sandman" will be from *The Golden Pot and Other Tales*, trans. Ritchie Robertson, Oxford, 1992. Citations will be given by page number(s).

   b) Citations of Hoffmann's original German text of "Der Sandmann" will be from *Poetische Werke*, 12 vols., ed. Walter Wallerstein, Berlin, 1957, III, 3–44. Citations will be given by page number(s).

Acknowledgments

Part of the argument of this book is that Freud understood the process of looking back as the recognition of a debt incurred. But while Freud saw such a debt as a burden and its recognition as potentially traumatic, the recognition of a debt can also be the cause for the expression of gratitude. And so, as I look back to the various debts I have incurred over the many years in which this book has taken shape, I would like now to express my gratitude to those who have offered special guidance: Lisa Schnell, Todd McGowan, Steve Schillinger, Molly Rothenberg, Loka Losambe, Tony Bradley, and Gabriel Moyal. I would also like to thank the University of Vermont's College of Arts and Sciences and its Department of English for other forms of support. And I would like finally to thank Andrew Kenyon and Charles Shepherdson at SUNY Press for their efficiency and helpfulness in guiding the manuscript through the various stages of the publication process. I dedicate the book to my children who are now and have always been the source of joy and wonder.

Introduction

> It is very unhappy, but too late to be helped, the discovery we have made that we exist. That discovery is called the Fall of Man.
>
> —Ralph Waldo Emerson, "Experience"

> What stakes are raised by these questions? One doesn't need to be an expert to foresee that they involve thinking about what is meant by living, speaking, dying, being and world as in being-in-the-world or being towards the world, or being-with, being-before, being-behind, being-after, being and following, being followed or being following, there where *I am* . . . It is too late to deny it. . . . I must once more return to the malaise of this scene. . . . I will do all I can do to prevent its being presented as a primal scene. . . . [W]e shall have to ask ourselves, inevitably, what happens . . . when a son is *after* his father.
>
> —Jacques Derrida, "The Animal That Therefore I Am"

I

For a study so foundationally concerned with the problem of origins, it would seem appropriate to offer an initial reflection on its own literal starting point. And so I begin with the book's cover art: Magritte's "La Reproduction interdite" (1937).[1]

A male figure stands looking into what appears to be a mirror. We assume it is a mirror because we see the cover of a book (Poe's *The Narrative of Arthur Gordon Pym*) and a partially revealed mirror image of that cover in the lower-right corner of the painting. Given the position of the foregrounded figure relative both to the mirror and to our own point of view, we would expect to see a frontal image (face and torso) looking back at us from the mirror. But what we see instead is the figure's backside: back of the torso, neck, back of the head. In other words, what we see reflected in the mirror is precisely the same back view we have of the figure itself. In short, an impossible image.

The painting obviously aims to compel us to ask questions to which we have no immediate answers: Is this actually a mirror? Is what we see in the mirror what the front of the figure looks like or is this an illusion, an artist's trick? More to the point, the painting thematizes (and enacts) its own unreadability in a specific context: what we think a mirror should unequivocally make available to us, our very capacity to know ourselves through an experience of reflection.

Looking at the foregrounded figure, we expect to see his (hers? its?) identity clearly revealed. We also expect that the figure's point of view—and in having a point of view, however obscured, the figure is, in a sense, the viewer's double—will not only establish the correct object of perception (his own reflected face staring back at him) but also, and perhaps more importantly, permit us to trust the very act of seeing and the site from which it originates. In most situations involving the seeing-knowing subject, such self-si(gh)ting would typically, and quite literally, be out-of-sight. It is only in the particular case of an original looking at its mirror image that the origin of seeing and knowing becomes visible at all. Minimally, then, Magritte makes present to us what is typically invisible and all the more reliable for that: the epistemological and ontological priority of the subject relative to the objects of its perception; or, more simply, the subject's own position as the starting-point of knowledge. But in making us consciously, even disconcertingly, aware of a position we normally take for granted, Magritte also problematizes the entire process of knowing—and here explicitly self-knowing—by confronting us with an absence at that very origin. Even in its newly visible, if *dis*figured, form, the constitutive act of the seeing-knowing subject is represented here as mediated through the mirror image itself and thus as strangely belated. The perspective that should logically come before the very object of perception is what we see *subsequently* and then only as an absent cause that we infer after the fact.

If my phrasing here might be taken as deliberately imposing some notion of temporality upon the painting's spatial configuration, I choose to do so because the painting's composition (we might almost call it a rhetoric) encourages that blurring. For what the painting can only depict in spatial terms figures a temporal condition: knowing's relation to being, self and other, cause and effect, before and after. *Qua* two-dimensional image, of course, the painting can only visualize a before-and-after in spatial terms (in front or behind). The image we see, both the foregrounded figure and its reflection, produces a dislocated sense of what precisely constitutes the before and what the after: if we stand *in front* of a mirror are we not also *behind* the image? (Here especially the "original" appears to be behind its own mirror image.) But that very confusion infiltrates our sense of our own position. Were we looking at the painting in the Museum Boijmans Van Beuningen in Rotterdam we would say that we were standing in front of it. But especially in the context of viewing the foregrounded figure as our surrogate, we see ourselves from behind. And to the extent we also then see ourselves *seeing from behind*, our spatial coordinates, vexed as they are, become temporal coordinates as well precisely because the painting makes us conscious of our own seeing as an activity that has duration, one *taking place over a space of time*. (Normally such phrases would be employed metaphorically, but here they are something more than metaphor.) The word that perhaps best captures this duality—and thus the word that perhaps best describes the viewer's position here—would be *after* since that word, as either preposition or adverb, can designate either a spatial or a temporal positioning relative to something else.

It is worth giving even more consideration to that *after* because, as a preposition, that word can also mean "in consequence of," which might lead us to ask just what is at stake in the viewer's state of afterwardsness.[2] If we think of the whole experience of viewing the painting in the context of the (self-)knowledge made available in and by a mirror, we might imagine that Magritte's aim here is to destabilize the entire Cartesian edifice by calling attention, even too much attention, to the confused relationship between thinking and being: which actually comes first in *cogito ergo sum*?[3] Here, it is as though neither knowing nor being is where we think it should be. Indeed, what the painting leaves us with is the uncanny sense that we do not know whether the knowing self, especially that self that would know itself, is the cause or the effect of its very act. How can we know ourselves if we cannot tell where knowledge, especially self-knowledge, even begins? And what, then, are the origins of knowledge and, more pressingly, of the self who would know?

Magritte's painting thus interrogates us with an impossibility that might now appear as all too real: we are somehow absent from the origin of our own knowledge and from ourselves as the origin of our knowledge. That origin seems to begin elsewhere, in a place that we cannot see because, for some reason, it has left us behind. In *Moses and Monotheism*, his last major work and whose first two sections were published in the same year Magritte completed his painting, Freud would write that "everything new must have its roots in what went before" (22). In special accord with Freud's musing in a text deeply vexed by its own crisis of origins, Magritte seems also to be saying that, in its very effort to see where it begins, the subject discovers that it can never catch up. In searching for its very origin, as the painting seems intent on reminding us, the subject necessarily discovers that it always already comes too late.

II

This introduction's two epigraphs, from Emerson and from Derrida, point to different perspectives on the problem of belatedness, perspectives that, taken together, form the interpretive foundation of my study. For Emerson, the self-knowledge that comes "too late to be helped" is the "discovery we have made that we exist."[4] In the immediate context of the essay, this gnomic utterance suggests that the burden of discovery—a discovery seemingly coincident with self-consciousness itself—is our awakening to lived reality as shadowed by a kind of epistemological loss, the distance constitutive of all acts of reflection.[5] "Ever afterwards we suspect our instruments," Emerson continues, for what "we have learned [is] that we do not see directly, but mediately, and that we have no means of correcting these colored and distorting lenses which we are." At times, Emerson appears to locate this loss in the simple fact that nothing is quite real or that things just don't last: "we live amid surfaces" (261), "the world is all outside; it has no inside" (263); "life is a flitting state, a tent for a night" (264). But more often he laments that we are actually close to reality without ever fully touching it or being touched by it:

> Souls never touch their objects. (256)

***

> There are moods in which we court suffering, in the hope that here at least we shall find reality, sharp peaks and edges of truth. But it turns out to be scene-painting and counterfeit. (256)

***

> The Indian who was laid under a curse that the wind should not blow on him, nor water flow to him, nor fire burn him, is a type of us all. . . . Nothing is left us now but death. We look

to that with grim satisfaction, saying, There at least is reality that will not dodge us. (256–57)

***

[T]his evanenscence and lubricity of all objects . . . lets them slip through our fingers when we clutch hardest. (257)

***

Spirit is matter reduced to an extreme thinness: O *so* thin! (258)

For Emerson in this mood, what we discover in existence is that, for some reason, we can only intuit without ever being able to arrive at some deeper, more lasting reality, a reality that is screened from us and thus remains inexplicably inaccessible.

This screening effect appears to have something to do with our time-bound nature. Thus, the notion of a fall into self-consciousness is inseparable from a stumbling into a mysterious before-and-after. Among other things, that is, the discovery of existence includes the awakening to the fact that there can be a time before such a discovery, a time in relation to which the discovery itself necessarily comes after; paradoxically, we can exist without knowing that we do. In this context I would venture that Emerson's phrase, "*Ever afterwards* we suspect our instruments," points more particularly to the problem of mediation as something to be understood in temporal terms. The "ever afterwards," that is, does not just locate us in time as responding to an earlier event but is rather a condition of being. The lag in knowing—a discovery "too late to be helped"—refers not simply to the act of discovery as itself belated but also to the very content of that discovery. The Fall, that is, is not just coincident with the discovery that we exist but resides also in our failure to have recognized this fact earlier. What we discover includes the recognition of an inexplicable failure to have recognized, of an earlier missing, and thus of a belatedness (the "too late") that appears not simply to describe the "when" but also the "what" of discovery: to exist and to exist "after" (and then to discover later that we do) are inextricably intertwined.

Thus, Emerson plaintively begins his essay: "Where do we find ourselves? In a series of which we do not know the extremes . . . We wake and find ourselves on a stair; there are stairs below us, which we seem to have ascended; there are stairs above, many a one, which go upward and out of sight." And then again: "We are like millers on the lower levels of a stream, when the factories above them have exhausted their water. We too fancy that the upper people must have raised their dams" (254–55). In both, a spatial image (moving on stairs, the flow of a river) suggests a temporal condition. In the former image, we appear trapped in some undefined place, at once located and dislocated; in the latter image, we are downstream in time, and the upper levels of the river (the past) mark the present as lacking, exhausted, depleted because coming after the fullness of the before. And later in the essay, Emerson will reflect on what it feels like to encounter this "something before"—some force, vital and true, outside the self—that necessarily defines the perceiving perspective as inescapably too late: "every insight from this realm of thought is felt as initial, and promises a sequel. I do not make it; *I arrive, and behold what was there already*" (267; my emphasis). That which mediates or screens us from the reality we desire and would possess exists within and is time itself. The movement of time seems to be loss itself draining away meaning whose reality exists somewhere before us but which is no longer available.[6] For Emerson, the discovery of existence (the Fall of Man) takes place in the beginning (the subject's g/Genesis) because in our finding out we must confront the very problem of beginnings as the predicament of coming after something else. In the temporality of loss—in the loss that is temporality—the self's origin is what can never be claimed as its own.

III

In "Experience," Emerson paradoxically imagines this crisis of afterwardsness from the perspective of the one who comes *before*, the father who mourns his dead son (though even here, it is worth noting, the father comes after the son who has passed before him).[7] But my second epigraph repositions the crisis from the perspective of the one who, in the normal scheme of things at least, comes *after*: "[W]e shall have to ask ourselves, inevitably, what happens . . . when a son is after his father." And, as Derrida's first sentence aptly puts it, we must also ask "what stakes are raised" by such a question.[8]

More explicitly than Emerson, Derrida defines the crisis of coming too late as a content: *what* we confront in our belatedness—"what is meant by living, speaking, dying, being and world as in being-in-the-world or being towards the world . . ."—rather than *when* we confront it. If Derrida's language is more philosophical than religious in the way Emerson's had been, it also hints at a situation open to psychoanalytic investigation. For not only is the crisis defined in relational terms (and a particularly Freudian relation at that: the son's belated relation to the father), but it is also grounded in a specific psychical process, denial (though, tellingly, the predicament is precisely "*too late* to deny"). Most obviously, if Emerson uses a biblical reference to draw us back to the crisis as one of beginnings (the Fall of Genesis 3), Derrida draws our attention to a definitively Freudian starting point: the primal scene. Whatever such a scene might entail—and we shall consider it in more detail in a moment—it is for the one who comes upon it as much after-the-fact ("too late") as Emerson's discovery of existence.

Before taking up how the Freudian primal scene is a particular example of the crisis of belatedness I have been sketching, we might take one final look at "Experience" to consider how Emerson in a more indirect way represents afterwardsness from the perspective of the son rather than from that of the father. The unnamed son who barely makes an appearance in the essay proper (even in mourning, Emerson rather infamously never even names his dead son[9]) is, in effect, restored before the essay actually begins in the poem Emerson uses as his epigraph:

> The lords of life, the lords of life, —
> I saw them pass
> In their own guise,
> Like and unlike,
> Portly and grim, —
> Use and Surprise,
> Surface and Dream,
> Succession swift and spectral Wrong,
> Temperament without a tongue,
> And the inventor of the game
> Omnipresent without a name, —
> Some to see, some to be guessed,
> They marched from east to west:
> Little man, least of all,
> Among the legs of the guardians tall,
> Walked about with puzzled look.
> Him by the hand dear Nature took;
> Dearest Nature, strong and kind,
> Whispered, "Darling, never mind!
> Tomorrow, they will wear another face,
> The founder thou; these are thy race!" (254)

Whatever else is going on here, a confused sense of temporality, priority, and authority attends the figure of the "little man" (a child-Adam?). For, as the poem reaches its conclusion, what he would have naturally assumed to come before him—his "guardians" (the "lords of life")—turn out to have derived from him: "The founder thou; these are thy race!" Still, even as he eventually comes to know that he is the founder (the cause?) of his guardians, the little man yet must have his priority revealed to him by another figure, "Nature," whose own place relative to his "Darling" and to the lords of life remains unclear. Just what relation is Nature to the little man? Did one create or "found" the other, and if so when and in what order? The little man seems to have discovered himself in some dislocated present, the origin lost sight of, uncertain, misplaced. Although he is told that he precedes what he sees before him (in both senses), he appears belated without perhaps knowing why. And he certainly shows no signs now of remembering what he previously founded, as though he were absent from a moment he must have been present for. As in Emerson's brief account of the Fall in the essay proper, self-consciousness seems constituted by loss. Here, we intuit the loss in the little man's discovery that he has failed to recognize some situation that has preceded him, has necessarily included him, and yet one that he cannot truly call his own.

With Emerson's poem in mind, what then does it mean for Derrida to suggest that the son's coming "after the father" is particularly related to the Freudian primal scene? We shall return to Freud's own formulation of that concept at the beginning of chapter 4, but for now we might just deal with some basics. In general, Freud understands the primal scene as a moment in infancy or early childhood when the infant/child observes an act of sexual intercourse, usually, though not always, between the parents.[10] Although such an observation might produce a certain amount of sexual excitation, at this early life-phase the infant/child has virtually no context to assign meaning either to the sex-act itself or to its own feelings in response; as Freud puts it in the *Interpretation of Dreams*, "what we are dealing with is a sexual excitation with which their [children's] understanding is unable to cope" (V, 585).[11] Precisely because it comes too early to be translated into meaning, what inheres of the experience remains psychically disorganized, neither a memory nor something repressed in the unconscious. It is, rather, as Freud might say, an ontogenetic or perhaps even a phylogenetic inheritance from the past of the child that is carried forward in life where it awaits reengagement of some kind.[12] As William Kerrigan aptly observes in a study we shall have reason to revisit in chapter 5, it is as if with the "advent of meaning" that is the primal scene "a traumatic future enters the world of the child, but defers announcing itself."[13]

For that reason, the child's first real meaningful (and meaning-making) encounter with the primal scene is delayed (via *Nachträglichkeit* or deferred action), usually until the emergence of a more defined sexual identity, which would normally mean after the onset of the Oedipal phase. At this point, some other event triggers the child's memory of the original event, and the child's (typically male's) emergent sexualization of its relationships with his parents (already complexly bound up with the struggle of ego-differentiation) now retrospectively confers meaning on that original event so that its impact is experienced for the first time.[14] It isn't just that the developing psyche registers what is sexual in parental intercourse, but it also experiences its own exclusion from what it desires—a relationship with the mother now interrupted by the father's taking his place and so forming the fully triangulated terms of the Oedipus complex.[15] To the extent this process creates for the child "a scene of . . . intolerable anxiety" (especially as the complex leads toward castration anxiety), the child's openness to retrospective interpretation means, as Kerrigan adds, that it is "ready all at once to experience and disavow the entrance" into consciousness of the primal scene.[16] This complex psychical balancing at once relocates the original experience to the Unconscious (via repression) and permits its expression in various substitutions or conversion-symptoms.[17]

Understood in these terms, the term "primal scene" is a bit misleading in the sense that it refers at once to the original viewing of parental intercourse (which may not even be an actual event) and the later perspective from which the original event comes to be invested with meaning in the first place.[18] As Jean Laplanche and Jean-Bertrand Pontalis put it, in the case of the Wolf Man in particular, although Freud "is concerned to establish the reality of the primal scene, he is already laying stress on the fact that it is only through a deferred action (*Nachträglichkeit*) that it is grasped and interpreted by the child."[19] In other words, even as a *later* interpretive reworking the deferred moment in some sense yet has conceptual priority because, though "after" in chronological time (assuming the original event even happened), it creates the primal scene's very priority and invests that priority with meaning. To put this another way, the later event of retrospective meaning-making produces what is "primal" in the primal scene even as its own *conceptual* priority or precedence is thereby converted into a lateness, a lateness then (re)enacted in various substitutions.[20]

Just as important, if the moment of conceptual priority thereby functions as and is (re)located to an "afterwards," it necessarily discovers itself as shadowed by a something before and, more to the point, a something just beyond its grasp. As Laplanche and Pontalis write in their entry on "deferred action," "it is not lived experience in general that undergoes a deferred revision but, specifically, whatever has been impossible in the first instance to incorporate fully into a meaningful context" (112). Not even fully available as a memory but only as a retroactive conferral of meaning on an event that might be more fantasy than reality, what Laplanche and Pontalis call "unassimilated experience" is, of course, what demands the revisionary work in the first place. But the unassimilable is also, effectively, what renders the primal scene traumatic. For the sense of identity bound up in this complex interpretive process is grounded in a kind of originary loss. That is, at the heart of this process, the self becomes newly aware of itself as necessarily linked to something earlier that yet remains obscure, inaccessible, at least partially lost or hidden even as there is some corresponding recognition, however fleeting, of the (too) familiar: simultaneously some known within the unknown and something unknown within the known; something that reveals even as it conceals; something that includes even as it excludes.

But just what sort of wound is this?[21] Thinking of the primal scene in broadly existential terms, Kerrigan makes the important observation that "the image of parental intercourse . . . foretells the end of narcissism in the knowledge of contingency and createdness: the imaginer is as nothing before the truly revealed meaning of his image—there in the image, he was not. . . . All one is stems from a contingent event during which one was as nothing, nowhere to be found."[22] The subject's terrifying experience of being "as nothing, nowhere to be found" suggests that Kerrigan sees the "intolerable anxiety" at the heart of the primal scene as a retrospective discovery of the problematic nature of the origin itself in which the mere fact of being created entails an impossible absence (as in Magritte's painting, the act of seeing paradoxically cannot locate the see-er). The primal scene becomes intolerable, if inescapable, because it traverses an impoverishment at the beginning, a beginning that can be grasped only after-the-fact.

That said, despite his provocative sense of how this debilitating "knowledge of contingency and createdness" vexes the psyche of the child who stumbles across it, in the end Kerrigan can do no more than restate Freud's own understanding of what this anxiety involves. That is, Kerrigan follows Freud in claiming that the crisis of self-consciousness at stake in the primal scene necessarily involves a sexual(ized) identity, an identity fully created through the working out of the Oedipal economy.[23] But what if we took Kerrigan's initial insight more seriously and let it stand apart from Freud's own formulation? What if the crisis of "contingency and createdness" were less about one's immersion in the Oedipus complex or about the full emergence of the sexualized identity related to this complex? What if Freud's Oedipal interpretation of the primal scene were itself understood as just another instance of a retrospective conferral of meaning that aimed at displacing, even explaining away, the real source of intolerable anxiety, the experience of the subject as "nothing, and nowhere to be found"?[24]

To open this line of inquiry, we might note that, even in the possibility that the infant/child actually did witness an act of parental intercourse, within the full interpretive economy of retrospection that moment is itself late. In other words, the primal scene—the original moment in this long process—already comes *after* a more original moment, but one which, tellingly, is impossible to see in any form. The very impossibility of seeing this moment is marked by Freud's not even noticing just how missing it is from his own analytical and theoretical work. Focusing on how the dream of the four-year-old Wolf Man looks back to an occurrence some two and a half years earlier, Freud writes that "behind the content of the dream lay some . . . unknown scene—one, that is, which had already been forgotten at the time of the dream" (XVII, 33); here, the "unknown" is what has been "forgotten," a trajectory suggesting that at an earlier point the Wolf Man's mind had possessed some rudimentary trace of the original event.[25] Freud acknowledges that the interpretive process is never so clean. Doubtful of "forming a clear picture of the origin and development of the patient's illness," he concludes that, "we must be content with having clearly recognized the obscurity" (XVII, 104–05). But he continues to hold out the hope that, even through the primal forgetfulness that appears to place the origin under perpetual concealment, there is yet some psychical record of the event that formed or at least opened the door to the future neurosis (if only fully shaped retrospectively).[26]

Ned Lukacher's account of Freud's very radicality is instructive in this case. Comparing Freud to Nietzsche in their shared "problematization of the question of the origin," Lukacher writes:

> Instead of Nietzsche's "active forgetfulness" of the origin, Freud develops a strategy for speculating on the incalculability of the event. Like Nietzsche, Freud acknowledges the insurmountable unfamiliarity that conceals the origin; unlike Nietzsche, . . . he wants to go on to construct a narrative about what precedes the event . . . by moving back before the origin, back to the point prior to the presencing of the origin. Freud wants to tell a story about what is prior to presence and what has always already been forgotten. Instead of simply celebrating the concealment that forgetfulness brings, he wants to construct a story about what forgetfulness conceals.[27]

There is much to praise in this summation, but Lukacher confuses as much as he explains in his rather curious imprecision regarding his words "event," "origin," "precede," "moving back," "prescencing," "forgotten"/"forgetfulness," and "conceals." In the first place, Lukacher is conflating Freud's two different concepts of an origin. There is both the original event that Freud understands by the term "primal scene" and the beginning of the neurosis that emerges at the moment of retrospective investment of that earlier event. So when Lukacher writes that "Freud acknowledges the insurmountable unfamiliarity that conceals the origin" and then that "he wants to go on to construct a narrative about what precedes the event," "origin" and "event" refer to those two different starting points. It would be more accurate to say that, for Freud, a complex constellation of later meaning-possibilities (what he calls an "inexhaustible variety of new shapes") makes it difficult, almost impossible, to claim the original determinative event (or even to define the precise nature of that scene, as real event or as fantasy); and he wants to construct a backward-looking narrative from the event (the advent of interpretive meaning *and* symptomology) to what precedes it (its origin or cause: the primal scene). Thus, when Lukacher concludes that "Freud wants to tell a story about what is prior to presence" ("prior to the prescencing of the origin"), he misleadingly suggests that what Freud is searching for as "prior" (prior to presence/prior to the origin) *precedes even the primal scene.*[28] But, for Freud, "prior to presence" would mean "before the beginning of symptoms," that which is the origin or cause of those symptoms even if it is only the revision of the original event that truly causes a neurosis to emerge. In that context, when Lukacher uses the phrase "construct a story about what forgetfulness conceals," he is more precisely pointing to Freud's analytical-therapeutic drive to construct an account that coincides with memory (or can stand in its place where true recollection is impossible) to reclaim the primal scene from the concealment of primal forgetfulness.[29]

Of course, the very notion of forgetfulness presumes a memory formed in relation to some earlier event and the "witnessing" or "possession" of that event in the mind, however fleeting such possession might be.[30] What is forgotten must, in some sense, have actually been experienced (remembered and only subsequently forgotten). But if we really want to think about what is "prior to presence" as something that actually precedes the primal scene, then we must take a different approach. Or we must at least modify Lukacher's promising beginning: the primal scene resides within "the crisis of interpretation that emerges when the question of the origin becomes at once unavoidable and unanswerable, when the origin must be remembered but memory fails utterly, when all the evidence points toward an origin that nevertheless remains unverifiable." Lukacher does understand the primal scene as caught up in an experience of knowing and self-knowing that is yet bound to a "fundamental and insurmountable concealment." But he also imagines the crisis of inaccessibility at the origin to be a problem of interpretation that has no origin: "the primal scene . . . becomes the name for the dispossessive function of language that constitutes the undisclosed essence of language" (24); or, again, it is "a kind of historical 'event' that cannot be thought outside the question of intertextuality," an intertextuality so radical that "it does not have a subject" at all (13–14; original italics deleted). In short, what is most important for Lukacher is the groundlessness of the act of interpretation rather than what precisely constitutes the absence at the origin, an absence he understands as figural in any event: an expression of a postmodern skepticism about meaning itself—"deferred action" becomes Derrida's *différance*.[31] But to the extent Lukacher, following Freud, is still caught up in the language of presence, memory, and forgetfulness, he is yet imagining some "there" at the origin along with a subject who can only be dispossessed of what he in some mysterious fashion already possessed.[32] And so we might rephrase Lukacher's statement—"the origin must be remembered but memory fails utterly"—to refer to that part of the past the awareness of which is necessary to self-consciousness (the Emersonian discovery of our own existence) but that is truly missing, absent, unavailable, inaccessible, but not "forgotten" because beyond the possibility of memory in the first place: in short, what truly precedes the primal scene.

Lukacher provocatively ventures that Freud aims to "bring . . . his patient, and his readers, to the threshold of an insurmountable concealment"; and he adds that the "primal scene is the preexistent trace underlying the possibility of distinction between presence and absence" (27). But in what sense can we not move beyond this boundary? How does presence become absence? If, despite the lack of an actual memory, we can yet imagine a child witnessing of an act of parental intercourse, to the extent such an act involves the child at all it is because parental intercourse is the "cause" of the child: the act has a procreative and not just a sexual-pleasure function. And that the child could have witnessed the act at all means that he (for Freud, typically male) was already positioned *after-the-fact*: the sex-act that was most crucial—most determinative—isn't what is present before him (Freud's primal scene) but is, rather, always earlier, impossibly hidden away in time. To put this another way, if the child can see (or even just imagine seeing) his parents having sex, then he is reminded (though perhaps only at a later moment of retrospective interpretation or inference) of a necessarily earlier instance of parental joining: the union that brought the child into being. The child can only even see the sex now (this "now" already belonging to a time that cannot even be remembered but is reconstructed at a later time) because he already exists to see it.[33] And he already exists—the now is already "after"—only because of the earlier sex-act he does not see and could not see and will never be able to see because it forever resides across that "threshold of insurmountable concealment": the origin of origins, the moment from which the belated child was absent even though, in a different sense, undeniably present.

And so we return to Kerrigan's insight: in the primal scene "the imaginer is as nothing before the truly revealed meaning of his image—there in the image, he was not." If to that terrifying image of the subject's self-absence we add the problem of origins defined in terms of a temporality of loss, then we have the idea that is at the heart of this study. Addressing how the primal scene is caught up in such a temporality, Lukacher writes that from the vantage of belated interpretation "nothing can halt the process of deferral in which the notion of the origin and the etiology of the event are caught" (141). Lukacher is referring to the way in which the deferral forever displaces the scene of interpretation itself (a symptomology of chronic substitution).[34] Against this view, I suggest that we read the deferral of etiology more literally as an always pushed back absence at the scene of the origin. It is this absence that constitutes the subject's traumatic knowledge of contingency and createdness, the crisis of the "was not."

In this context, we might return then to Laplanche and Pontalis's statement that what "undergoes a deferred revision . . . [is] whatever has been impossible in the first instance to incorporate fully into a meaningful context" and juxtapose that with the following from their entry on the "primal scene": "what Freud wants to uphold" in his notion of the primal scene, "particularly against Jung, is the idea that this scene belongs to the . . . past of the individual and that it constitutes a happening which may be of the order of myth but which is *already given* prior to any meaning which is attributed after the fact" (336). What Freud appears to have meant is that, whether as actual event or retrospective fantasy, the primal scene effectively comes before the later conferral of meaning as a reality to be interpreted (the "*already given* prior to any meaning which is attributed" to it). But I would argue, by contrast, that what is "attributed after the fact" is that the self—the very self who interprets—is constituted as the "already given" where both parts of that phrase are necessary. The self is *already* given in the sense that there is some crucial part of the self that exists *before* itself; the self is founded in some temporal gap of before and after and inhabits a place of temporal belatedness. And the self is already *given* in the sense that it exists in passive relation to what precedes it and thus has priority over it (its giver). What I want to argue, then, is that it is precisely the self's uncanny discovery of itself as "already given" that is "impossible . . . to incorporate fully into a meaningful context." What comes into being as an attribution after-the-fact is precisely the Emersonian discovery of existence, the discovery (too late to be helped) of the self who exists in and as a condition of belatedness in relation to an origin it cannot claim as its own. In a way similar to the situation of Magritte's viewer whose self-knowledge can never quite catch up with itself, the primal scene marks a failure to have recognized something when it was happening. It thus marks the necessarily belated recognition of a terrible paradox: that the self was absent from the scene of its own origin, an origin that, forever after, can only be that self's own and not its own simultaneously.

IV

In his 1955 seminar, "The Psychoses," Lacan made the almost passing observation that "we always have to come back to disturbances of memory to know what the point of departure for psychoanalysis was."[35] We assume that Lacan is referring here to how an analyst struggles with such disturbances within any particular analysis: situations, times, places, people, events, the past itself are all buried under, behind, and within consciousness and from that location disrupt the mind. Yet it is essential that the analyst attempt to retrieve what the analysand's thought has concealed: some sort of missing resides at the origin of memory, and that missing must be filled in.

Such a view of how traumatic incidents are retained in the mind and then retrieved through the psychoanalytic process is, of course, traceable to the very beginnings of Freud's project. As Freud and Breuer wrote in "Preliminary Communication" (1893), "we have found . . . at first, that each individual hysterical symptom immediately and permanently disappeared when we had succeeded in *bringing clearly to light the memory of the [traumatic] event* by which it was provoked . . . and when the patient had described that event in the greatest possible detail" (II, 6; my emphasis). Over the course of his career, Freud would problematize the notion that an initial trauma is available as memory, but he never gave up on the notion of a definitive etiology of neurosis that the analyst endeavored less to reconstruct than to unearth.

That said, Lacan's phrase "to know what the point of departure for psychoanalysis was" might more subtly suggest that psychoanalytic discourse developed in the context of its own disturbances of memory, difficulties of recollection that are central to the discourse itself and not just a problem of analytical practice. And to the extent that "the point of departure for psychoanalysis" was Freud himself, we might also imagine that Lacan is pointing to Freud's particular disturbances as though his own struggle to remember, to work through (and perhaps even his failure to do so), remains at the heart of both his own thought and of the entire psychoanalytic enterprise.

We might return in that context to my earlier suggestion that Freud's Oedipal interpretation of the primal scene can be understood as an instance of belated revision of the kind he associates with the Wolf Man's retrospective conferral of meaning upon the scene. In a way analogous to the Wolf Man's "repudiation" of the primal scene, Freud's revisionary work (the Oedipus complex itself) might be understood, that is, as aimed at defending against—screening, displacing, disavowing, censoring—the source of an intolerable anxiety regarding the origin of his own project. It is conceivable, then, that the origin of psychoanalysis—its own primal scene—constituted a trauma in relation to which Freud's subsequent writings formed a fantasy response, both revealing and concealing how it all began, but a beginning that remained hidden, elusive, never directly available to proper theorizing. We might then apply as an apt description of Freud's entire Oedipal model the same description he applies to the Wolf Man's retrospective fantasizing: such "phantasies . . . correspond . . . exactly to the legends by means of which a nation that has become great and proud tries to conceal the insignificance and failure of its beginnings" (XVII, 20). Freudian psychoanalysis, I want to argue, is itself crossed by the shadow of a loss—a crisis of the origin, "a failure of its beginnings" (and *about* beginnings)—it could never quite confront.

It is the central argument of this study that Freud both grasped this crisis and struggled to bring it into clear theoretical focus (if he did not precisely disavow it). To the extent he most consistently formulated its presence in psychical life in the son's deeply ambivalent relationship to his father, Freud never veered very far from the central issue: that concern emerges in his writing as early as 1896 (in the wake of the death of his own father, Jacob Freud) and was still central to his thinking in his final major work, *Moses and Monotheism*. But for complex reasons having to do with his early insistence on sexual explanations for the etiology of neuroses, even before the *Interpretation of Dreams* Freud imposed upon filial ambivalence—a son's response to parental and especially paternal priority and authority and thus centrally caught up in the condition of belatedness—an Oedipal framework. Thus, in an October 15, 1897 letter to Wilhelm Fliess, Freud describes his eureka moment:

> Only one idea of general value occurred to me. I have found love of the mother and jealousy of the father in my own case too, and now believe it to be a general phenomenon of early childhood, even if it does not occur so early as in children who have been made hysterics. . . . If that is the case, the gripping power of *Oedipus Rex* . . . becomes intelligible. (*Origins*, 223)

Gradually articulated as the Oedipus complex, the motive force of the son's ambivalence toward his father is explained in terms of *sexual* rivalry. In sum, I understand the privilege Freud gives to the Oedipus complex in the psychical development of the human (male) subject as his attempt to ascertain the cause of the ambivalence he felt in response to his father's death a year earlier. But the chief effect of this theory was to evade many of the more disturbing elements of that ambivalence.

To follow this interpretive path is not to reject Freud's thought outright, for even his failures often register powerful insights. This study, in fact, aims to reclaim what Freud himself lost sight of in his own work by recognizing that many of his best ideas are often buried under the weight of his interpretive apparatus. I thus want to restore those ideas by working from the inside, through what, following Elizabeth Bellamy, we might call the method of "immanent critique, or a critique from within, conducted on the terms Freud laid down himself."[36] It is precisely within that framework that I make the concept of *Nachträglichkeit* (deferred action or afterwardsness) central to my line of inquiry.

Freud himself gave no particular theoretical attention to this concept.[37] But because he referred to it several times in relation to his formal elaboration of the term "primal scene," it is worth reminding ourselves of the original link. As we have noted, even in its most traditional sense the primal scene is suggestive of how psychical development is caught up in the experience of some sort of absence. And to the extent the primal scene is associated, more specifically, with the delayed advent of meaning through *Nachträglichkeit*, the very notion of a primal scene can be understood as a crucially self-defining experience that is yet shadowed by a mysterious missing at the point of origin.[38] This missing, moreover, includes the uncanny sense of a failure to have grasped something while it was happening. A belated discovery thus becomes a discovery of belatedness, a dawning awareness of one's own lateness relative to an origin that belongs elsewhere. It is the wager of this study that what Freud tries to grasp through the notion of deferred action is conceptually equivalent to Emerson's discovery of existence, one "too late to be helped": that belatedness is the very condition of being, at once enabling and disabling. And what we might call the afterwardsness of existing entails the beginning of self-consciousness in our awakening to the fact that what is most important about ourselves lies forever beyond our grasp. For this something beyond resides not just in the past but in a past not truly available and which, though familiar in some inexplicable way, is yet defamiliarized. It is a part of the self that the self can never lay claim to (even if, as we shall see, others can).

Part I of this study aims to document Freud's formulation of this concept and his own strained relationship to it primarily through extended discussions of *Beyond the Pleasure Principle* (chapter 1) and *Inhibitions, Symptoms and Anxiety* (chapter 2), the latter read as a response to Otto Rank's *The Trauma of Birth*. Grappling in those texts with a host of issues related to the problem of origins, Freud yet reveals, against his own explicit intentions, a kind of experience that cannot be meaningfully rendered in terms of a deferred unconscious response to an earlier traumatic episode because what has come earlier was not properly experienced at all. It is only known in the afterwards of recognition that is simultaneously a recognition of a constitutive afterwardsness: it must have happened to me yet, inexplicably, I wasn't there. To put this another way, I am interested in exploring how Freud's speculations illuminate the problem of the subject's belatedness as that experience shows many of the same traits, without actually being the same, as the deferred action by which the Unconscious absorbs and symptomatically responds to an event that "happened" earlier.

While the issues addressed in part 1 will remain central to the study as a whole, parts II and III will take a different approach. There, I will try to illuminate two key Freudian texts—"The Uncanny" (part II) and *Moses and Monotheism* (part III)—by juxtaposing them with non-Freudian writings: Shakespeare's *Hamlet* and E. T. A. Hoffmann's short-story, "The Sandman" (part II), selections from Genesis and Exodus and Milton's account of the fall of Satan in *Paradise Lost* (part III). In offering this broader interpretive framework, I need also to revisit my earlier claim to be approaching Freud through an immanent critique, "or a critique from within, conducted on the terms Freud laid down himself." For in drawing on theoretical concepts already at work in these other texts, I am necessarily pursuing a revisionary perspective from outside of Freud's own writings and indeed from outside of psychoanalytic discourse generally.

My immanent critique might be better understood then in terms of what Shoshana Felman once referred to as the interpretive labor of "generat[ing] implications" between psychoanalysis and other domains of thought. Felman is explicitly imagining such mutual implications working between psychoanalysis and literature, but whether the other writings drawn into this interdisciplinary dialogue are precisely literary or not (that is an open question when it comes to biblical texts), we might apply the same kind of repositioning of interpretive authority to all types of psychoanalytic/non-psychoanalytic encounter as Felman does to the particular one between psychoanalysis and literature. Noting that the etymological sense of "implication" is to be "folded within," Felman argues that literature maintains "a relation of *interiority*" with psychoanalysis in the sense that literature provides much of the "constitutive texture of [psychoanalysis's] *conceptual* framework, . . . the language which psychoanalysis uses in order to *speak of itself* in order to *name itself*. Literature is therefore not simply *outside* psychoanalysis, . . . since it is the *inherent reference* by which psychoanalysis names its findings."[39] Viewed from that perspective, the work of generating implications between psychoanalysis and literature simply represents a different method of carrying out an immanent critique, for the mode of writing used to reconceptualize psychoanalysis is already at work *within* it.

In parts II and III, then, I embrace Felman's paired notions that the non-psychoanalytic maintains "a relation of interiority" to the psychoanalytic and that this relation is almost of necessity confrontational in some way.[40] My discussions of certain biblical texts, *Hamlet*, "The Sandman," and *Paradise Lost* are thus all aimed at showing not only that these texts anticipate Freud's thought (which is why he looks back to them in the first place) but also that they proleptically correct the very claims he retrospectively imposes on the insights they provided him with, insights he registered only to swerve away from in order to champion other ideas. As previously outlined, that is, Freud comes up with the theory of the Oedipus complex in an effort to explain (with the effect of explaining away) the son's vexed relation to father. But this effort to read the son's hostility toward the father, or, more accurately, the son's ambivalence, in terms of Oedipal rivalry misstates the nature of that ambivalence. For filial ambivalence has much less to do with sexual rivalry than with the existential dilemma that Derrida calls the primal scene, the question of "what happens . . . when a son is *after* his father." In short, Freud's Oedipal theory imposes psychoanalytic discourse—a psychoanalytically conceived narrative—on an existential crisis of coming after, a crisis in which the son's defiance is directed at that figure whose priority can never truly be overcome.

While my readings of non-Freudian texts in parts II and III will necessarily draw on certain Freudian insights, I am more interested in reconstructing their proto-psychoanalytic self-conceptualizations as these can then be (re)directed to Freud's writings. In those dialogic encounters, I will attempt to generate moments of mutual implication between texts that anticipate Freud and Freud's own texts as these effectively lose sight of the very ideas that initially drove them. What I want to examine, in short, are key insights that Freud refused without precisely abandoning. When I turn to "The Uncanny" (chapter 4) and *Moses and Monotheism* (chapter 6) I will thus attempt to demonstrate that Freud powerfully spoke beyond the limits of his own Oedipal theory in ways he did not recognize. My other point is that what he said without recognizing was already recognized and indeed actively conceptualized in the other writings I consider.

It should be evident then that I do not aim to produce Freudian readings of these other writings. If Felman is right to suggest the possibilities of a mutually informing negotiation between literature and psychoanalysis, Freud's thought can still be a productive starting point if not the endpoint. Despite the fact that Freud is often off the mark, indeed perhaps because of his interpretive waywardness, his writings often permit us to hear the questions that other writings are already posing. These questions and whatever answers are offered can then be brought into productive exchange with psychoanalysis. Freud may have obscured many of these ideas or even buried them under the heavy weight of theories he could never part with. But that interpretive complexity just makes the exchange with what is not psychoanalysis all the more important. As I will try to show, these other writings prompt us to hear the questions Freud forgot or simply failed to register. The goal of this study, then, is to document a counter-stream in Freud's vision we would do well see, or see again, even if only belatedly.

PART I

The Refusal of Being Born

Psychoanalysis, Belatedness, and Existential Trauma

We were born without our own knowledge or choice, by our parents coming together.

—Justin Martyr, *First Apology*

In terms of psychoanalysis, one could say that violence is the refusal of being born.

—Sartre, *Notebooks for an Ethics*

Introduction to Part I

Why Are We Born?

Inversion in Freud's "Theme of the Three Caskets"

> Men must endure
> Their going hence, even as their coming hither.
> —Shakespeare, *King Lear*

I

Each at about the age of five, though some eight years apart, my children Emma and Ian had terrible epiphanies, the kind that parents would hope to spare their children if they could. But, alas, we know we cannot. These epiphanies need to be recognized as existential crises of the kind that are the subject of this book.

First for my eldest, Emma, now twenty-one-years-old as I write this. At a Good Friday service at Burlington Vermont's Episcopal Cathedral in the spring of 1999, Emma suddenly awoke to the meaning of the words from the Gospel of John: "Crucify him, crucify him." What made this moment worse was that the story was being read aloud, almost performed, by the whole congregation, so that people Emma loved and who, as she had every right to believe, protected her, were implicated in her young mind in the clamor for Jesus's death. What exactly clicked in her head we will never know for sure, but she said she felt sick in her stomach, that she needed to go to the washroom. Once there, she didn't cry, but, close to inconsolable and barely coherent, she stammered her terror in the form of a question: "Why are we even born at all if we just have to die?"

It's a testament to the radical evolution (or devolution) of some types of Christianity that neither my wife nor I thought to console Emma with explicit, traditional Easter promises. And yet Emma had heard at least some of those about ten months earlier at the funeral of her sister Claire, younger by three years (to the day), who, at eighteen months, had died of a fatal brain malformation called lissencephaly. It was impossible not to read into Emma's outburst some release of pent up fears and anxieties about Claire, yet it might also be true that it took a certain kind of cognitive development (perhaps normally appearing at about age five) for Emma to extrapolate from Claire to Jesus to herself. Claire wasn't just gone from our lives, and that little gravesite we visited wasn't just a place with a beautiful view of Lake Champlain. Jesus was going to die too (or had died already), and dying wasn't pretty. It was horrible, if not always violent, and there was suffering involved even for those who didn't experience the immediate physicality of death for themselves. What Emma realized was that death was necessary, inevitable for all, and that although it might be linked to some cosmic principle such a connection hardly proved that the cosmos had our best interests at heart. Since life might have been designed in a way that wasn't so horrible and terrifying, it only made sense to conclude that someone had it in for us. And, in Emma's transformed consciousness, that "us" was now all of us: her parents too would die someday as she would herself.

One wonders, however, if what Emma experienced was really a fear or even an anticipatory awareness of real death. Although in *Totem and Taboo* he would follow Schopenhauer in venturing that "the problem of death stands at the outset of every philosophy" (XIII, 87), in later pondering the nature and origin of the fear of death in his *Inhibitions, Symptoms and Anxiety* (1926), Freud would observe that "the unconscious seems to contain nothing that could give any content to our concept of the annihilation of life. . . . [N]othing resembling death can ever have been experienced; or if it has, as in fainting, it has left no observable traces behind" (XX, 129–30). But here Freud is wondering about the fear of death in those who have never witnessed it (perhaps they've seen something analogous, like fainting, but not an actual death). Emma wasn't present when Claire died, but she twice saw Claire's dead body, first at our home just a few hours later and again the next evening at the funeral parlor when Claire had been formally laid out. Would such contact count for Freud as "content" for "our concept of the annihilation of life"? That is, did Emma recognize the actual annihilation of life in Claire (or in Jesus for that that matter), and did she fear that? Or had she stumbled across something else?

What was troubling my son Ian had nothing to do with death and everything to do with being born. For several weeks before his fifth birthday he had been telling us, sometimes tearfully, sometimes angrily, that he didn't want a birthday at all. He had clearly come to register some connection between having birthdays and growing up, a concern seemingly linked to his sense that the baby of the family got preferential treatment. At one point during his moping he chanced to notice a picture of my wife and me with Emma and Claire, taken when we lived in a different house. He recognized his parents and he recognized his oldest sister, but he didn't know who "that baby" was. He somehow knew, perhaps it had just occurred to him, that whoever "it" was—this other baby in the family—wasn't himself. Beyond that recognition, the picture, which had always been in plain view, captured his attention in a strange way, as though it finally dawned on him that he had never fully appreciated its implications. Where were we and why wasn't he in the picture, he wanted to know. Why hadn't he lived in that house (or at least why couldn't he remember living there), and where was this sibling that he had never known? And why did he have no memories of her? Most of all, he seemed to be saying (at least as angry as confused), how could there have been a time and a place we had all been without him? How could there have been a time or a place before Ian?

Originally, it had seemed to me only by chance that Ian first considered the picture around the same time as he complained about the necessity of birthdays. But perhaps the link wasn't so accidental. Indeed, while, as I said, it had seemed to my wife and me that the main source of his disgruntled state of mind was that he didn't want to do anything to jeopardize his status as youngest child (and simply getting a year older appeared to put that status at risk), it occurred to me sometime later that birthdays are emblematic of what he was registering in response to the picture, registering for the first time: we can be absent from the world and even preceded by others who know much more about everything (including ourselves) and who don't actually ask us if we want to be brought into it. Or, to put this another way (and I am here anticipating my extended discussion in chapter 5), Ian experienced something of the same tortured discovery Milton represented in his character Satan: that, despite what the God of *Paradise Lost* argues, rather unconvincingly it might be added, we are not "authors" to ourselves (*Paradise Lost*, 3.122); rather, we are authored by others.

By the verb "to author" I intend here something of what Giorgio Agamben means in the passage that will serve as a kind of conceptual touchstone throughout this study:

> In Latin, *auctor* originally designates the person who intervenes in the case of a minor (or the person who, for whatever reason, does not have the capacity to posit a legally valid act), in order to grant him the valid title that he requires. . . . It is thus possible to explain *the sense of the term auctor . . . as the general meaning of "setting into being"* . . . The act of the *auctor* completes the act of an incapable person, giving strength of proof *to what in itself lacks it and granting life to what could not live alone*.[1]

To the extent *auctoring*/authoring is an act that one person (an author[ity]) imposes upon another, the person receiving this originating—authorizing act is, in some paradoxical sense, absent from it: "set into being," "granted life" before actually possessing being or life. Being authored, in that sense, means that we are compelled to recognize our inhabiting of a life we cannot—could not, could never—claim on our own.

I will address this concept in more detail subsequently, but for now I would just like to build on the study's introduction to suggest that such compulsion—or perhaps more accurately the compulsion to recognize—should be understood as the primal scene: that is, the subject's belated recognition of its very exclusion from the scene of its own origin. To put this idea back into the family narrative I've been sketching, Ian's moment of recognition just prior to his fifth birthday—his discovery of his missing sister and everything his own "missing" of her implied—was his primal scene. To (come to) know of a time before one "was" is to be forced to acknowledge the condition of being absent and thus also of being preceded, to witness one's own necessary *afterwardsness*. Such an absence, moreover, must also mean that it is possible to have an origin about which one knows nothing. Or, perhaps worse, it is an origin about which one knows at once nothing and now too much: too much about parents—or some other force: nature? god(s)?—who are more powerful and mysterious than we might have otherwise believed, who grant us a life we never even knew about, who threw us into an existence we did not and could not choose for ourselves. And we also now know that it is too late to go back and change that fact. For the primal scene is precisely the discovery—a discovery that itself necessarily comes too late—that we are forever belated in relation to our own existence.

To return to Emma's crisis, it is possible that her confrontation with mortality was more closely related to Ian's than first appears. We might especially see a link if we feel that Freud's intuition is right: the fear of death at once masks and reveals a fear of something else. The very logic of Emma's question—why are we born at all if we just have to die?—suggests as much. For what Emma was asking had as much to do with being born as with dying. Indeed, the five-year-old Emma seemed to be recognizing death simply as a fact. And she wasn't asking why we die; that was clear enough: we die because we are born. But that stark reality just begged the real question: why are we born, or why do we come into existence in the first place, if our lot is to die?

Emma's insight, as such an insight is available to a child's mind, has something in common with the following passage from Nietzsche's *Birth of Tragedy*, a passage we shall have cause to revisit in chapter 2:

> An old legend has it that King Midas hunted a long time in the woods for the wise Silenus, companion of Dionysos, without being able to catch him. When he had finally caught him the king asked him what he considered man's greatest good. The daemon remained sullen and uncommunicative until finally, forced by the king, he broke into a shrill laugh and spoke: "Ephemeral wretch, begotten of accident and toil, why do you force me to tell you what it would be your greatest boon not to hear? What would be best for you is quite beyond your reach: not to have been born, not to *be*, to be *nothing*. But the second best is to die soon."[2]

Viewed in the context of this passage, Emma's question suggests that she has taken on the unvoiced perspective of King Midas *after* he has heard Silenus's answer. That is, despite her "why are we born at all?" she wasn't faced with an absence of meaning or too little meaning; rather, she has too much meaning already: Silenus's answer. Or, in Nietzsche's sense, Emma wasn't experiencing confusion; rather, she was experiencing a deep sense of the fundamentally problematic nature of existence as grotesque, absurd, nonsensical. For Silenus, death is precisely a solution (admittedly, a second best one) rather than a problem, a solution to having been born at all. But under what compulsion must we come into existence in the first place? Despite the initial context of Emma's terror, her problem, like Ian's, seems to have been less about endings than about origins.

The earlier, rather passing reference to Freud's *Inhibitions, Symptoms and Anxiety* is not incidental. Following the logic of the passage from Sartre I have used as the second epigraph for part I, the remainder of this introduction and the subsequent two chapters will take up the problem of origins (for Sartre "the refusal of being born") precisely in relation to certain psychoanalytic concepts. Chapter 1 will give special attention to how the problem of the origin is at the heart of Freud's concept of the death drive as formulated in *Beyond the Pleasure Principle*, a text I will (re)read in relation to Cathy Caruth's famous revisionary theory of Freud's idea. In part to demonstrate how Freud's own ideas had unleashed metapsychological possibilities he was unwilling to accept, chapter 2 will then consider both Otto Rank's 1924 *The Trauma of Birth* and Freud's response in his *Inhibitions, Symptoms and Anxiety*. One of my key points is that, in the 1926 text, Freud (re)imposes his Oedipal model even against his own earlier and indeed more compelling insights. In so doing (as he will throughout his career), he uses the Oedipus complex and castration anxiety to explain—or explain away—the existential crisis of belatedness his own earlier work had so powerfully theorized.

Before we get to those later writings, I would like to take up a short earlier text, the 1913 "Theme of the Three Caskets." Besides demonstrating something of Freud's habits as a literary critic, that essay introduces us to how psychoanalysis might grapple with the Sartrean first-cause of violence, the refusal of being born. More especially, I want to use this essay to suggest that, for Freud, Emma's and Ian's problems were one and the same: the problem of dying is always already the problem of being born. To put this another way, the recognition of mortality is just another expression of the primal scene, the acknowledgment of the origin we did not and could not choose for ourselves.

II

In "Theme of the Three Caskets," Freud works through the mythic material underlying several texts, including Shakespeare's *Merchant of Venice* and *King Lear*. As Freud construes them, these stories recount moments of choice faced by male protagonists (in Shakespeare's plays Bassanio and Lear) that, in direct or indirect ways, involve choices concerning women. More specifically, sifting through what he sees as a series of inversions, he reconstructs stories that feature a woman choosing among three male suitors (as Portia does in *Merchant of Venice*) as disguising the opposite scenario: a man choosing among three women (as *King Lear* does).[3] Freud goes on to observe, moreover, that the courtship theme is itself a kind of distortion. In *King Lear*, for example, the three women are the man's daughters—part of the change by which Shakespeare gives us an *old* man rather than a lover, and, as an old man, a man close to death, "a dying man" as Freud provocatively suggests, even "a doomed man" (255–56).[4] And because, in this context, we now have daughters of the same father, the three women are necessarily sisters. The particular detail is critical for Freud because the presence of three sisters helps him to establish the etiological underpinning of later revisions of the original myth. Through a series of associations with the other versions he analyzes, Freud comes to understand the third sister (variously pale, silent or even mute, concealed, symbolized by a lead casket) as a dead woman. This identification is itself a displacement, one "not infrequent," he tells us, wherein the "qualities that a deity imparts to men are ascribed to the deity himself" or in this case *her*self. The dead woman, then, "may be something else," Freud concludes, "Death itself, [or] the Goddess of Death" (250).[5]

Reading this (re-)identification of the youngest sister/daughter through subsequent revisions of the myth, Freud argues that these revisions are typically built on two new inversions that, taken together, constitute a compensatory rhetoric against the fear of death: (1) a conceptual reversal from a necessary passivity before destiny, a destiny in which we are chosen, to the representation of our own agency through the act of choosing (as Bassanio and Lear choose among the three objects/women); and, (2) a substitution for the thing we would never choose (death) by the thing we willingly choose, the beloved or, in the mythic revisions, variously the "Goddess of Love, . . . one comparable to the goddess, . . . the fairest and wisest of women, . . . the one faithful daughter" (252). Here is Freud's summary of this process of inversion:

> [E]very time in this theme of ours [when] there occurs a free choice between the women, . . . the choice is thereupon to fall on death—that which no man chooses, to which by destiny alone man falls a victim. . . . [But through inversion,] choice stands in the place of necessity, of destiny. Thus man overcomes death, which in thought he has acknowledged. No greater triumph of wish-fulfillment is conceivable. Just where in reality he obeys compulsion, he exercises choice; and that which he chooses is not a thing of horror, but the fairest and more desirable thing in life. (253–54)[6]

And near the close of the essay, Freud then interprets the emotionally shattering ending of *King Lear* through this lens: "The free choice between the three sisters is, properly speaking, no free choice, for it must necessarily fall on the third if every kind of evil is not to come about, as in *Lear*. . . . Cordelia is death. Reverse the situation and it becomes intelligible and familiar to us—the Death-goddess bearing away the dead hero from the place of battle . . . Eternal wisdom, in the garb of primitive myth, bids the old man renounce love, choose death and make friends with the necessity of dying" (254, 256).

In short, as a prime example of "reaction-formation"—what he here defines as those "forces in mental life tending to bring about replacement by the opposite" (253)—Freud comes to read mythic representations of the "theme" as a reaction-formation against death. Thus, believing he now has the key to reading the revisions' distortions, he triumphantly declares that he has succeeded in his major aim, declared at the outset of the essay, of tracing this "ancient theme . . . back to its origin" (245):

> The Moerae [Fates] were created as a result of a recognition which warns man that he too is part of nature and therefore subject to the immutable law of death. Against this subjection something in man was bound to struggle, for it is only with extreme unwillingness that he gives up his claim to an exceptional position. We know that man makes use of his imaginative faculty (phantasy) to satisfy those wishes that reality does not satisfy. So his imagination rebelled against the recognition of the truth embodied in the myth of the Moerae, and constructed instead the myth derived from it. (253)

In this most potent of all reaction-formations, then, death ceases to be something that chooses us and becomes instead something we choose and choose precisely because we desire rather than fear it. To put this idea in its original form, we fear death not simply because we fear mortality generally but because we recognize our helplessness against it: we have no agency in the face of this inexorable force or, more precisely even, in the face of this force in relation to which we are stripped of our capacity to choose.

Of course, as we noted above, in his later *Inhibitions, Symptoms and Anxiety* Freud will argue that "the unconscious seems to contain nothing that could give any content to our concept of the annihilation of life. . . . [N]othing resembling death can ever have been experienced; or if it has, as in fainting, it has left no observable traces behind." It is worth pondering whether this same thought is already active in Freud's thought some thirteen years earlier. That is, in "Theme of the Three Caskets" is Freud already beginning to theorize that the fear of death stands in for something else? In this context we might see a fourth key inversion in the essay, one that Freud addresses without fully acknowledging (though it is more accurate to refer to this inversion, in its initial form at least, as an equivalence).

Noting the "double nature" of the third sister, her "alteration between the ugly and the beautiful" (254n1), Freud observes that this alteration is in line with an "ancient ambivalence" that had once viewed the Goddess of Love (of Fertility) and the Goddess of Death as "identical": "The great Mother-goddesses . . . all seem to have been both founts of being and destroyers; goddesses of life and fertility, and death-goddesses." But here too we may have more of an inversion, one that emerges through a process of substitution. For despite the fact that Freud understands "the replacement by the wish-opposite . . . in our theme"—(the Goddess of) Death becomes (the Goddess of) Love—as "built upon an ancient identity" (254), in his earlier summary of how the three Fates ("personifying . . . the inevitable doom" we call death) mythically developed "in connection with other divine [sister-] figures, to which the Moerae are clearly related" (the Hours), he suggests not only an evolution more than an original identity but also that the very concept of the necessity of human death evolved from its opposite, from the concepts of life and natural fertility: "The Hours are originally goddess[es] of the waters of the sky, dispensing rain and dew, and of the clouds from which rain falls . . . In the sun-favored Mediterranean land it is rain on which the fertility of the soil depends, and thus the Hours become the goddesses of vegetation. The beauty of flowers and the abundance of fruit is their doing, and man endows them plentifully with charming and graceful traits. They become the divine representations of the Seasons." Only later, according to Freud, did these "weather goddesses" become "goddesses of destiny": when, in short, a "knowledge of nature reacted on the conception of human life," the life-giving "aspect of the Hours . . . found expression in the Moerae, who watch over the needful ordering of human life as inexorably as do the Hours over the regular order of nature. The implacable severity of this law, the affinity of it with death and ruin, . . . was now stamped upon the Moerae, as though mankind had only perceived the full solemnity of natural law when he had to submit his own personality to its workings" (251–52).

At the very end of the essay, Freud will then combine identity with something like temporal evolution in mapping this mythopoeic material onto a deeper psycho-mythic structure, one in which man's (and the gendered meaning here is not merely incidental) entire life-narrative is representable as a series of encounters with real or symbolic female-figures:

> The regressive treatment he [the poet or myth-maker] has thus undertaken with the myth, which was disguised by the reversal of the wish, allows its original meaning so far to appear that perhaps a superficial allegorical interpretation of the three

> female figures in the theme becomes possible as well. One might say that the three inevitable relations man has with woman are here represented: that with the mother who bears him, with the companion of his bed and board, and with the destroyer. Or it is the three forms taken on by the figure of the mother as life proceeds: the mother herself, the beloved who is chosen after her pattern, and finally the Mother Earth who receives him again. But it is in vain that the old man yearns after the love of woman as once he had it from his mother; the third of the Fates alone, the silent goddess of Death, will take him into her arms. (256)

Freud might be anticipating his concept of the death drive as formulated in *Beyond the Pleasure Principle* (1920) in his quasi-Oedipal suggestion that man longs for the embrace of death as a substitute for the lost mother. But development of that particular concept lies in Freud's future. Here, we are faced more directly with Freud's intuition that mythic distortions about man's (men's) encounter with the threat of dying evince a deep and troubling association between death and birth: the Goddess of Death is *Mother* Earth and so just a later version of "the figure of the mother as life." For the male psyche at least, the powerful link between death and birth is forged by an association between being born and being destroyed as both the creative and destructive powers are wielded by or in the maternal presence. The "silent Goddess of Death" merely completes a process initiated at the point of origin when the man is delivered from the body of his biological mother.

The gender-implications of this anxiety deserve more attention than I can give here.[7] What is crucial for our purposes is that Freud's formulation enables us to imagine in a very general way that the (male) fear of death, the cause of which is so remarkably untheorized in "Theme of the Three Caskets," has its origins precisely in origins rather than in endings. Freud understands Lear as "an old man . . . a dying man" (255), but despite his viewing the Fates—"personifying . . . the inevitable doom" (251) we call death—as inverting an original personification of fertility in the Hours, he does not take the next logical step: a dying man figuratively stands in for a man being born. In this context, our fearful confrontation with death might be better understood as a confrontation with an anxiety-riddled beginning. Freud himself views death less as an endpoint in itself than as the conclusion of a sequence that begins at birth: the moment an existence is given to or even imposed upon us by some enigmatic Other, something that is there before us. Thus, where, for example, Freud reads Lear's story as the (male) fantasy of (re)claiming the capacity to choose in relation to his death, we might counter that account with one final reversal: it is not that he wishes to be able to choose when or how he will die; rather, as the four-year-old Ian's crisis suggests, he wishes to have been able to choose when or how or even why he was born.

As we shall see in greater detail in relation to *Beyond the Pleasure Principle* (chapter 1) and *Inhibitions, Symptoms and Anxiety* (chapter 2), the problem of death (the ending) becomes the problem of birth (the beginning) precisely because one has no choice about coming into existence in the first place. This crisis of origins is thus the crisis of the primal scene because, as we observed in the study's introduction, the primal scene is the moment of recognition of having been absent from the scene of one's own origin. And, as Freud intuits in "Theme of the Three Caskets" without quite recognizing, what in particular is absent at the origin is choice itself. Revising Freud, we might say that what is (re)enacted in the image of Lear carrying the dead body of Cordelia in his arms (Cordelia as the Goddess of Death and the Goddess of Life simultaneously) is less what Freud had called an old man's "mak[ing] friends with the necessity of dying" (256) than his making his own choice to exist, a choice denied him at birth.

What this all means is that, as early as 1913, Freud is beginning to explore how death anxiety expresses an anxiety of the origin precisely because it is in relation to our origin that we are compelled to confront most powerfully our existential helplessness. If, as Freud explicitly notes in "Theme of the Three Caskets," the reaction-formation against death turns the very sign of that helplessness—our lack of choice—into a sign of our power (our choosing), it is in that essay that Freud first formulates a matrix of ideas he will develop later without ever fully crediting his own insight: as he will put it seven years later in *Beyond the Pleasure Principle*, at the origin we are helpless before "a force of whose nature we can form no conception" (XVIII, 38). If in the primal scene we discover not some repressed knowledge but a reality of our lives that, paradoxically, we never even experienced, that very missing locates us in an ever-afterwards we can never escape: a being chosen by what necessarily precedes us.

"It is very unhappy," Emerson writes in his essay "Experience," "but too late to be helped, the discovery we have made that we exist." Emerson doesn't explain in that cryptic utterance how there can be a time in life before such a discovery. Emerson would not have used a Freudian vocabulary, of course, but that discovery of existence—what he calls the Fall of Man—is less a religious event than, as Freud might have recognized, a traumatic one. More to the point, Emerson hints that the experience of belatedness (what is "*too late* be helped") is central to that trauma. But the "too late" does not simply mark trauma's delayed appearance or deferred impact. Rather, the belatedness speaks to what Cathy Caruth, following Freud, sees as a latency inherent in the original experience: despite being present, the subject yet misses it. But as I will try to argue *against* Caruth, there is one trauma—Emerson's Ur-trauma as existential crisis—in relation to which the latency is constituted not by what Caruth means by *missing*, a being there that is always already forgotten (through dissociation). Rather, it is constituted by an actual absence, the very space in which we can come into existence without knowing that we do.

It is in this context that we might give special attention to this statement from "Remembering, Repeating, and Working-Through": "In these [psychical] processes it particularly happens that something is 'remembered' which could never have been 'forgotten' because it was never at any time noticed" (XII, 149). By "something . . . 'remembered' which could never have been 'forgotten,'" Freud means something experienced and then immediately repressed (so "never at any time noticed"). But here and throughout this study I take Freud's statement more literally. There are things we come to accept as part of our pasts that we cannot actually remember. These are things that "could never have been forgotten" because, while they most certainly happened—they had to have happened—we did not actually experience them while they were happening. Especially in relation to the origin, it is possible, paradoxically, to have been absent from things that happened to us. Chapters 1 and 2 aim at providing a fuller examination of what this issue might have meant to Freudian psychoanalysis.

1

"Awakening is itself the site of a trauma"
Rethinking Caruth on Freud

> There is a brute contingency to all origins as such.
> —Harold Bloom, *Ruin the Sacred Truths*

I

In discussing the impact of traumatic experience on the workings of memory, Bessel van der Kolk and Onno van der Hart challenge one of the central tenets of Freudian psychoanalysis—the concept of repression—at least as it relates to trauma. Like Freud, especially from the writing of *Beyond the Pleasure Principle* (1920) onward, van der Kolk and van der Hart are interested "in the role of overwhelming experiences on the development of psychopathology."[1] But against Freud's theory of repression as a response to trauma, they offer a new way of understanding what it means for the traumatized psyche not to be able to lay claim to a past experience in the form of a conscious relation to it.

Concerned both with how, in general terms, "memories are stored in the mind" and, more particularly, with the "disruptive impact of traumatic experiences" on the storage and retrieval of memories (158), van der Kolk and van der Hart argue that trauma's disabling of the mind has less to do with repression as an active refusal of an experience—its forced relocation to a hidden region that escapes conscious attention—than with dissociation, a process whereby the mind, faced with an incomprehensible experience, fails to organize that experience within an unfolding temporal order, fails, that is, to assign it narrative coherence.[2] Where such coherence is lacking, they argue, the mind cannot assimilate an experience into a broader life narrative. In this model, trauma renders experience inaccessible to conscious thought through the failed psychic integration of that experience: the experience cannot be assimilated into the broader cognitive patterns that are central to memory and, through memory, to the possibility of continuous or narrative selfhood. One might say that, for van der Kolk and van der Hart, trauma and narrative inaccessibility or incomprehensibility are one and the same.[3]

Nevertheless, even as they disagree with Freud on the mental process that governs trauma, van der Kolk and van der Hart implicitly accept a key element of Freud's thought. If in the formation of trauma the role of conscious thought in engaging experience is somehow bypassed, the mind yet latches onto this experience at a different level. Thus, even as they reject Freud's use of the term repression in the context of trauma, van der Kolk and van der Hart still imagine some subconscious storehouse where the experience will be retained:

> With regard to trauma, [Freud's] use of the term "repression" evokes the image of a subject actively pushing the unwanted traumatic memory away [later, they will write "pushed downward into the unconscious"].... [But] contemporary research has shown that dissociation of a traumatic experience occurs as the trauma is occurring ... There is little evidence for an active process of pushing away of the overwhelming experience; the uncoupling seems to have other mechanisms. Many trauma survivors report that they are automatically removed from the scene; they look at it from a distance or disappear altogether, *leaving other parts of the personality to* suffer and *store the overwhelming experience.* ... [W]hen a subject does not remember a trauma, *its "memory" is contained in an alternate stream of consciousness.* (168; my emphases)

Although van der Kolk and van der Hart are no doubt right at the technical level to note that "traumatic memories cannot be both dissociated and repressed," they yet share with Freud the notion that trauma creates, indeed is essentially coincident with, an experience that goes underground and that subsequently disrupts consciousness "during traumatic reenactments" (168–69), that is, through repetition compulsion. The traumatic event may not be accessible to consciousness, but the mind retains a remnant, however distorted, of some part of an actual experience.[4]

Without trying to resolve the debate here (trauma as repression or trauma as dissociation), in the remainder of this chapter I would like to offer another possibility for understanding the formation and continuing impact of trauma (at least one type of it). And I would start with this simple observation: it is not self-evident that the psychical material marking a trauma must always be viewed as the remnant of an event that we actually experienced. As previously noted, van der Kolk and van der Hart appear to agree with Freud that, as an ongoing experience, trauma is the repeatedly expressed trace of such an event. But what if the experience of trauma registers an absence rather than a dislocated presence? What if the traumatic remnant is inaccessible precisely because it is not stored somewhere else in the mind? What if there is nothing to repress or what if there is nothing there to be transformed even into traumatic memory because there was no original experience to be remembered? Is it possible, then, to imagine that one could be traumatized precisely by what has *not* been experienced?

In the subsequent discussion I want to suggest that this possibility is hinted at (though only hinted at) in Cathy Caruth's seminal study, *Unclaimed Experience*. But whereas Caruth builds on Freud's related notions of fright, repetition compulsion, and deferred action (Freud's *Nachträglichkeit*) to explore trauma as an ethical crisis, I will attempt to show that at key points Caruth misstates Freud's original argument and so imposes new, sometimes questionable meanings on certain Freudian concepts (most notably the death drive). More to the point, while in the final section I will briefly revisit the notion that trauma has an ethical aspect, I will argue that, whether or not Freud fully understood it this way, his original formulation represented trauma in its relation to the death drive less as an ethical situation than as an existential crisis.

II

Before we consider how Caruth's study might help us to rethink trauma, it is instructive to observe how, like van der Kolk and van der Hart, she yet retains a critical aspect of Freud's theory even as she reworks other parts of it. Focused explicitly on how trauma persists—and how especially it is re-experienced in the form of repetition compulsion—Caruth never addresses the precise mechanism through which an original traumatic event becomes embedded in the psyche. But her descriptions of such an original event suggest that she would incline more to van der Kolk and van der Hart's view than to Freud's:

> [T]he wound of the mind—the breach in the mind's experience of time, self, and the world—is not, like the wound of the body, a simple and healable event, but rather an event that . . . is experienced too soon, too unexpectedly, to be fully known and is therefore not available to consciousness until it imposes itself again, repeatedly, in the nightmares and repetitive actions of the survivor. . . . [T]rauma is not locatable in the simple violent or original event in an individual's past, but rather in the way that its very unassimilated nature—the way it was precisely *not known* in the first instance—returns to haunt the survivor later on. . . . [Trauma] is always the story of a wound that . . . addresses us in the attempt to tell us of a reality or truth that is not otherwise available. This truth, in its delayed appearance and its belated address, cannot be linked only to what is known, but also to what remains unknown in our very actions and our language.[5]

Caruth is more concerned here with the circumstances under which trauma is formed than with the specific process by which an initial event becomes disruptive psychic residue. But even as she goes on to write that "traumatic experience, as Freud indicates suggestively, is an experience that is not fully assimilated as it occurs" (5), to say that such an experience "is not fully assimilated *as it occurs*" leans toward van der Kolk and van der Hart's position. For example, as previously noted, they observe how "contemporary research has shown that dissociation of a traumatic experience occurs *as the trauma is occurring* . . . There is little evidence for an active process of pushing away of the overwhelming experience [Freud's repression]; the uncoupling seems to have other mechanisms" (my emphases). More generally, Caruth's claim that trauma is a "breach in the mind's experience *of time*" accords with van der Kolk and van der Hart's sense that the traumatic remnant is inaccessible to conscious thought because unassimilated into the mind's normal temporal ordering of experience.[6]

That said, though hardly explicit about it, Caruth appears to share with van der Kolk and van der Hart the Freudian notion that the traumatic remnant is something retained in the psyche as a record or trace of an actual occurrence. She notes, for example, that the experience of trauma "stubbornly persists in bearing witness to some forgotten wound" (5). That the wound is *forgotten* suggests that it has been lost to or in the mind only after it has first been retained: if now forgotten it must previously have been remembered (even if in unassimilated form), and this memory points to something that really happened in the past. While that original experience may not be "*fully* assimilated as it occurs," something *is* assimilated at that initial occurrence; if there is a "*delayed* appearance," that appearance yet points to the original event or at least to our response to the original event.

Still, as we have noted, Caruth insists that the relation between the trauma and the original event is governed by incomprehensibility. Because the original event "is experienced too soon, too unexpectedly," it is "precisely *not known* in the first instance" and so "not available to consciousness." And when it is available at all, it is only in the form of "belated address" or through "belated impact." Indeed, for Caruth, "the story of trauma" is "the narrative of belated experience" (4, 7). Such a narrative is precisely that experience of bearing witness subsequently to what, we might say, is always already forgotten. Belatedness is thus, for Caruth, coincidental with repetition compulsion: trauma's "belated address" or "belated impact" or "delayed appearance" resides in the temporal afterwards from which the mind looks back, repetitively, longingly, futilely, on an event it experienced but never truly knew.[7]

Perhaps it is just a quibble to note the paradox of Caruth's wording: how can something be belated or delayed if it is experienced "too soon?" No doubt, Caruth uses the phrase "too soon" to figure the perspective of the mind relative to an event rather than to situate a subject's actual temporal relation to that event. In other words, the original event is experienced *before* the mind is ready to encounter and assimilate it. The subsequent "afterwards"—the time of the belated impact—would thus refer to when the mind *is* ready even as the delay would mark the breach in time that dislocates the original experience. Caruth sees the full force of trauma as operating belatedly in the sense that the subject experiences a delayed onset of symptoms: this notion of belatedness is best understood as equivalent to Freud's *Nachträglichkeit* or "deferred action," what "returns to haunt the survivor *later on*" (4). But, as we have noted, Caruth is just as interested in the *initial condition* of incomprehensibility (the "unassimilated nature" of an experience, "the way it was precisely not known in the first instance"). And when she writes that, in traumatic experience, "the most direct seeing of a violent event may occur as an absolute inability to know it; that *immediacy, paradoxically, may take the form of belatedness*" (91; my emphasis), she hints that belatedness is not just a statement of the temporal positioning of the response (its delayed appearance) but is also, and perhaps more crucially, descriptive of some quality in the original experience itself.

Indeed, if for Caruth trauma is "an event that . . . is *experienced too soon*," in her subsequent discussion that "too soon" will become precisely its opposite. Borrowing from Freud's key distinctions between fear, fright, and anxiety as laid out in *Beyond the Pleasure Principle*, Caruth notes that the "breach in the mind" characteristic of trauma is caused by "the lack of preparedness to take in a stimulus that comes too quickly" (here it is the stimulus that comes "too soon"). And "the threat is recognized as such by the mind *one moment too late*. The shock . . . is thus not the direct experience of the threat, but precisely the *missing* of this experience, the fact that, not being experienced *in time*, it has not yet been fully known" (62).[8] This notion of traumatic belatedness as the subject's coming *too late* rather than too soon helps us conceptualize the possibility of an experience of an initial seeing that fails to see, a presence that is also an absence, the inexplicable missing of what could not possibly have been missed. That is, what Caruth calls the "central enigma" of Freud's contextualizing of trauma in terms of the unexpected or accidental ("for instance, a train collision," as Freud puts it) might point to a different way of understanding belatedness. It "is not so much the period of forgetting that occurs after the accident, but rather that the victim . . . was never fully conscious during the accident itself." The deferral, or what Freud in *Moses and Monotheism* will call "latency," within the experience of trauma "would thus seem to consist," Caruth concludes, "not in the forgetting of a reality that can hence never be fully known, but in *an inherent latency within the experience itself*" (17; my emphasis).[9]

Nevertheless, this notion of belatedness is still figurative rather than literal: the subject was "there" but, inexplicably, missed the experience. But what if the initial encounter is not a presence dislocated in the mind but precisely a true originary absence, an experience in relation to which the traumatized subject was never and could never have been "there"? Caruth observes that much within trauma "defies . . . our witness" and "defies . . . our understanding" (5). But perhaps in some cases trauma defies understanding because the event that prompted it was never witnessed at all. Could "precisely not known in the first instance" mean, in some circumstances at least, that there was no such original event or, even if there were, that this event was not actually experienced, never actually remembered (even in dissociated form), and so never actually forgotten?

In short, what if we were to take the notion of "coming too late" literally rather than as a figurative description for that initial experience of incomprehensibility? Caruth is undoubtedly correct to suggest of trauma's relation to repetition compulsion that what is experienced in "traumatic neurosis . . . [is] the unwitting reenactment of an event that one cannot simply leave behind" (2). In some instances, however, it may be that the reenactment or obsessive return occurs precisely because, at the time of the original event, the subsequently traumatized subject was already left behind in the sense of not having been present. For the remainder of this chapter, I want to pursue this interpretive trajectory. On the one hand, I will follow Caruth in arguing that the ghostly reality of the real event, a reality the traumatized subject inexplicably missed, fixes belatedness not just as a temporal lag in the registering of an event (the "delayed appearance" of trauma) but also, and more crucially, as a formative condition of trauma. On the other hand, I want to revise Caruth by arguing that, for a particular kind of trauma (one first theorized by Freud and subsequently appropriated by Caruth), the subject does not just "miss" the event but is in fact absent from it. Indeed, the event as constituted requires the subject's absence. It is to an exploration of this possibility that we now turn.

III

This section, which has much to do with the concept of origins, has its own origin in Freud's justly famous account of the dream of the burning child (*Interpretation of Dreams*, chapter 7), a dream that Freud felt compelled to interpret twice. Here is Freud's account of the setting of the dream and of the dream itself:

> A father had been watching beside his child's sick-bed for days and nights on end. After the child had died, he went into the next room to lie down, but left the door open so that he could see from his bedroom into the room in which his child's body was laid out, with tall candles standing round it. An old man had been engaged to keep watch over it, and sat beside the body murmuring prayers. After a few hours' sleep, the father had a dream that *his child was standing beside his bed, caught him by the arm and whispered to him reproachfully: "Father, don't you see I'm burning?"* He woke up, noticed a bright glare of light from the next room, hurried into it and found that the old watchman had dropped off to sleep and that the wrappings and one of the arms of his beloved child's dead body had been burned by a lighted candle that had fallen on them.

Freud begins his interpretation by noting how the dream can be read in terms of the fundamental processes of dream-work he has previously described. Although there seems to have been an external reality to which the dream makes direct reference, the main terms of the dream—the child's words to the father—show evidence of the two primary dream-processes, condensation and displacement:

> [T]he words spoken by the child must have been made up of words which he had actually spoken in his lifetime and which were connected with important events in the father's mind. For instance, "*I am burning*" may have been spoken during the fever of the child's last illness, and "*Father, don't you see?*" may have been derived from some other highly emotional situation of which we are in ignorance. (V, 509–10)

Freud recognizes that the very explicit connection between the dream and an external reality is atypical of dreams, and he "wonder[s]" at first "why it was that a dream occurred at all in such circumstances, when the most rapid possible awakening was called for." It is, therefore, the delay in the father's response—that is, the force of dreaming that postpones an awakening urgently demanded—that arouses Freud's interpretive interest.

Despite the dream's direct reference to an external reality, because the details of the dream yet "can be inserted into the chain of the dreamer's psychical experiences," Freud initially interprets the dream as a instance of his theory of wish-fulfillment:

> [H]ere we shall observe that this dream, too, contained the fulfillment of a wish. The dead child behaved in the dream like a living one: he himself warned his father, came to his bed, and caught him by the arm, just as he had probably done on the occasion from the memory of which the first part of the child's words in the dream were derived. For the sake of the fulfillment of this wish, the father prolonged his sleep by one moment. The dream was preferred to a waking reflection because it was able to show the child as once more alive. (V, 510)

Freud does not say this in so many words, but the fact that the dream takes place in the context of an actual external reality to which it appears to refer directly (though it is not, of course, a simple reflection of that reality) provides even more evidence for the complex rhetoric of the dream-work. For the external reality of the light is reconfigured in the dream as an indirect representation, both metaphorical and metonymical, of the child's death ("don't you see I'm burning?"). And the very ambiguity of that representation (why is the child burning? where is he burning? where is the father?) serves the ends of wish-fulfillment: a burning child who can yet speak is precisely not a dead child. Freud adds that "if the father had woken up first and then made the inference that led him to go into the next room, he would, as it were, have shortened his child's life by that moment of time." Following a logic more in line with Freud's own observations concerning the solipsistic nature of dreams, we might turn this remark around to say that, had he woken up immediately, he would have shortened his own *fatherly* life by that moment of time. That is, dreaming that his child yet lives (even if suffering), the father extends the time in which he has not yet failed in his chief paternal duty, to protect his own child from harm.

Freud's first answer then to the problem of the delay in waking up is completely in line with his theory of dreams. But Freud seems unsatisfied with this interpretation, and, later in the chapter, without rejecting that initial interpretation, he adds a secondary motive:

> [W]e may assume that a further motive force in the production of the dream was the father's need to sleep; his sleep, like the child's life, was prolonged by one moment by the dream. "Let the dream go on"—such was his motive—"or I shall have to wake up." In every other dream, just as in this one, the wish to sleep lends its support to the unconscious wish. (V, 570–71)

The phrase "wish to sleep" might suggest that the presence of a second wish just goes to prove that the relation of dreaming to wish-fulfillment is overdetermined: because dreams are efficient, more than one wish can be accommodated in a single dream. But it is curious that Freud distinguishes the wish to sleep from "the *unconscious* wish" to prolong, even for just a moment, the life of the child. In other words, it is not clear if the wish to sleep is a "wish" in the way the theory of dreams understands wish-fulfillment as the release through the censoring mechanisms of the psyche of desires created under the pleasure principle. Is there simply a bodily *need* for sleep that is facilitated by the drive of the Unconscious to engage in wish-fulfillment or is there an *unconscious* wish for sleep, that is, a desire for sleep that can be understood in terms of the urgings of the Unconscious? And, if the latter, why would the wish for sleep need to be unconscious in the first place?

We might even ask if any part of the psyche is aware of a need or desire to sleep. Earlier in the *Interpretation of Dreams*, Freud appears to answer in the affirmative but not without some ambiguity: "All dreams . . . serve the purpose of prolonging sleep instead of waking up. Dreams are the GUARDIANS of sleep and not its disturbers. . . . Thus *the wish to sleep (which the conscious ego is concentrated upon . . .)* must in every case be reckoned as one of the motives for the formation of dreams, and *every successful dream is a fulfillment of that wish*" (IV, 233–34; my emphases; original emphases deleted). On the one hand, Freud says explicitly that the wish to sleep is related to "the conscious ego"; on the other hand, the fact that the prolonging of sleep marks the fulfillment of a wish (an instance of the generalized process that governs all dreams) suggests that, like other wishes, it derives from the Unconscious. But it isn't clear how the conscious ego "concentrates upon" the wish to sleep. Does this wish emanate from consciousness or does it come from someplace else and only thereafter come to the attention of consciousness?

In her analysis of Freud's dual interpretation of the dream of the burning child, Caruth notes that the father's wish for sleep is "more profound and enigmatic" than his wish to sustain a fantasy that his child yet lived "because . . . it comes not only from the body but from consciousness itself, which desires somehow its own suspension." "[C]ommon to all sleepers," Caruth adds, this desire "represent[s] . . . the wish fulfillment of consciousness itself" (96). Caruth's phrasing in a certain way repeats the ambiguity of Freud's original account, and we must ask, again, what sort of wish emanates from consciousness. What makes this notion truly profound and enigmatic is that it offers the possibility that consciousness is not simply to be distinguished from the Unconscious but that consciousness itself has its own unstated or unknowable or even forbidden desires.

What we need to ask then is just what is this forbidden desire of the wish to sleep that consciousness can face only in the form of a dream. I quoted Caruth's observation that "consciousness itself . . . desires somehow its own suspension"; she goes on to note that the "wish of consciousness to sleep" is, in some form, "the desire of consciousness as such not to wake up." Attempting to gloss this notion, Caruth, who still sees the "desire of consciousness as such *not to wake up*" very much in the context of the father's emotional struggle over his child's death, comments that "it is not the father alone who dreams to avoid his child's death, but *consciousness itself* that, in sleep, is tied to a death from which it turns away" (97). The phrase "tied to a death from which it turns away" appears to mean the death of the child, the death the grieving father cannot yet accept. But to the extent that, in Caruth's curious formulation, the desire of consciousness to sleep is bound up with its turning away from the child's death, we might rightly ask if the idea of "the desire of consciousness not to wake up" can be anything other than a metaphor for wish-fulfillment itself. That is, if sleeping as opposed to waking marks the father's turning away from his child's death, what sleep both enacts and represents is simple disavowal, the resistance to waking up to a reality the conscious mind does not want to admit. And when Caruth then concludes by noting that "Freud seems to suggest [that] something in reality itself . . . makes us sleep" (97), we might respond that this something is precisely reality itself, in other words, the reality principle in opposition to the pleasure principle. This tautology does not advance our understanding very far.

Perhaps we can redirect the inquiry by asking a different question. Let us return to Caruth's statement that "it is not the father alone who dreams to avoid his child's death, but *consciousness itself* that, in sleep, is tied to a death from which it turns away." As I noted, the death from which consciousness turns away here appears to be the death of the child. The father's consciousness of this death—or at least an awareness within consciousness that this death marks a reality to which it does not want to awaken—is thus a response to a very specific setting, the death of this particular child of this particular grieving father. What can it mean then to suggest, as Caruth does, that the experience of consciousness itself "desir[ing] somehow its own suspension . . . refers to a desire *common to all sleepers*?" Caruth appears to be imagining an experience different from a shared need (bodily or otherwise) to sleep. The experience is rather, as she suggests, a desire within consciousness not to wake up. But this desire cannot be as specific as a disavowal of a child's death for the simple reason that this particular situation of grief is *not* common to all sleepers. We are thus left with another, as yet unexplained possibility. If "the desire of consciousness as such not to wake up . . . is tied to a death from which it turns away," is there another death from which this father and all sleepers turn away? In other words, perhaps the death we are considering is not the death of this particular child but precisely the death that is *common to all*: our own death.

To explore this possibility in more detail, I want to pick up on a line of inquiry that Caruth hints at only to set aside in favor of an ethical reading of the dream. Discussing Lacan's account of the dream in his Seminar XI as yet another revision of Freud's original dream-interpretation, Caruth observes how the complex dream-work of the dream of the burning child suggests that "awakening . . . is itself the site of a trauma" (100; original emphasis deleted). And the trauma that Caruth imagines as arising from the father's experience is "the necessity and impossibility of responding to another's death." It is this failure of response to another, and in particular to another's death, that Caruth sees as definitive of trauma and might even, she ventures, "represent the very nature of consciousness itself" (96).

This nexus of trauma, death, and consciousness leads Caruth, briefly, to set aside her focus on what she calls "the story of an urgent responsibility" (102)—a responsibility both to bear witness to and to acknowledge the impossibility of ever bearing witness to the true otherness of someone else's death—to recall an earlier section of her study in which she considers Freud's analysis of trauma in *Beyond the Pleasure Principle*. In chapters 4 and 5 of that path-breaking study, Caruth observes, Freud

> moves from a speculation on consciousness that explains trauma as an interruption of consciousness by something . . . *that comes too soon to be expected*, to an explanation of the origins of life itself as an "awakening" from death that precisely establishes the foundation of the [death] drive and of consciousness alike. This peculiar movement therefore traces a significant itinerary in Freud's thought from trauma as an exception, an accident that takes consciousness by surprise and thus disrupts it, to trauma as the very origin of consciousness and all of life itself. (104)

As if concerned that this way of reading Freud will take her too far afield of her main concern, Caruth immediately drops this line of inquiry (one that, as we shall see in a moment, she has previously pursued). She goes on to argue instead that the "global theoretical itinerary" unveiled in *Beyond the Pleasure Principle* (the relation of trauma, death and the death drive, and the simultaneous origin of consciousness and life) is best understood by Lacan's *revision* of Freud's dream-interpretation, especially Lacan's "suggestion that the accidental in trauma is also a revelation of a basic, *ethical dilemma* at the heart of consciousness itself insofar as it is essentially *related to death, and particularly to the death of others*" (104; my emphases). What is amiss in Caruth's argument is that her understanding of Freud's own expansion of the scope of trauma (from "trauma as an exception, an accident" to "trauma as the very origin of consciousness and all of life itself") ends up defining the death drive as though it took its original orientation from the death of another. Caruth acknowledges later that this view of the death drive is at most only hinted at in Freud and that the true source of this idea is not Freud but Lacan.[10] In any event, we are reminded here of precisely what failed in her analysis of the father's wish-fulfillment: "the story of a sleeping consciousness figured by a father unable to face the accidental death of a child" (102) cannot "refer to a desire *common to all sleepers*" (that is, to consciousness's desiring "its own suspension") because the accident of a child's death is not common to all people. In other words, despite what Lacan or Caruth might think, the trauma that arises in response "to the death of others" is precisely what is the exception and therefore should not be substituted for Freud's "global theoretical itinerary," a theory of the origins of trauma as something common to all.[11]

In short, in considering Caruth's earlier discussion of *Beyond the Pleasure Principle*, we recognize that, "insofar as" what is common to all people "is essentially related to death," the death in question has little to do with the death of another. Perhaps even more important, as Caruth herself appears to recognize initially, this shared experience is "related to death" only to the extent death is itself related to something else entirely. To understand what this might mean, let us return to Caruth's attempt to reconstruct one of Freud's fundamental claims in *Beyond the Pleasure Principle*:

> In this work, Freud . . . moves from a speculation on consciousness that explains trauma as an interruption of consciousness . . . to an explanation of the origins of life as an "awakening" from death that precisely establishes the foundation of the [death] drive and of consciousness alike. This peculiar movement . . . traces a significant itinerary in Freud's thought from trauma as an exception, an accident that takes consciousness by surprise and thus disrupts it, to trauma as the very origin of consciousness and all life itself.

As I have noted, Caruth is here referring to a section from *Beyond the Pleasure Principle* she had previously addressed. Freud's key statement reads as follows: "The attributes of life were at some time awoken in animate matter by the action of a force of whose nature we can form no conception. . . . The tension which then arose in what had hitherto been an inanimate substance endeavored to cancel itself out. In this way the first drive came into being: the drive to return to the inanimate state."[12] In line with her core argument, Caruth substitutes "awoken" for the *Standard Edition*'s "evoked"—hers is a much better rendering of *erweckt*—and in that context she goes on to suggest that Freud himself locates the "beginning of the [death] drive" not in any encounter with death "but rather [in] the traumatic 'awakening' to life." But when she immediately adds that "life itself, says Freud, is an *awakening out of a 'death'* for which there was no preparation" (65; my emphasis), her argument begins to go awry. In the first place, at this point in her discussion she does nothing to establish that trauma has its origin in the death of another. Second, and more important, even if Freud is here imagining the "awakening to life" as a traumatic experience that is shared by all, he does not in fact say that this is the equivalent of an awaking "out of a death."[13] What he says rather is that life is awoken (*erweckt*) from an "inanimate state," a state that is linked to what we call death only in the sense that the death drive marks an urge to "return" to that state.[14]

Caruth's misrepresentation is significant because it forms the basis of her unsubstantiated extension of Freud's theory: "the origin of the [death] drive is thus precisely the experience of *having passed beyond death without knowing it*" (65; my emphasis). While this assertion anticipates and lays the groundwork for her subsequent reading of the dream of the burning child, the "experience of having passed beyond death without knowing it" is precisely *not* Freud's way of articulating the origin of the death drive. Indeed, as we have just noted, although Freud views the death drive as an instinctual response to the trauma of awakening (to life and to consciousness), that awakening is "out of a death" only to the extent that death might be taken as a metaphor for an inanimate state (Freud himself does not call that state "death"). Thus, Caruth's "having passed beyond death without knowing it" can really only mean coming into being or experiencing the origin of life and consciousness—or, perhaps more accurately, moving from an inanimate to an animate state—without understanding how or why. And this is precisely how Freud himself puts it: "The attributes of life were at some time evoked [awoken] in animate matter *by the action of a force of whose nature we can form no conception*" (XVIII, 38; my emphasis).

Within his speculative history of organic life, Freud does see the movement from an inanimate to an animate state as occurring without the organism fully knowing that it is undergoing this transition. Any knowledge of the origin would therefore be after the fact, partial and retrospective at best. In short, this "discovery" of existence (to borrow from the Emersonian phrasing I have discussed in the study's introduction) is belated ("too late to be helped," as Emerson puts it). Freud's main contention, in fact, is that, from this impossible perspective in which we come to consciousness too late to have been truly present, we simply cannot understand the force that can act on us in this way. What force exists that can awaken us from our inanimate state and drive us into our new animate one? What is this force that comes *before* and so locates us forever after in the afterwardsness?

While waking up (being "awoken"/*erweckt*) is a reasonably expressive metaphor for the experience of this origin—the coming into the consciousness of one's being—the notion of being "evoked," while a poor translation of the German, more fully captures Freud's sense that we are passive recipients of an action performed by something outside and temporally prior to ourselves.[15] Thus, as Freud has previously noted, "it follows that the phenomena of organic development must be attributed to *external* disturbing and diverting influences" (XVIII, 38; my emphasis). And to the extent that, for Freud, this "process [is] similar in type to that which later caused the development of consciousness in a particular stream of living matter" (XVIII, 38), we might now revise Caruth's statement yet again: "having passed beyond death without knowing it" more reasonably means, for a higher-level organism, coming into the consciousness of being while yet being faced with the mystery of its own origin, that force external to itself about "whose nature we can form no conception."

Caruth is thus correct in observing that, for Freud, any particular traumatic experience both marks an "enigmatic testimony . . . to what . . . resists simple comprehension" (6) and replicates, even as it derives from, an "awakening to life," "the very origin of consciousness . . . itself." But because Caruth misrepresents this traumatic awakening by locating it in an experience of death, she goes astray in viewing the central enigma of trauma as the *survival* of consciousness rather than as the *origin* of consciousness. For example, despite the fact that she understands what we might call the Freudian Ur-trauma as related to the *origins* of life and consciousness, Caruth invariably uses a language that equates this moment with *continuation* rather than with *beginning*:

> What Freud encounters in the traumatic neurosis is not the reaction to any horrible event but, rather, *the peculiar and perplexing experience of survival*. If the dreams and flashbacks of the traumatized thus engage Freud's interest, it is because *they bear witness to a survival that exceeds the very claims and consciousness of the one who endures it*. At the heart of Freud's thinking in *Beyond the Pleasure Principle* . . . is the urgent and unsettling question: What does it mean *to survive*? . . . *The problem of survival, in trauma, thus emerges specifically as the question: What does it mean for consciousness to survive?* (60–61; my emphases; original italics deleted)

Caruth here cites *Beyond the Pleasure Principle* precisely to establish how any particular trauma is akin to, even a repetition of, an original "*waking into consciousness*" (64). But her notion that "the dreams and flashbacks of the traumatized" (precisely those instances of repetition compulsion that are the symptoms of trauma) "bear witness to a *survival* that exceeds the very claims and consciousness of the one who endures it" doesn't make much sense in the context of an organism that has just awoken. What can survival even mean at such a moment?[16] Even more to the point, to the extent that trauma necessarily marks what "exceeds the claims and consciousness of the one who endures it," what this experience "bears witness to" at the moment of first awakening can be nothing other than what consciousness cannot claim for itself: the knowledge of how and why it came into being in the first place. What consciousness is thus forced to endure is the burden of its own incomprehensibility, its sense of having been evoked elsewhere. What Caruth fails to grasp, in short, is that the origin of trauma is precisely the trauma of origins.

IV

As we noted in the study's introduction, in the Emersonian Fall of Man belatedness (what is "too late to be helped") marks an absence, the very space in which we can come into existence without knowing that we do. Read in relation to Freud's notion of trauma, the "origins of life and consciousness" come too late to be helped precisely because, from the start, we were helpless before it; or, rather, we were helpless because the event necessarily came before us. Latency inheres in the trauma of origins because, as the primal scene reminds us, we were, in some paradoxical way, absent from the scene of our own creation, a scene marked, as Justin Martyr anciently observed in a passage I used as an epigraph to part I, precisely by the impossibility of choice, a perspective oddly echoed in Freud's "Theme of the Three Caskets." At the origin, we did not and could not choose for ourselves because we were chosen instead and chosen, so Freud notes in *Beyond the Pleasure Principle*, by "a force of whose Nature we could form no conception." In short, what is absent at the scene of creation—the latency inherent in this event—is precisely our choosing because the moment of choosing necessarily preceded us.

Even as an existential crisis, traumatic belatedness yet resides in an ethical situation because, as Jean Laplanche writes, it "is inconceivable without a model of translation: that is, it presupposes that something is proffered by the other, and this is then afterwards retranslated and reinterpreted." He adds that this "something that comes before" is precisely "the [other's] implantation of [an] enigmatic message."[17] Laplanche is thinking here of an exchange that takes place during an actual if unintelligible and so unassimilated encounter (a child breastfeeding, for example).[18] But even as it presupposes an originary event (precisely *the* originary event), the trauma of origins is founded on an exchange that exists only at the later discovery, a discovery that points to the irresolvable mystery of the other's place in my own identity.

Although for reasons we have seen Caruth's explanation of this mystery is quite different, her phrasing is instructive: "The peculiar temporality of trauma" includes "the sense that *the past it foists upon one is not one's own*," a "perspective," she adds, that may "be understood in terms of a temporality of the other" (143n10; my emphasis).[19] In his *On the Psychotheology of Everyday Life*, Eric Santner similarly considers the ethical implications of Freud's thought in the context of otherness. Writing that Freud permits us to "rethink what it means to be genuinely open to another human being . . . and to share and take responsibility for one's implication in the dilemmas of difference," Santner argues that, in its "psychoanalytic conception," an ethics of "communality is granted on the basis of that fact that every familiar is ultimately strange and that, indeed, I am even in a crucial sense a stranger to myself." While Santner reads this "internal alienness" optimistically, I would counter that the experience of self-estrangement might take different forms. At a minimum, to the extent that being a stranger to myself means that my origin lies elsewhere, the experience of internal alienness—its recognition—must be understood as profoundly traumatic.[20] This is so because, in the Emersonian context at least, if such self-estrangement includes the discovery of existence then it is an experience that necessarily comes after the fact. And absence—especially the absence of my own ethical act, my choosing—thereby becomes constitutive of my identity because that identity exists in relation to what must come before, the enigma of the other's choice of me. To know the impossibility of having been there will ever after be what cannot be helped: to discover existence precisely as the burden of always coming too late.

That said, to the extent that Santner views the "ethical consideration of . . . 'everyday' life" as "pertaining to my answerability to my neighbor-with-an-unconscious"—the other "is a stranger . . . not only to me but also to him- or herself"—the trauma of origins as existential crisis need not be the end of the story. For, tracing out Santner's logic, we might envision an ethics arising precisely from our recognition that the Other (first and foremost our parents) is also the subject of a trauma because it did not choose its origins: our parents had parents and so they too, as Justin Martyr anciently reflected, "were born without . . . knowledge or choice."[21] As Santner provocatively, and hopefully, suggests, "against [the] background" of how the self shares its estrangement with the Other, "the very opposition between 'neighbor' and 'stranger' begins to lose its force."²² What Caruth calls "the temporality of the other" would thus also include the Other in its infinite regress, and the trauma of belatedness could come to function ethically to the extent we might recognize that all of us are wounded from the beginning.

As we shall see in chapter 2, however, this sense of connection to the ethical connection—an obligation to or the recognition of the very otherness of the Other—is yet crossed by the possibility of violence, or what Sartre calls "the refusal of being born." To the extent an ethical connection might also entail a conferral of responsibility to the other, such an ethics also marks an imposition, even a sense of indebtedness (what a child might owe to its parents). And that experience of owing the other might be as anxiety-riddled as it is morally enabling. While fuller discussions of that situation will come in chapters 3 and 5 (especially in relation to Shakespeare's *Hamlet* and Milton's *Paradise Lost*) I will conclude part I with some reflections on how Freud, in response to his disciple Otto Rank's understanding of the trauma of the origin (the birth trauma), engages this issue even as he effectively explains it away by reasserting the Oedipal economy (in particular castration anxiety) as the source of hostility that problematizes the child's relation to the parents, which for Freud invariably means the son's vexed relationship toward his father.

2

Owing Life

The Birth Trauma and its Discontents (Rank and Freud)

> . . . in thy sight to die, what were it else
> But like a pleasant slumber in thy lap?
> Here could I breathe my soul into the air,
> As mild and gentle as the cradle-babe
> Dying with his mother's dug between its lips.
>
> —Shakespeare, *2 Henry VI*

I

As a way of beginning this final chapter of part I, I would like to return briefly to "Theme of the Three Caskets" to explore another way that essay grapples with the crisis of origins. While this particular line of inquiry differs markedly from my own way, as an alternative it does open a door to the discussion of a curious episode in the history of the psychoanalytic movement that culminated in Freud's rejecting many of the insights he had recently formulated in *Beyond the Pleasure Principle*. We will come back to that rejection later, but, first, we revisit the 1913 essay.

Particularly sensitive to its gender-implications, Julia Reinhard Lupton and Kenneth Reinhard have interpreted the essay's concern with what we might call the temporality of loss as centrally related to the (male) subject's inscription within a life-sequence dominated by female figures. Building on Freud's statement that the "theme" represents "the three inevitable relations man has with woman[,] . . . the mother herself, the beloved who is chosen after her pattern, and finally the Mother Earth [death] who receives him again," Lupton and Reinhard argue more particularly that the sequence marks the subject's psychical movement from a pre-Oedipal unity with the mother in earliest infancy to an Oedipal phase in which the mother becomes the (male) child's chief object of desire, and, finally, to a post-Oedipal phase in which the experience of maternal loss is reconfigured as a danger to be overcome, even to the point of equating the too-powerful mother with death.[1] In this context, Lupton and Reinhard understand the subject's experience of belatedness (its "*nachträgliche* constitution" [156]) in relation to the view of trauma as based on the retroactive investment of an earlier event with symbolic meaning rather than on a simpler determinist model, which typically views the delayed onset of traumatic experience in terms of an incubation-period within the psyche.

The main point here is that the male subject's move toward his endtime has a relation to his origin precisely as a regressive movement: the movement back from the third to the first casket marks an interpretive return to the pre-Oedipal state of "maternal unity" (Lupton and Reinhard, 152).[2] From this perspective, the male subject's crisis of origins has less to do with his discovery of existence as a necessarily belated condition than with a forced separation from the mother and the inescapable but impossible effort to overcome that separation. Within the full temporal sequence, in the wake of castration anxiety (in particular the male subject's simultaneous perception and disavowal of maternal castration), negativity toward the mother is asserted, at first, to form a kind of barrier and so to bolster the male ego. That is, maternal loss must be disavowed as what the son must choose in order to protect himself from what is now perceived as her annihilating presence. But that negativity is subsequently reimagined as loving embrace so that death itself can be transformed from a terrifying imposition into something willingly chosen (the dying King Lear carrying the body of his beloved Cordelia in *his* arms). Still, the fantasy of reclaiming the lost origin yet retains in remnant form aspects of the other two phases, the son's object-love for the mother (Oedipal) and the understanding of the mother as danger (post-Oedipal).[3] Especially in regard to the regressive "movement between the third and the first caskets," what begins in "the image of the nurturing mother figured in the first casket represents at once a fantasy of original oneness and, contaminated by the specter of mother-as-death, signals the constitutive fracture of the pre-Oedipal by loss . . . [and] aggression" (153–54).

It is not my purpose here to dispute this reading of "Theme of the Three Caskets." In fact, although we come at it from different angles, I agree with Lupton and Reinhard that Freud's essay should be read as centrally concerned with a crisis of origins.[4] What is of more interest to my argument is that their portrayal of this crisis in terms of the male relation to maternal loss effectively repeats, even as it updates in Lacanian terms, an understanding of originary trauma as first formulated just a few years after Freud published *Beyond the Pleasure Principle*. Just as important, in response to this formulation Freud himself felt compelled to return to the Oedipal economy as the origin of psychical unsettlement precisely because he would not, or could not, accept where his own thought was being taken (or perhaps even where it was taking him).

The catalyst for Freud's failure of nerve was Otto Rank's 1924 *The Trauma of Birth*. Although this study makes no direct reference to *Beyond the Pleasure Principle*, Rank appears to be picking up on the new direction in Freud's thought as laid out in that treatise of four years earlier. In particular, Rank is sensitive to Freud's novel way of linking traumatic experience to the problematic nature of the origin. Rank, however, went his own way with these ideas. *The Trauma of Birth* is primarily concerned with the emergence of the male subject's separation-anxiety as coincident with birth itself and his subsequent struggle either to overcome that anxiety or to relive it. (In this sense, Rank anticipates later notions of a constitutive relationship between pre- and post-Oedipal phases.) Subsequently, perceiving that Rank's ideas contradicted some of his most cherished and influential formulations or, worse, made those very ideas look like mere afterthoughts to the new theory, Freud responded by rejecting not only Rank's argument about birth trauma but also, and more to the point, even his own insights as set out in *Beyond the Pleasure Principle*. It was as though part of the effect of Rank's study (dedicated to Freud himself) was to make Freud feel that his own new ideas were too radical, too much of a departure from established Freudian thought. In 1926, then, Freud will publish *Inhibitions, Symptoms and Anxiety* both as a counter to Rank and as a reassertion of many of the core elements of his own earlier theorizing, especially the Oedipus complex and castration anxiety. To put this sequence in clearer relationship to my main argument, Freud (re)imposes the Oedipal model on the as yet tenuous ideas that *Beyond the Pleasure Principle* had just recently articulated; *Inhibitions, Symptoms and Anxiety* thus aims to contain this emerging concept of existential belatedness. In so doing, the 1926 treatise effectively reimagines the link "Theme of Three Caskets" had made between dying and being born as just another instance of the Oedipal crisis: object-love for the mother, sexual rivalry with the father, and loss of the mother in the wake of the threat of castration.[5]

II

To understand Freud in 1926, we must first understand Rank in 1924. At its heart, Rank's birth trauma (what he also calls the "primal trauma") is the wound of human individuation as effected by an originary differentiation and, in consequence of, the discovery of one's selfhood as an essential otherness.[6] As it passes out of its paradisal intrauterine existence at the moment of birth, the newborn experiences the actual physical separation from its mother, a separation that, as it becomes a psychical event, is (re)experienced as a trauma.[7] That trauma, which, as Rank describes it, retains some strange recollection of the intrauterine condition itself, is forever after the defining condition of human life:

> [A]ll forms and symptoms of neurosis [are] expressions of a regression from the stage of sexual adjustment to the pre-natal primal state, or to the birth situation, which must be thereby overcome. . . . [I]n the child's biological adjustment to the extrauterine situation, in the normal adjustment of civilized man, as well as in his compensatory superproductions of art (in the widest sense), the same striving to overcome the birth trauma enacted in similar forms, the only essential difference being that the civilized human being and still more the "artist" can reproduce this objectively in manifold, strictly determined forms, fixed by the primal trauma, whilst the neurotic is compelled again and again to produce it in a similar way only on his own body. But the essence of most pathological processes seems to rest on this compulsive "return of the same" product on one's own body. The neurotic is thrown back again and again to the real birth trauma, whilst the normal and supernormal throw it . . . forwards and project it outwards, and are thus enabled to objectify it. (210, 212–13; original emphases deleted)

On the one hand, through all its stages—from newborn to infant to child to adult—the human psyche ceaselessly attempts to reclaim the primal happiness of the womb.[8] On the other hand, it is compelled just as ceaselessly to relive the traumatic separation from the mother; this separation is repeated, for example, through the process of weaning and later, after the more pronounced development of infantile sexuality, by castration anxiety which effectively replaces the mother with the father as the source of the trauma, a point to which we shall return especially in relation to Freud's response.⁹ Even a person in a state of relative psychical health is at best constantly struggling to overcome the wound of separation and to reclaim himself (for the subject is always imagined as male) against the overwhelming if now mostly internalized maternal presence.

These subsequent experiences or repetitions manifest as anxiety, a situation that can take both normal and neurotic forms. As Freud himself will summarize without endorsing Rank's point, "those people become neurotic in whom the trauma of birth was so strong that they have never been able completely to abreact it" while "the more intensely a . . . person reproduces the affect of anxiety [in such a way as to master it] the more closely will he approach to mental health" (*Inhibitions, Symptoms and Anxiety*, XX, 151). In short, in Rank's view neurotic symptoms (attacks of anxiety, for example) represent the psyche's struggle to abreact the original trauma. In that context, such symptoms are at once manifestations of a neurotic condition and the mechanism of working through that condition. To the extent neurotics are those who either cannot overcome their longing to return (in)to the mother or cannot master the terror of the primal separation, they are doomed to repeat one or both experiences rather than moving beyond the birth trauma to a self-mastering maturity.

Rank's use of a passage from Nietzsche's *Birth of Tragedy* as his study's epigraph is thus meant to call attention to an existential crisis that he subsequently contextualizes in psychoanalytic terms:

> An old legend has it that King Midas hunted a long time in the woods for the wise Silenus, companion of Dionysos. When he had finally caught him the king asked him what he considered man's greatest good. The daemon remained sullen and uncommunicative until finally, forced by the king, he broke into a shrill laugh and spoke: "Ephemeral wretch, begotten of accident and toil, why do you force me to tell you what it would be your greatest boon not to hear? What would be best for you is quite beyond your reach: not to have been born, not to *be*, to be *nothing*. But the second best is to die soon."¹⁰

If for Nietzsche's Silenus it is better not to be born because we are doomed to suffer (existence *is* suffering), Rank's theory of birth trauma is intended to provide an explanation for that suffering. Or, perhaps more precisely, the theory aims to show that suffering is really just a manifestation of neurosis but a neurosis from which, in ways similar to the generalized suffering Silenus refers to, no one can ever truly escape. Indeed, as Rank sees it, even for a reasonably well-adjusted adult the experience of being alive necessarily entails the acknowledgment that we can never reclaim the lost and longed-for origin (the maternal womb) whose memory ever after haunts us. As Silenus suggests, moreover, the discovery of that reality already comes too late. Still, to the extent there is any compensation here, it is precisely the psychical force of separation that creates, or is at least coincident with, the emergence of, the human consciousness. So Rank writes: "It would seem that the primal anxiety-effect at birth, which . . . is from the very beginning not merely an expression of the new-born child's physiological injuries . . . but in consequence of the change from a highly pleasurable situation to an extremely painful one, immediately acquires a 'psychical' quality of feeling. *This experienced anxiety is thus the first content of perception*, the first psychical act, so to say, to set up barriers; and in these we must recognize the primal repression against the already powerful tendency to re-establish the pleasurable situation just left" (187; my emphasis). We might say that, for Rank, human consciousness is formed as at once the site of otherness (one's own in relation to the mother) and a defense against both that relation and the traumatic longing for reunion it generates.[11]

III

In *Inhibitions, Symptoms and Anxiety*, Freud will claim that his own earlier work laid the foundation for Rank's theory of the birth trauma: "Rank's contention—which was *originally my own*, [is] that the affect of anxiety is a consequence of the event of birth and a repetition of the situation then experienced" (XX, 161; my emphasis). We can trace Freud's thinking on this point all the way back to the second edition of the *Interpretation of Dreams* (1909). There, as part of a new section added to his discussion of *déjà vu* dreams ("these places [where one has been before] are invariably the genitals of the dreamer's mother"), he observes that a "large number of dreams, often accompanied by anxiety and having as their content such subjects as passing through water, are based on phantasies of intra-uterine life, of existence in the womb and the act of birth" (V, 399).[12] Having just analyzed the latent-manifest content of "Oedipus dreams" (V, 397–98) and going on to note that in at least one case the dream-fantasy of intrauterine existence should be understood from the perspective of the son's "intra-uterine opportunity of watching his parents copulating" (V, 400; see also "Fragment of an Analysis of a Case of Hysteria," VII, 80), Freud is yet insistent on the primarily sexual nature of the womb-fantasy. That is, he reads the fantasy as a displacement of the fetus's original privileged position (inside the mother), a particular transvaluing of the perspective on the primal scene that will be so central to his analysis of the Wolf-Man ("From the History of an Infantile Neurosis," XVII, especially 29–47). If Freud is holding out for the primacy of the sexual (whereas Rank makes the sexual a later development that marks a return to the birth trauma), Freud's own 1909 footnote appears to grant a certain primacy to a nonsexual aspect of the fantasy even to the point of suggesting his own radical revision of the Oedipal theory and its corresponding castration complex: "It was not for a long time that I learned to appreciate the importance of phantasies and unconscious thoughts about life in the womb. They contain an explanation of the remarkable dread that many people have of being buried alive; and they also afford the deepest unconscious basis for the belief in survival after death, which merely represents a projection into the future of this uncanny life before birth. *Moreover, the act of birth is the first experience of anxiety, and thus the source and prototype of the affect of anxiety*" (V, 400–01n3; emphasis in original). Apart from the fact that Freud here imagines a return to the mother that is not explicitly sexualized (it is the womb and not the genitals that matter), we might also note in anticipation of Freud's subsequent revisions that "unconscious [i.e., repressed] thoughts about life in the womb" mark something akin to a memory of the intrauterine state, an "uncanny" connection to "life before birth." Be that as it may, over the next fourteen years, Freud will occasionally come back to this undertheorized speculation.[13]

Nevertheless, in broad terms *Inhibitions, Symptoms and Anxiety* will mark a shift in Freud's thinking, a determination to withdraw his support for Rank while clarifying his own position on the form and causes of anxiety. In other words, in 1926 Freud revises his own earlier position, one that, as we have already seen, he recognizes as the basis Rank's theory (a fact Rank himself openly acknowledged). Still, Freud's position on Rank (or thus on his own earlier idea) is not always clear. Throughout *Inhibitions, Symptoms and Anxiety* he will make assertions that, on the surface at least, encourage the reader to believe that he is still open to the possibility that Rank has helped to clarify by drawing out the implications of one of psychoanalysis's foundational insights. Without explicitly mentioning Rank, Freud will observe, for example, that "there is much more continuity between intrauterine life and earliest infancy than the impressive caesura of the act of birth would have us believe" (XX, 138). And in the opening chapter he will write, in ways that are more directly related to Rank, that "in man and the higher animals it would seem that the act of birth, as the individual's first experience of anxiety, has given the affect of anxiety certain characteristic forms of expression" (XX, 93).

That said, here Freud is only addressing the "forms of expression" characteristic of anxiety-attacks (breathlessness, palpitations of the heart). Thus, despite some occasional uncertainty in regards the issue, on the whole he decisively moves away from Rank's global position on the birth trauma as the prototype of anxiety that all later manifestations of anxiety merely repeat. In the study's second chapter, for example, he will write, "I do not think that we are justified in assuming that whenever there is an outbreak of anxiety something like a reproduction of the situation of birth goes on in the mind" (XX, 94).[14] And later in the study, where he will explicitly mention Rank, he will raise more pointed objections, ones directed more at Rank than at his own earlier formulations.

Three of these objections merit special attention since they will have bearing on my own efforts to retheorize Freud's thinking on the issue of traumatic origins.[15] First, as Freud notes, Rank's theory appears to suggest that humans carry around with them something akin to a *memory* of birth and even of their intrauterine state (see *Trauma of Birth*, 196; this is a position that, as we have seen, Freud himself had imagined in earlier work). Freud will now reject that view, at least as it suggests recollection of the actual moment of birth. He starts by observing that the fetus does not have the requisite distance from the mother to form a memory: "birth is not experienced subjectively as separation from the mother, since the foetus, being a completely narcissistic creature, is totally unaware of her existence as an object" (XX, 130).[16] Later, he will be more specific about the memory issue even as he makes explicit reference to Rank's study for the first time:

> In his book on the trauma of birth, Rank (1924) has made a determined attempt to establish a relationship between the earliest phobias of children and the impressions made on them by the event of birth. But . . . he assumes that the infant has received certain sensory impressions, in particular of a visual kind, at the time of birth, the renewal of which can recall to its memory the trauma of birth and thus evoke a reaction of anxiety. This assumption is quite unfounded and extremely improbable. It is not credible that a child should retain any but tactile and general sensations relating to the process of birth. (XX, 135)

In short, Freud argues against Rank that, because birth is something experienced only in its sensory immediacy, it is not something that can subsequently be remembered in any life-phase: newborn, infant, child, or adult.[17]

Building on, if perhaps slightly contradicting, this first objection, Freud's second line of attack is that, even if there were something like primal memory, Rank's theory is not always consistent in its portrayal of how the newborn recalls its own past and how it relates to what might be considered traumatic within this past:

> In considering these later anxiety-situations Rank dwells, as suits him best, now on the recollection of its happy intra-uterine existence, now on its recollection of the traumatic disturbance which interrupted that existence, which leaves the door wide open for arbitrary interpretation. There are, moreover, certain examples of childhood anxiety, which directly traverse his theory. When, for instance, a child is left alone in the dark one would expect it, according to his view, to welcome the re-establishment of the intra-uterine situation; yet it is precisely on such occasions that the child reacts with anxiety. And if this is explained by saying that the child is being reminded of the interruption which the event of birth makes in its intra-uterine happiness, it becomes impossible to shut one's eyes any longer to the far-fetched character of such explanations. (XX, 65)

Put another way, Freud is calling attention here to how Rank shifts the focus of the psyche's attention (whether as newborn, infant, child, or adult) to whichever part of the process best supports the theory: at times, the psyche longs for the womb; at other times it anxiously recollects (and/or attempts to disavow) the trauma of separation. Sidestepping the question of whether there is any recollection at all, Freud's most pointed comment on this issue comes in a 1924 letter to the Central Committee of the International Association. Against Rank's notion that the birth trauma not only interrupts but also puts up a barrier to the longing to return to the womb, Freud writes that "as a matter of counter-argument . . . it is not in the nature of an instinct to be associatively inhibited, as is the instinct to return to the mother through the association with the birth terror" (qtd. in Jones, *Life and Work*, III, 62). Adding that "there cannot be any ambivalent instincts, i.e. any accompanied by anxiety," Freud finds it implausible that birth would create both a longing to return to the womb and a reaction against that longing.

In that same letter of 1924, Freud begins to articulate his final major objection to Rank's theory, an objection that, while not always explicitly linked to Rank, will form the foundation of *Inhibitions, Symptoms and Anxiety*. In the letter, Freud's observation that it is "not in the nature of an instinct to be associatively inhibited" immediately follows a more detailed comment on how his own views diverge from Rank's:

> Now comes the point where I find the difficulties begin. Obstacles, which evoke anxiety, the barriers of incest, are opposed to the phantastic return to the womb: now where do these come from? Their representative is evidently the father, reality, the authority which does not permit incest. Why have these set up the barrier against incest? My explanation was a historical and social one . . . I derived the barrier against incest from the primordial history of the human family, and thus saw in the actual father the real obstacle, which erects the barrier against incest anew. Here Rank diverges from me. He . . . regards the anxiety opposing incest as simply a repetition of the anxiety of birth, so that neurotic repression is inherently checked by the nature of the birth process. This birth anxiety is, it is true, transferred to the father, but according to Rank he is only a pretext for it. Basically the attitude toward the womb or female genital is supposed to be ambivalent from the start. Here is the contradiction. I find it very hard to decide here, nor do I see how experience can help us, since in analysis we always come across the father as the representative of the prohibition. (qtd. in Jones, *Life and Work*, III, 62)

Although Freud concludes by observing that, "for the time being I must leave the matter open," in fact his "explanation" seems merely to repeat his standard position. That is, in rejecting Rank's displacement of the father as the central figure in the family romance, Freud shows that his main resistance to Rank comes in the fact that, if accepted, the theory of the birth trauma would effectively supersede the Oedipal-castration theory by rendering castration anxiety merely a repetition of the trauma of the newborn's separation from the mother, a repetition coming after (and in response to) the child's phallic phase.[18] In other words, Freud uses the occasion of his response to Rank to restore the full Oedipal economy to its central place in psychoanalysis.

Even before he mentions Rank in *Inhibitions, Symptoms and Anxiety*, Freud uses the question about the etiology of anxiety to review his own earlier studies of Little Hans and the Wolf Man, which, he now reminds us, are properly and exclusively intelligible in terms of Oedipal longing and castration anxiety. More generally, he takes every opportunity to restate his core position: that the threat of castration as embodied in the figure of the father is the chief cause of neurotic symptoms (see XX, 101–05, 124–31, 137–39). For example, as part of his initial discussion of Rank, he notes that a child's longing for an absent person (typically its mother) "turns into anxiety. This anxiety," he continues, "has all the appearance of being an expression of the child's feeling at its wits' end, as though in its still very undeveloped state it did not know how better to cope with its cathexis of longing. Here anxiety appears as a reaction to the felt loss of the object, and we are at once reminded of the fact that castration anxiety, too, is a fear of being separated from a highly valued object, and that the earliest anxiety of all—the 'primal anxiety' of birth—is brought about on the occasion of a separation from the mother." At this stage, Freud refers to the loss of the mother as a situation of danger, "of a *growing tension due to need*," and then suggests that all such situations are "analogous to the experience of being born" or "reminiscent of birth" (XX, 137–38). In other words, at first Freud seems to be taking a similar approach to that of Rank, and we might imagine here that even castration anxiety (as a situation of danger) is simply drawing the (male) child back to the birth trauma (since "castration anxiety, *too*, is a fear of being separated from a highly valued object"). Freud even appears to be taking Rank's approach that castration anxiety is a repetition of the birth trauma only after the onset of sexuality (see Rank, 192, 194): "The significance of the loss of object as a determinant of anxiety extends considerably further. For *the next transformation of anxiety*, viz. the castration anxiety belonging to the phallic phase, is *also a fear of separation* and is thus attached to the same determinant [a lost object]" (XX, 138–39; my emphases).

But in adding immediately that "in this case the danger is of being separated from one's genitals" (139), rather than endorsing Rank's theory Freud inverts its terms. For he makes it seem as though castration anxiety actually precedes the birth trauma, which itself is merely a retroactive-substitutive manifestation of the former. To put this another way, by holding on to his emphasis on sexual longing for the mother as the crux of the issue—what the (male) child desires is not to be restored to the intrauterine condition but to enter his mother sexually—Freud makes Rank's womb-fantasy appear "reminiscent" of Oedipal longing rather than the other way around, a longing that is then cut off, as it were, by the (paternal) threat of castration. Noting that "the high degree of narcissistic value which the penis possesses can appeal to the fact that that organ is a guarantee to its owner that he can be once more united to his mother," Freud imagines this (re)union in terms of fantasized sexuality: ". . . united to his mother—i.e. to a substitute for her—in the act of copulation. It may be added," he goes on, "that for a man who is impotent (that is, who is inhibited by the threat of castration) *the substitute for copulation is a phantasy of returning into his mother's womb*. . . . [W]e might say that the man in question . . . is now (in the phantasy) *replacing [his genital] organ regressively by his whole person*" (69; my emphases). In other words, Freud attempts to debunk Rank's birth trauma by arguing that the return to the womb is just a substitute-fantasy for failed sexual entry of the mother, the fulfillment of which is blocked not by birth itself but by the threat of castration.[19]

IV

The difference between Rank's and Freud's theories might be measured in part by their different ways of viewing the human reaction to death as something other than a fear of mortality itself, an issue that takes us back to my introduction to part I. For his part, Freud understands this reaction in terms of castration anxiety. Observing, first, that after the Great War many had come to the mistaken idea that an immediate threat of death ("a threat to the instinct of self-preservation") "could by itself produce a neurosis without any admixture of sexual factors and without requiring any of the complicated hypotheses of psycho-analysis," he goes on, in a passage we have previously considered, that

> the unconscious seems to contain nothing that could give content to our concept of the annihilation of life. . . . [N]othing resembling death can ever have been experienced; or if it has . . . it has left no observable traces behind. I am therefore inclined to adhere to the view that *the fear of death should be regarded as analogous to the fear of castration*. (XX, 129–30; my emphasis)

We shall look at this assertion in more detail subsequently, but for now we might simply take note of the phrase "analogous to." Freud appears to mean that the fear of death is a displaced form of castration anxiety because the instinct of self-preservation carries its own "sexual factor" (he refers to "the libidinal character" of this instinct). In other words, the threat of death is symbolically charged as a recollection or repetition of the fear of castration.

By contrast, initially at least, Rank understands what we might call death anxiety not in terms of a repetition of a trauma (for him, the primal separation from the mother) but precisely as an undoing of that trauma. As though anticipating Freud's remark that the unconscious "contain[s] nothing that could give any content to our concept of the annihilation of life," Rank comments that "the complete lack of negation *per se*—*i.e.*, the idea of death—belongs essentially to the character of the Unconscious."[20] But whereas for Freud the signifying content of this negation or annihilation is "analogous to the fear of castration," for Rank its content is the desire for union: "the child and its psychical representative, the Unconscious, knows only the situation *before birth*, given to it in experience, the pleasurable remembrance of which continues in the indestructible belief in immorality, in the idea of an everlasting life after death."[21] Thus, "what biologically seems to us the impulse to death, strives again to establish nothing else than the *already experienced condition before birth*, and the 'compulsion to repetition' arises from the unquenchable character of this longing, which exhausts itself again and again in every possibility of form" (196–97; my emphasis). In short, whereas for Freud death symbolically reenacts a painful separation—the loss of a highly cathected object—Rank's equivalent of the death drive ("the impulse to death") aims to overcome that pain: "This separation [death] is still easy for the Unconscious, as it is only a matter of giving up one substitute for the attainment of real blessedness" (197). In other words, in much the same way that in "Theme of the Three Caskets" Freud had depicted the theme's death fantasy in the image of the primal mother's once again taking her beloved son "in her arms," Rank similarly understands the "impulse to death" in terms of the (son's) longing to be restored to the maternal embrace, even for (re)enclosure within the womb. The forward movement of our lives is thus, for Rank, always a search to reclaim a lost origin or, perhaps more accurately, a refusal of that origin. "This process," Rank concludes, "is what biologically speaking we call 'life'" (196). Effectively accepting the logic of Nietzsche's Silenus, Rank might agree that, if the best thing a human could hope for would "not to be born at all," the second best would be to "die soon": in the first instance we would never be separated from the mother and in the second we would be restored to her as quickly as possible.[22]

Yet in other places Rank presents a more convoluted account of the impulse to death. Briefly addressing the idea of death in what seems more clearly Freudian terms, Rank notes that death is not always simply the fulfillment of a longing for reunion: "On the other hand, the fearful idea of death as a scythe-bearer, who severs one sharply from life, is to be traced back to the primal anxiety which man produces for the last time in the last trauma, in the last breath at death, and so gains from the greatest anxiety, namely, that of death, the pleasure of denying death by again undergoing the birth anxiety" (197–98). All the key phrases here—"fearful idea," "death as a scythe-bearer," "severs one sharply"—are suggestive of Freudian castration despite the fact that Rank does not use that term. More to the point, Rank's "on the other hand" returns us to one of Freud's chief objections to Rank's theory of the birth trauma, that Rank wants to have it both ways. For Rank, that is, birth at once marks the beginning of the longing to a return to the womb and a reaction against that longing, a defense aiming to fend off the traumatic nature of the primal separation. Rank thus sees the "fearful idea" of death as producing a perverse sort of "pleasure," that of "denying death by *again undergoing* the birth anxiety." Minimally, Rank here ventures that the human impulse to death is something more than a manifestation of the desire to return to the womb. For death is at once a fantasy of maternal reunion and an act of resistance of some kind.[23]

What seems to be a tension in Rank's thought suggests more fundamentally that the birth trauma marks for him a site of psychical ambivalence. And Rank eventually comes exactly to this position. Referring to it as the "primal ambivalence," he argues that "the primal tendency to re-establish the first and most pleasurable experience is opposed not only by the primal repression, acting as a protection against the most painful experience associated with it, but simultaneously by the striving against the source of the pleasure itself" (199). The "not only . . . but simultaneously" construction is instructive and, in fact, suggests that the "primal ambivalence" resides in more than one place. On the one hand, Rank acknowledges the primal repression that, as he puts it, aims at "the prevention of memory" of the "painful experience" of separation: "one does not wish to be reminded because [the most pleasurable experience: returning to the womb] must remain unattainable" (199). On the other hand, he observes a simultaneous "striving against the source of pleasure itself." In other words, even the resistance to maternal loss is experienced in a contradictory way: at once an anticipatory defense against a longing for return through the symbolic reenactment of the original trauma and some as yet unexplained pleasure—"the pleasure of denying death"—enacted in the refusal of (a "striving against") the original "source of pleasure."

Rank refers to the ego's defensive postures in relation to the primal separation as "reaction-formations against the breaking out of this fearful yearning to go back" (116). But given the distinction he makes between the two very different modes of defense, we might reasonably ask if the psyche experiences "fearful yearning" only because of the "painful memory of the birth trauma." Is it possible that the idea of return is "fearful," even traumatic, for another reason? Developing his understanding of what he calls the necessary "renunciation of the primitive mother," Rank observes not just "the fear of her caused . . . by the birth trauma" (89–90) but also, variously, an "anxiety of the mother" created in part as a "reaction against . . . infantile dependence on her" (92), a fear of being "bound by the navel string to the . . . mother" (92n1), the need of "protection from" the mother and especially the need to resist her "dominance" and dangerous "sexual power" (93), and a desire to be liberated "from the maternal prison" (94). Most concisely, in ways that might cause us to rethink his use of the passage from Nietzsche's *Birth of Tragedy* as his study's epigraph, Rank will suggest even more provocatively that the birth trauma and its subsequent manifestations in anxiety mark an awareness of the "painful share of woman in one's own origin" (96). Against the notion that the ego disavows the pleasure of return simply because it is unattainable, Rank now points to new source of anxiety: a fear *of* the mother that competes with and perhaps even predominates over the longing for the unattainable (to be [re]united with the mother), a fear whose object is the very possibility of that (re)union.[24]

How should we understand this second mode of resistance? As we previously noted, Freud's first comment on what would form the basis of Rank's theory came in a footnote added to the second edition of the *Interpretation of Dreams*: "It was not for a long time that I learned to appreciate the importance of phantasies and unconscious thoughts about life in the womb. They contain an explanation of the remarkable dread that many people have of being buried alive; and they also afford the deepest unconscious basis for the belief in survival after death, which merely represents a projection into the future of this uncanny life before birth." Setting aside the question of the precise content of those mysterious "thoughts about life in the womb," we might note a tension in Freud's own thinking. For while it might seem that our "belief in survival after death" would mark a special wish—precisely for our own continuation beyond the grave—Freud appears to imagine such survival as a kind of nightmare: "being buried alive." Minimally, we should note that, in this early context, Freud does not directly associate the fear of death with the severing of castration. But we might also wonder if the "remarkable dread" he imagined in 1909 is related to Rank's later image of the maternal prison. In other words, to the extent that, for Rank, the impulse to death opens up a different sort of pleasure—the pleasure of remaining free from this prison—should the possibility of reunion with the mother (going back to prison) be equated with Freud's "dread"? Does birth create our first ambivalence precisely because the longed-for return to the mother is psychically reconstructed as a kind of living death?

I would like to suggest here that Rank's concept of a "primal ambivalence" (directed toward the mother as both what is longed-for and what is dreaded) has less to do with the giving up of what can never be (re)attained than with an even more primal fear: the very possibility of restoration to the mother-as-prison fuels the emergent ego's terror of being trapped, annihilated, s/mothered. Another way of understanding the movement of ideas here would be to observe how a psychical situation described in Freud's 1913 "Theme of the Three Caskets"—a dying man's openness to death as a fantasized choosing to return to the embrace of the loving mother—is, by 1924, reimagined by Rank both as a much more generalized scenario (one need not be dying to have this fantasy) and, more to the point, as a site of intense ambivalence. Such ambivalence is precisely what Lupton and Reinhard's Lacanian reading of post-Oedipal experience understands in terms of Lear's "regressive fantasy" (his longing to return to the "idylls of infancy" [152]) as that fantasy is crossed by a remnant horror of maternal aggression. The point, of course, is that primal ambivalence emerges when a regressive fantasy—the traumatized subject's longing and ceaseless search for the origin—runs up against something terrifying at the beginning, what Rank provocatively refers to as the "painful share" another has "in one's own origin" (96).

V

How does *Inhibitions, Symptoms and Anxiety* engage these concerns? As we have already noted, in the opening chapters of the study, Freud reviews his own previous analyses of Little Hans and the Wolf Man with an eye toward reiterating the importance he accords the Oedipal situation generally and, more particularly, the centrality of the paternal threat of castration in the etiology of anxiety. Freud observes that in both cases the neurosis was focused on an animal—a horse in the case of Little Hans, a wolf in the case of the Wolf Man—that functioned as a father-substitute. More to the point, the animal itself was less of an issue in the formation of the neurosis than was the activity threatened by the animal: "as we know, 'Little Hans' alleged that what he was afraid of was that a horse would bite him"; "immediately after . . . , [the Wolf Man] had developed a fear of being devoured by a wolf." In the latter case, Freud observes that the Wolf Man's "fear of being devoured" was related to his father's playful "threat . . . to gobble him up," and he connects both fears (being bitten, being devoured) to another case in which a boy's neurosis was linked to the story "about an Arab chief who pursued a 'ginger-bread man' so as to eat him up. He identified himself with this edible person, and the Arab chief was easily recognizable as a father-substitute." Immediately after, Freud mentions the "idea of being devoured by the father [as] typical age-old childhood material. It has familiar parallels in mythology (e.g., the myth of Kronos)." At first baffled at how such a "strange" idea could "become the subject of a phobia," he then solves his own problem: "the idea of being devoured by the father gives expression, in the form that has undergone regressive degradation, to a passive, tender impulse to be loved by him in a genital-erotic sense." But as though he then realizes that Little Hans fear of being bitten would not immediately suggest the "impulse to be loved," Freud revises that statement: the phobia, he now surmises, covers a "hostile" instinctual impulse "against the father that is "transformed into it opposite[,] . . . aggressiveness (in the shape of revenge) on the part of his father towards the subject." And, to the extent that, in the case of Little Hans at least, "the process of repression" manifests "almost all the components of his Oedipus complex" (including his "tender impulses toward his mother"), Freud has no problem reading the biting-phobia as a "substitute . . . by distortion for the idea of being castrated" by his father (XX, 104–08).

Even as he admits that in the case of the Wolf Man the phobia as "expressed . . . contained [no] allusion to castration," Freud decides that the "motive force" on the onset of the phobia "was the same in both" cases: "it was from fear of being castrated, too, that the little Russian relinquished his wish to be loved by his father, for he thought that a relation of that sort presupposed a sacrifice of his genitals" (XX, 108).[25] But what if being bitten has more affinity with being devoured or gobbled up (as the wolf and Arab chief threatened and as, in myth, Kronos did in fact) than those images of being eaten have with being castrated? And what if the feelings toward the father mark something of the same ambivalence that Rank almost unwittingly uncovers in the son's relation with the mother: longing for a (nonsexual) bonding counterbalanced with the fear of being trapped in that maternal prison? In other words, are we necessarily looking at the fear of separation (in Freud's reading *separation-as-castration*), or is the real fear the fear of not being separate enough? For Rank the self can be trapped in the mother's womb, and for Freud it can be returned to the father's stomach. In this context, what Rank had called the "fearful yearning to go back" might suggest a deeper and more primal anxiety. For to the extent both images of return to the parental body suggest the reversal of birth, they also serve as reminders that one's birth belongs to someone else as much as to oneself. Perhaps what is really at stake in these accounts, then, is the child's primal ambivalence about having an origin at all and one that always and necessarily belongs to another.

Clearly, *Inhibitions, Symptoms and Anxiety* does not consciously make such an argument. But besides what Freud had previously articulated in "Theme of the Three Caskets" and *Beyond the Pleasure Principle*, there are other passages both in the 1926 treatise and in earlier writings that suggest this line of thinking. In chapter 5 of the *Ego and the Id* (1923), for example, just prior to asserting that the "dread of castration" is "the nucleus round which" the ego's fear of the superego ("of conscience") "has gathered," Freud describes this fear in a way that sounds like something very different from castration anxiety: "we know that the fear is of *being overwhelmed or annihilated*, but it cannot be grasped analytically" (XIX, 57; my emphasis).[26] *Inhibitions, Symptoms and Anxiety* will pick up this thread by making several references to a condition of "psychical helplessness" whose "prototype" is "the act of birth" (XX, 141–42; see also 144, 166–68). And that study's final chapter will take a broader perspective on this experience in linking this condition to what Freud calls the "traumatic situation."[27] In relating this helplessness to the "experience a being born," Freud sees the ego's struggle with a constantly increasing instinctual demand (the "situation of danger") as caused by "the loss of object," a loss he consistently defines in terms of the threat of castration even while acknowledging that the first such danger is "the absence of the mother" (XX, 137–38). But it is worth reminding ourselves that, as we saw in chapter 1, Freud's most provocative consideration of trauma (*Beyond the Pleasure Principle*) had treated the situation of danger—and its link to something we might call psychical helplessness—in a very different way, the confusion attendant upon being brought to consciousness from an inanimate state. This alternative way of viewing the primal trauma might also help us rethink what it means for the ego to be overwhelmed. Does that experience arise precisely because, at the primal scene, consciousness confronts its very belatedness in relation to its own existence and the "painful share" another has in its "own origin"?

To understand what such a confrontation might mean for Freud, we might consider his early work, "A Special Type of Choice of Object Made by Men" (the first of his "Contributions to the Psychology of Love" [1910]). There, in addressing what he calls the "parental complex," he observes that "when a child hears that he *owes his life* to his parents, or that his mother *gave him life*, his feelings of tenderness unite with impulses which strive at power and independence, and they generate the wish to return this gift to the parents and to repay them with one of equal value."[28] More to the point in anticipation to what we shall examine in part II, Freud then goes on to suggest that, even where the mother is involved, this ambivalence is particularly bound up with the son's hostile relationship to this father:

> It is as though the boy's defiance were to make him say: "I want nothing from my father; I will give him back all I have cost him." He then forms the phantasy of *rescuing his father from danger and saving his life*; in this way he put his account square with him. . . . In its application to a boy's father it is the defiant meaning in the idea . . . which is by far the most important; where his mother is concerned it is usually its tender meaning. The mother gave the child life, and it is not easy to find a substitute of equal value for this unique gift. . . . [R]escuing his mother takes on the significance of giving her a child or making a child for her, needless to say, one like himself. This is not too remote from the original sense of rescuing, and the change in meaning is not an arbitrary one. His mother gave him life—his own life—and in exchange he gives her another life, that of a child which has the greatest resemblance to himself. The son shows his gratitude by wishing to have by his mother a son who is like himself: in other words, in the rescue-phantasy he is completely identifying himself with his father. All his instincts, those of tenderness, gratitude, lustfulness, defiance and independence, find satisfaction in the single wish *to be his own father*. (XI, 172–73; emphases in original)

Apart from suggesting how a psychical situation originally created in relation to the mother might be transferred to the father—and it is worth noting that immediately after this passage he makes one of his earliest references to birth as "both the first of all dangers to life and the prototype of all later ones that cause us to feel anxiety"—Freud here provides a complex portrait about what is at stake in these fantasies in relation to one's parents. Striving "at power and independence" the son (I will follow Freud's gendered usage here) attempts defiantly to disavow that he "owes his life to his parents." In returning or repaying "this gift," he essentially switches places with his father: in fantasy, he either rescues his father from danger (his father now owes his life to *him*) or creates a new son with his mother (in either case, Freud suggests, the son "identif[ies] himself with his father"). But Freud's description of the mother-fantasy is especially intriguing. For if on the surface it seems to follow the logic of Oedipal longing (the son must copulate with his mother to produce this child), Freud's claim that the son "find[s] satisfaction in the single wish *to be his own father*" might be read in another way. While Freud almost certainly means that the boy longs to take his father's place (to identify with the father is to copulate with the mother), we might take the phrase "wish to be his own father" in a very different sense: this fantasy in which he fathers—that is, gives life—precisely by giving life *to himself* ("a child that has the greatest resemblance to himself") might suggest that to be his own father is a wish not so much to take his father's place (sexually) with the mother but actually not to have any father at all (or not any father who is not also himself). In other words, the son would most effectively disavow the fact that his parents "gave him life" by giving it to himself.

Such a wish is mere fantasy, of course. For the son to be his own father would mean that he must exist before he exists; he must, that is, always already reside at the time and place at which he can bring himself into existence. But the point of origin is, as Freud had speculated in *Beyond the Pleasure Principle*, "a force of whose Nature we can form no conception." And we can form no conception of a time and place from which we were always and necessarily absent. The son's disavowal of the "painful share" of the other in his own origin, is thus also, as Sartre might have recognized, a defiant refusal to be born, a refusal to have one's very existence imposed by another.

VI

By way of concluding both this chapter and part I as whole, I would say that what is most significant for the purposes of my larger argument is the following. Even as Rank's contortions concerning what he calls primal ambivalence point toward a different way of understanding what Freud means by linking the fear of death to the devouring father, that very revisionary perspective makes it possible to realign Freud's thinking in 1926 with his speculations on the death drive as a crisis of origins as he had formulated that position six years earlier in *Beyond the Pleasure Principle*. My reconstruction of the Rank-Freud debate also aims to show that, whatever the importance the mother might have in this crisis, for Freud the son's experience (and it is always the *son's* experience) necessarily comes back to his father. Freud's Oedipal economy is an attempt to explain the son's ambivalence toward the father: such ambivalence includes his identification and sexual rivalry with as well as his fear of castration at the hands of paternal authority. But what is primal in this ambivalence marks the existential problem *par excellence*.

"It is too late to be helped," Emerson writes, "the discovery we have made that we exist." And our belated awakening to that condition is the primal scene, a belatedness essentially disavowed, as Freud suggests, in the son's assertion that he owes nothing to his parents. Whether it is the maternal prison or the fear of being devoured by the father, Rank's birth trauma and Freud's castration anxiety might be better understood in the very Emersonian terms that vexed my son Ian just prior to his fifth birthday: we come too late to the scene of our beginning. More to the point, at the heart of this existential crisis we are forced to admit that there is a time and a place before us, that we were necessarily if impossibly absent from the scene of our own creation, and that what was absent most of all was our own choice.

To the extent this question is at the heart of my study, part II ("Tardy Sons") will be especially concerned with how it plays out in the context of filial ambivalence toward the father, an ambivalence that continues at once to reveal and to conceal Freud's engagement with the problem of belatedness. Chapter 3 will take up this topic primarily in relation to Freud's writings on mourning (first broached in relation to the death of his father, Jacob Freud, in 1896). Freud's own speculations will be conceptually channeled through one of his chief interpretive interests and what we might also quite reasonably understand as one of his chief interpretive models: Shakespeare's *Hamlet*. Chapter 4 will then both return to Freud and take up the issue of the son's crisis of belatedness more directly in a discussion of the 1919 essay, "The Uncanny." One of my own interpretive touchstones in that discussion will be Freud's almost passing reference in his 1909 *Interpretation of Dreams* to "this uncanny life before birth," a phrase I take to mean that what we experience as uncanny has some particular association with what we imagine of our life before birth, what in *Beyond the Pleasure Principle* Freud would understand as the inanimate condition preceding our living or animate state. But even in my critical reconstruction of the 1919 essay, Freud's precursors will still be important. Part of my aim in chapter 4 will be to demonstrate that, when read in conjunction with E. T. A. Hoffmann's "The Sandman" and Ernst Jentsch's theory of the uncanny, Freud's interpretation of Hoffmann's story can be seen often missing its own best insights. Moreover, as we shall see, in "The Uncanny" Freud often makes claims that are not only anticipated by Hoffmann and Jentsch but also proleptically corrected by them. Finally, chapter 4 will show, once again, how, when confronted with the problem of the son's origin as a crisis of belatedness, Freud invariably turns to the Oedipal economy to explain the son's vexed relationship to the father, an interpretive position that regularly explains away what for some reason Freud himself could never quite face.

PART II

Tardy Sons

Shakespeare, Freud, and Filial Ambivalence

The father and the son, is this not a history of the doubling of consciousness? Is it not also a struggle to the death?

—Paul Ricoeur, "Fatherhood"

3

"More than his father's death"

Mourning at Elsinore and Vienna

> For this book [*Interpretation of Dreams*] has a further subjective significance for me personally—a significance which I only grasped after I had completed it. It was, I found, a portion of my own self-analysis, my reaction to my father's death—that is to say, to the most important event, the most poignant loss, of a man's life. Having discovered that this was so, I felt unable to obliterate the traces of the experience.
>
> —Freud, Preface to the Second Edition

> O heavens, die two months ago, and not forgotten yet? Then there's hope a great man's memory may outlive his life half a year.
>
> —Shakespeare, *Hamlet*

I

One might imagine that, at the first performance of *Hamlet* (probably in late 1600), the audience at the Globe would have taken a certain delight in the *mise en abyme* of the following exchange:

HAMLET: My lord, you play'd once i' th' university, you say?

POLONIUS: That did I, my lord, and was accounted a good actor.

HAMLET: What did you enact?

POLONIUS: I did enact Julius Caesar. I was kill'd i' th' Capitol; Brutus kill'd me.

HAMLET: It was a brute part of him to kill so capital a calf there. (3.2.98–106)

Shakespeare's *Julius Caesar* had opened at the Globe one year earlier, and it is likely that Shakespeare is making a nod here to the community of London theatergoers by referring to a play many of them had recently seen. The actors playing Hamlet and Polonius may also have performed the roles of Brutus and Caesar. If so, the exchange becomes, in part, a joking reminder that stage violence has no lasting effects: the actor killed in the Roman Capitol one day can come back the next as a high-ranking Danish civil servant.

These are but possibilities, of course. Yet, taken together, they suggest that in *Hamlet* Shakespeare is interested in the relationship between memory and repetition. If we consider his particular metatheatrical marking of this relationship, then we might also infer that Shakespeare wants to explore it in a deliberately oblique, if playful, way: we remember that we've been here before, but the "here" is the space of representation itself, the space of repetition with a difference. There is something twisted in Shakespeare's toying with his audience's memory when what we recall of the past is precisely what is present before us in altered form. Is this memory after all or a reminder that it is always now in the theater? And if it is always now, what then is our relationship to the past, whether the past of ancient Rome, of medieval Denmark, or of the Globe of the previous year? How does the past stay alive in the present and to what effect?

We might note that *Hamlet*'s explicit references to *Julius Caesar* in certain ways problematize any notion of memory as a simple connection to the past. Faced with the unintelligibility of the Ghost in the play's opening scene, Horatio views the Ghost as a "usurpation" of the present by the past: "the same figure like the King that's dead" (1.1.41, 46). Even as it seems to offer a forewarning of what is to come, this figure (more repetition than memory) can only be rendered intelligible by remembering the past; thus Horatio must explain to the guards (and so also to the audience) that the present preparation for war is in anticipation of an invasion that would attempt to undo a state of affairs created some thirty years previously (1.1.80–107). Just as significantly, Horatio's scholarly mind attempts to justify his explanation—less causally than analogically—by recourse to the situation in Rome on the eve of Caesar's assassination:

> In the most high and palmy state of Rome,
> A little ere the mightiest Julius fell,
> The graves stood tenantless and the sheeted dead
> Did squeak and gibber in the Roman streets.
> As stars with trains of fire, and dews of blood,
> Disasters in the sun; and the moist star
> Upon whose influence Neptune's empire stands
> Was sick almost to doomsday with eclipse.
> And even the like precurse of fear'd events,
> As harbingers preceding still the fates
> And prologue to the omen coming on,
> Have heaven and earth together demonstrated
> Unto our climatures and countrymen. (1.2.113–25)[1]

Although Horatio is never represented as anything other than decent and intelligent—hence, we have little reason to doubt his initial assessment—the first act of *Hamlet* appears to suggest not only that the scholarly exegesis here is wrong but also that it is wrong *because* of Horatio's failure to properly read the lessons of the past: despite his detailed recall of what he no doubt learned at school, Horatio fails to remember that the chief lesson of history is that history repeats itself. Thus, while Horatio infers from the Ghost's presence that an invasion is imminent (young Fortinbras's attempt at once to repeat and to reverse his father's exploits), by the end of Act 1 we would be hard-pressed not to believe that the Ghost signifies less a threat from outside than a rottenness within. In other words, the enemy you know, close at hand, already inside the gates is precisely what the Roman lesson should have taught the astute reader.

Even more than Horatio, it is Polonius whose questionable interpretive skills make him complaisant and dangerously overconfident. Indeed, if he had only recognized the Brutus who stood before him in the person of Hamlet he might never have thought that he could escape his destiny by hiding behind an arras. Still, as different as they are, Horatio and Polonius, taken together as dramatic mnemonics of an earlier play that, in some inexplicable way, haunts the present one, suggest Shakespeare's interest in how memory and repetition are complexly enmeshed in the human failure to know, whether that knowledge is directed at the world, at the past, at the other, or, finally, at ourselves.

These strange and strained relationships between present and past, self and other, memory and repetition, will be played out most pointedly in Hamlet's relationship to his dead father (where the son's very name, because of a change Shakespeare made to his sources, repeats the father's).[2] That relationship will be the main focus of this chapter. But before we get to that fuller discussion, it is worth briefly considering how the (Prince) Hamlet–(King) Hamlet link also remembers and repeats *Julius Caesar*.

Although Caesar's ghostly visitation to Brutus before the battle of Philippi (*Julius Caesar* 4.3) had its own theatrical precedents (a similar scene in 5.3 of *Richard III*, for example), what is new in *Julius Caesar* is the close relationship between Caesar and the man his ghost now haunts: Brutus was, or at least was believed to be, Caesar's illegitimate son.[3] The appearance of Caesar's ghost in 1599 thus sets the stage for another haunting, one year later, of a tragic son by his murdered father, the scene we know as 1.5 of *Hamlet*. Although Prince Hamlet is not King Hamlet's murderer, at one point he appears to make that allegation against himself (4.4.56–57). More broadly, Hamlet will reenact part of Brutus's central experience: the almost impossible burden of a son trying to shed the authority of the dead but still potent father.[4] Indeed, if Brutus's suicide (precisely what Hamlet contemplates and, for Freud at least, actually achieves) marks an attempt to lay to rest his father's restless spirit, it also marks a strange moment of the son's identification with his dead father (Brutus killed Caesar; Brutus kills himself), a mode of interaction—or repetition—that will similarly complicate the tragic plot of *Hamlet*.[5]

My reference here to Freud is not incidental. As the chapter's first epigraph reminds us, while writing the *Interpretation of Dreams* Freud himself may have been repeating much of Hamlet's struggle, working through his relationship to his own recently deceased father, Jacob Freud.[6] In this chapter's Afterword, I will reflect in more detail on my particular use of the terms of Freudian psychoanalysis to reconstruct meaning in an early-modern text. For now, I wish simply to make two related points. First, although I explicitly formulate the various relations among memory and repetition, past and present, in Freudian terms (especially in the context of a son's mourning his father's passing), what follows is less a Freudian reading of *Hamlet* than an attempt to put Freud in dialogue with *Hamlet*. Second, the possibility of this sort of dialogue leans heavily on, without fully endorsing, Stephen Greenblatt's suggestion that "psychoanalysis is at once the fulfillment and effacement of specifically Renaissance insights." Elaborating on this assertion, Greenblatt writes:

> If psychoanalysis was . . . made possible by (among other things) the legal and literary proceedings of the sixteenth and seventeenth centuries, then its interpretive practice is not irrel-

evant to those proceedings, nor is it exactly an anachronism. But psychoanalytic interpretation is causally belated, even as it is causally linked. . . . [P]sychoanalysis can redeem its belatedness only when it historicizes its own procedures.[7]

Although a full-scale attempt to historicize psychoanalysis is well beyond the scope of this chapter, I do want to suggest that one cannot merely apply Freudian insights to *Hamlet* precisely because, while Freud's reflections permit us to recognize what is at stake in the play, those reflections only permit us to hear the questions that the play is already asking. Moreover, and more in line with Greenblatt's assertions, this chapter attempts, in a very modest way, to historicize psychoanalysis in its belated relation to the Renaissance precisely by demonstrating why *Hamlet*—that is, why *Hamlet* in particular—should be understood as the starting point of psychoanalysis in ways Freud both did and didn't see. If Freud's thinking helps us understand mourning as a process that structures the plot of *Hamlet*, *Hamlet* in turn anticipates Freud and even, in some mysterious way, corrects Freud's own neurotic refusal to see what was in front of his own eyes. *Hamlet*, in short, helps us understand what is at stake in mourning—how does the past stay alive in the present?—even beyond what Freud himself could recognize. And if what is at stake is experienced as ambivalence toward the deceased, the true motive force of that ambivalence (for both Hamlet and Freud directed at the dead father) resides in an existential more than in a purely psychological question: what does it mean to be one's own and not one's own simultaneously?

II

I begin the historicizing of Freud's thought with a passage that comes from a letter to Wilhelm Fliess (November 11, 1896) in which Freud recounts a "very pretty dream" he had on the "night after" his father's funeral:

> I found myself in a shop where there was a notice up saying:
>
> > You are requested
> > to close your eyes.
>
> I recognized the place as the barber's to which I go every day. On the day of the funeral I was kept waiting, and therefore

arrived at the house of mourning rather late. The family were displeased with me, because I had arranged for the funeral to be quiet and simple, which they later agreed was the best thing. They also took my lateness in rather bad part. The phrase on the notice-board has a double meaning. It means "one should do one's duty toward the dead" in two senses—an apology, as though I had not done my duty and my conduct needed overlooking, and the actual duty itself. The dream was thus an outlet for the feeling of self-reproach which a death generally leaves among the survivors. (*Origins*, 171)

Apart from the general ways in which the problems and procedures of a fully developed psychoanalytic discourse are coming into focus here, I am particularly interested in how Freud himself revised both his description of this dream and its interpretation when, four years later, he recounted it a second time in the *Interpretation of Dreams*:

> During the night before my father's funeral I had the dream of a printed notice, placard or poster—rather like the notices forbidding one to smoke in railway waiting rooms—on which appeared either
>
>   'You are requested to close the eyes'
> or,   'You are requested to close an eye.'
>
> I usually write this in the form:
>
> $$\text{'You are requested to close} \begin{array}{c} \text{the} \\ \text{an} \end{array} \text{eye(s).'}$$
>
> Each of these two versions had a meaning of its own and led in a different direction when the dream was interpreted. I had chosen the simplest possible ritual for the funeral, for I knew my father's own views on such ceremonies. But some other members of the family were not sympathetic to such puritanical simplicity and thought we should be disgraced in the eyes of those who attended the funeral. Hence, one of the versions: 'You are requested to close an eye,' i.e. to 'wink at' or 'overlook.' Here it is particularly easy to see the meaning of the vagueness

expressed by the 'either—or.' The dream-work failed to establish a unified wording for the dream-thoughts which could at the same time be ambiguous, and the two main lines of thought consequently began to diverge even in the manifest content of the dream. (IV, 317–18)

Some of the changes might leave us scratching our heads. Why, for example, does Freud shift the date of the dream from the night *after* the funeral to the night *before*? And why is there no reference in the revision to Freud's visit to the barbershop? In the original, having been kept waiting at the barber's, Freud "displeased" the family by arriving late at the house of mourning. Freud then shifts the source of the displeasure to the funeral arrangements themselves (". . . displeased because I had arranged for the funeral to be quiet and simple"), even though the family members later agree that this "was the best thing." As befits its specific focus on the ambiguity of dreams, the revision, by contrast, emphasizes the "either—or" structure of the dream-work (he even replicates this typographically), but this new emphasis effectively covers over the attention originally given to the displeasure Freud himself had elicited from his family. Thus, when in the revision Freud does get to the source of his family's displeasure, the focus is exclusively on the inadequacy of the funeral arrangements (their "puritanical simplicity"). Not only is Freud's lateness in arriving not mentioned in the revision, but also, in a more general way, his central role in the account is diminished, while the disagreement within the family as a whole takes center stage. In short, in the revision Freud's key role in causing displeasure is doubly displaced: first, it is not his lateness that matters (it isn't even mentioned—an effect of changing the night of the dream); second, even though it was Freud himself who had chosen the arrangements, the family is less displeased with him than concerned over how others might judge the family as a whole: they "thought *we* should be disgraced in the eyes of those who attended the funeral."

We might observe, moreover, that Freud's understanding of the dream's ambiguity changes as he moves from his account in the 1896 letter to the fuller, more technical interpretation in 1900. In the original, although Freud seems reluctant at first to acknowledge that his lateness is the cause of the family's displeasure with him, he does eventually get to a point where he interprets the (single) wording of the notice as a kind of reproach, one directed at him exclusively: "The phrase on the notice-board has a double meaning. It means 'one should do one's duty toward the dead' in two senses—an apology, as though I had not done my duty and my conduct needing overlooking and the actual duty itself." What Freud, rather reluctantly, offers here shows a more nuanced sense of ambiguity in that the problem is not familial embarrassment over the inadequacy of the ceremony but rather Freud's own lack of filial respect to the dead: he had come late to the house of mourning and had arranged for a funeral whose sparseness did not, as it does in the revision, accord with his father's preference.

In the original, in fact, Freud interprets his dream's double meaning as an indication of emotional ambivalence: the "self-reproach which a death generally leaves among the survivors." But that generalized view of the problem appears to displace the more particular cause of self-reproach on display here: his failure properly to perform his filial duty. It is clear, moreover, that the revision covers over the original's sense of self-reproach even more completely. In short, building on a process of evasion already in evidence in the original account, the revision is like a dream itself, censoring (displacing, denying) unconscious feelings of hostility toward the dead it does not want to acknowledge.[8] For what the failure of filial duty in coming late and in arranging such a "quiet and simple" ceremony appears to point to is not simply survivor guilt but Freud's uneasiness about admitting an insult to his father's memory. Freud introduces the dream in his letter to Fliess by relating how much he valued his father, how his "peculiar mixture of deep wisdom and imaginative light-heartedness" meant to him. But the death that stirs the "whole past . . . within one," the death that reveals "obscure routes behind the official consciousness" that affect us deeply, even as a tree "torn up by the roots" (*Origins*, 170), these are what the dream and its interpretation, even in the original account, can only half reveal. And that obscure route to the past that can yet reveal what stands beyond consciousness, that past that can help us understand what is at stake in Freud's disavowing dream interpretation, brings us now to *Hamlet*.

III

Like Freud's dream, *Hamlet* is much concerned not just with grief over the deaths of loved ones (King Hamlet, Polonius, Ophelia, Hamlet himself) but also with the way such grief is ritualized in what Laertes calls "ceremony" (5.1.223). Shakespeare may have picked up a cue here from the sources of the play. Recounting the combat between Orvendil (Hamlet the Elder, general of Rørik's Danish armies) and Koller (Fortinbras the Elder, King of Norway), Saxo Grammaticus cites Koller's insistence that the winner properly "observe our obligations to the dead." "Let our sense of duty then,"

Koller continues, "make this stipulation, that the victor should conduct the last rites of the vanquished." After defeating Koller, Orvendil keeps his promise: "He honored their agreement by giving him a regal funeral, constructing an ornate tomb and providing ceremony of great magnificence."[9] In Shakespeare's version, at play's end young Fortinbras will return the favor to the slain Hamlet.

Beyond whatever hints Shakespeare might have picked up from his reading, the play's central concern with the ritualization of grief suggests, as Greenblatt has noted, "something deeper . . . at work in Shakespeare."[10] Greenblatt and Robert Watson have both argued that this "something deeper" is at once personal and cultural: personal, to the extent the loss of Hamnet Shakespeare and the impending loss of John Shakespeare might have opened as yet unhealed wounds in Shakespeare's psyche; cultural, to the extent that the Protestant dismantling of the Catholic cult of the dead produced a psychosocial condition in which a mourner's very capacity to sustain a sense that the "dead were [not] beyond . . . earthly contact" was strained to the breaking point. Greenblatt concludes that "the death of [Shakespeare's] son and the impending death of his father—a crisis of mourning and memory—constitute a psychic disturbance that may help to explain the explosive power and inwardness of *Hamlet*."[11]

If mourning and memory together form the play's central crisis, the dramatic force of that crisis derives, in part at least, from the way in which Shakespeare's initial conflation of remembrance and vengeance in the Ghost's command to Hamlet ("*Revenge* his foul and most unnatural murther" / "Adieu, adieu, adieu! *remember* me" [1.5.25, 91]) slowly comes undone. It is worth dwelling on this conflation/separation for a moment because the creative tension between vengeance and memory is one of the many subtle alterations Shakespeare made to his sources, alterations that, among other things, had the effect of radically altering the Elizabethan revenge-tragedy genre. Thomas Lodge's famous recollection that an earlier Hamlet-play featured what, from the perspective of Shakespeare's version, appears as a rather stock charge ("Hamlet, revenge") suggests that Shakespeare added the ghostly charge to remember because he was not satisfied with the simple, if dramatically proven, action of revenge as the core of the story.[12] The complexity of Shakespeare's version, including the otherwise unexplained delay in Hamlet's killing of Claudius, turns on the way Hamlet experiences revenging and remembering as opposing actions rather than as paired aspects of a single action. Thus, as Greenblatt continues, "Hamlet does not sweep to his revenge, and it turns out that remembering his father—remembering him in the right way, remembering him at all—is far more difficult to do than he imagined."¹³ Whether vengeance could or should be understood as a possible resolution to the crisis of mourning that inhabits the play, in Greenblatt's suggestive phrasing Hamlet (or Shakespeare himself) faces this crisis of mourning because of a failure of memory, a failure marked in Hamlet's inability to remember his father "in the "right way" or to remember him "at all."

Although the phrase "a crisis of mourning and memory" suggests that mourning and memory refer to slightly different experiences, in his account as a whole the failure of memory and the failure of mourning, taken together, point to a crisis of "ceremony" that Greenblatt, in good New Historicist fashion, puts at the center of his cultural reading of the play.¹⁴ I would like to suggest, however, that mourning and memory need to be distinguished more clearly and that the reason they need to be distinguished can only be fully grasped in psychoanalytic terms, though a psychoanalysis given back to history or at least to biography. To the extent we can draw on psychoanalysis here, the distinction points us toward a critical insight of Freud's mid-career, an insight that moves him beyond the Oedipus complex and so beyond the pleasure principle.¹⁵

In *Beyond the Pleasure Principle* (1920), Freud writes that one of the first solutions to what he calls the "therapeutic problem" is "to oblige the patient to confirm the analyst's construction from his own memory" in such a way that "what was unconscious should become conscious." The difficulty in so doing, however, is that "the patient cannot remember the whole of what is repressed . . . , and what he cannot remember may be precisely the essential part of it. Thus he acquires no sense of conviction of the correctness of the construction that has been communicated to him. He is obliged to *repeat* the repressed material as a contemporary experience instead of, as the physician would prefer to see, *remembering* it as something belonging to the past" (XVIII, 18). What Freud calls the "ratio between what is remembered and what is repeated" thus becomes the site of psychoanalytic investigation and intervention. On one side, repetition is aligned with the Unconscious and repression, where everything related to the situation is experienced as happening in the present. On the other side, proper memory permits the patient to gain some perspective on the situation ("some degree of aloofness"), and this perspective is understood in terms of the patient's ability to achieve a kind temporal gap between present reality (the experience in the present) and how that reality "is in fact only a reflection of a forgotten past" (XVIII, 18–19). Freud constantly hints that the effort to move from repeating as a marker of repression to memory as a marker of emotional control or detachment is central to the work of mourning. *Beyond the*

Pleasure Principle views the problem of a patient's repeating rather than remembering as a manifestation of trauma that is linked to an inability to mourn or the failure to mourn properly.[16]

Although Shakespeare's *Hamlet* will provide much of my subsequent evidence for this claim, we can get a partial measure of where Freud's thought is going in 1920 by considering how he got there. Two texts in particular offer key insight into how Freud will later attempt to triangulate mourning, memory, and repeating. Written and published in late 1914, the first of these texts, "Remembering, Repeating, and Working-Through," provides an early version of the distinction between memory and repetition that Freud will develop in *Beyond the Pleasure Principle*. As he will again in 1920, Freud positions remembering as kind of therapeutic alternative to repeating. Indeed, despite the fact that Freud employs various versions of the word "forget" throughout the essay, in psychological terms remembering is not the opposite of forgetting; rather, remembering is the opposite of repeating, even though repeating is, paradoxically, often the patient's sole "way of remembering" (XII, 150).[17] This paradox is a reminder that both remembering and repeating constitute some relationship between the patient's present and the past. In cases of neurosis, however, repetition displaces memory because the effect of repression is to prevent the patient from seeing the past as the past: "repetition is a transference of the forgotten past . . . *to all . . . aspects of the current situation*. We must be prepared to find, therefore, that the patient yields to the compulsion to repeat, which now replaces an impulsion to remember . . . in every . . . activity and relationship which may occupy his life *at this time*" (XII, 151; my emphases).[18] One of the chief effects of repression, in other words, is to make it difficult for the patient to *remember* the past, to relate to it with detachment ("aloofness") by seeing it as belonging to a different time. The notion of "working-through," then, is closely linked to the therapeutic effect of remembering. It is a term for describing how one manages to escape from the trap of repetition, the experience of the past as though it were still present.[19] In the bizarre world of neurosis, the patient must remember not to forget.

The second and more famous text, "Mourning and Melancholia," was published in 1917 but composed simultaneously with "Remembering, Repeating, and Working-Through."[20] This essay never explicitly addresses the distinction between memory and repetition Freud was then developing, but it is very much taken up with mourning ("normal mourning" and "pathological mourning" or melancholia) as a special kind of "work." Indeed, what Freud here calls the "work of mourning" might be understood as test-case for the more general process of "working-through." Or, to put the relationship between the two essays another way, "Remembering, Repeating, and Working-Through" is completed in "Mourning and Melancholia" to the extent that the latter is interested in some of the key motive forces that give rise to the processes described in the former.

Throughout the second essay, Freud cannot decide whether mourning and melancholia are two separate experiences or two different manifestations of the same experience. But to the extent he does finally distinguish them, the key distinction is between a patient's conscious connection to a lost love-object—and in "normal mourning" this almost always means "a real loss of the object . . . by its death" (XIV, 256)—and an unconscious or repressed connection. More precisely, in melancholia, the patient experiences not just the loss but also a particularly vexed relationship to what is lost even to the point of confusion over precisely what is lost: "the patient is aware of the loss . . . but only in the sense of *whom* he has lost but not *what* he has lost in him" (XIV, 245).[21] The confusion in melancholia, including the role that repression plays in it, derives, Freud concludes, from "conflict due to ambivalence" (251). And though expressed most directly in terms of antagonism toward the self (feelings of self-reproach and unworthiness, self-criticism, even, finally, suicidal tendencies), this ambivalence bespeaks a vexed relationship towards the lost love-object (typically the deceased).

In describing the confused feelings toward the object, Freud is in many ways providing an extended gloss on his 1896 dream of his dead father, which was, as we have seen, a complex expression of ambivalence. The motive force of this ambivalence is hinted at in one of the few places in "Remembering, Repeating, and Working-Through" that addresses situations occasioning these processes: in this case, resistance to "parents' authority" (XII, 150). In earlier texts, Freud had considered this resistance more precisely in the context of the death of a parent. In a draft of a letter to Fliess (dated May 31, 1897), for example, Freud writes that hostile impulses toward our parents (especially toward the parent of the same sex) "are repressed at periods in which pity for one's parents is active, at times of their illness or death. One of the manifestations of grief is then to reproach oneself for their death . . . or to punish oneself . . . by putting oneself into their position with an idea of retribution," an action Freud there terms "identification" (*Origins*, 207). And in the *Interpretation of Dreams*, he sees the patient's hostility (or ambivalence) explicitly in the relation to the father. Noting there both how "absurdity is . . . one of the methods by which the dream-work represents a contradiction" and that the clearest instances of the absurdity-contradiction nexus arise "in dreams related to a dead father," Freud goes on to provide the following explanation for the contradictory feelings: "The authority wielded by a father provokes criticism from his children at a very early age, and the severity of the demands he makes upon them leads them, for their own relief, *to keep their eyes open* to any weakness of their father's; but the filial piety called up in our minds by the figure of the father, *particularly after his death*, tightens the censorship which prohibits any such criticism from being consciously expressed" (V, 434–35; my emphases). The pressure to keep his eyes open to paternal weakness is, in a sense, what Freud's two interpretations of the funeral dream aim to defend against, a defense in which the shows of filial piety function as a kind of censor.

What Freud had observed almost in passing in 1896 as "the feeling of self-reproach which a death generally leaves among the survivors" is thus theorized by 1914 as an inverted act of resentment toward the lost love-object, the deceased parent, the dead father: "So we find the key to the clinical picture . . . that the self-reproaches are reproaches against a loved object which have been shifted away from it on to the patient's own ego" (XIV, 248).[22] As I have suggested, this argument harkens back to a much earlier formulation in the 1897 draft-letter to Fliess, which also addresses Freud's observations concerning self-reproach, the desire to punish oneself, and the disavowal of hostility through identification. It is worth noting that this draft-letter contains some of the first hints of what will become Freud's theory of the Oedipus complex. That is, attempting to understand the repressed feelings of antagonism toward his deceased father, Freud will begin to develop a notion of sexual rivalry in relation to the mother.[23] But by 1914 that theory has disappeared from Freud's account, and the explanation we get instead for what Freud calls the "mental constellation of revolt" (XIV, 248) is something more primal. In his typically understated way, Freud refers to this situation as a "disturbance in self regard" or a feeling of "loss in regard to . . . [the] ego" (246–47). More poetically, Freud remarks how "the shadow of the object [falls] upon the ego" (249). A person suffering pathological mourning thus "displays . . . an extraordinary diminution in his self-regard, an impoverishment of his ego on a grand scale"; or again, "the complex of melancholia behaves like an open wound . . . emptying the ego until it is totally impoverished" (246, 253). Although, as I have noted, Freud claims that "the patient cannot consciously perceive what he has lost in" the love-object, this confusion now appears to stem from repressed resentment toward the one whose presence, even in death, can so impoverish the ego. Read in conjunction with his 1896 dream, Freud's articulation of the threat posed to the ego appears to be the anxiety of a son who finds his own life inexplicably diminished in the wake of his father's passing, as though it only just occurred to him that his very selfhood was dependent on that of another.

Two final points need to be made about "Mourning and Melancholia." First, while Freud does not deal directly in the essay with the distinction between memory and repetition, he does at certain points hint that we should understand the difference between normal mourning and pathological mourning in terms of this distinction. For example, his twice-made observation that normal mourning is typically "overcome after a certain lapse of time" (XIV, 244, 252) is linked to another twice-made observation about the role of memory in that process: "Each single one of the *memories* . . . which demonstrate the libido's attachment to the lost object is met by the verdict of reality that the object no longer exists; and the ego, confronted as it were with the question whether it shall share this fate, is persuaded by the sum of the narcissistic satisfactions it derives from being alive *to sever its attachment to the object that has been abolished*" (XIV, 255; my emphases).[24] Normal mourning, we might say, is not just something that occurs "after a certain lapse of time"; rather, it is a way of dealing with time as lapse, as distance between the present and the past.[25] Memory is the mechanism by which the distance is created and sustained, not simply to produce a gap in time but also, and more importantly, to "sever attachment" to another whose continuing force in the present impoverishes the ego. In other words, memory structures a relationship to time and within time that also marks the assertion of self against the demands of a dead other. In pathological forms of mourning, by contrast, the patient's relation to the past fails to function as memory in the normal way: "in analyses it often becomes evident that first one and then another *memory is activated*, and that the laments which always sound the same and are wearisome in their monotony nevertheless take their rise . . . in some . . . unconscious source" (256; my emphasis). This observation that memory operates in relation to the Unconscious is a reminder of Freud's basic distinction between mourning and melancholia. And the form these melancholic memories take is precisely repetitive: "laments which always sound the same and are wearisome in their monotony." Although Freud himself doesn't register the significance of this point, he is implicitly relating the mourning-melancholia distinction to the distinction he was then formulating between remembering and repeating: in melancholia, the patient remembers only through repetition (his sole "way of remembering" [XII, 150]) and so cannot sever his attachment to the deceased, even though that attachment is vexed by repressed hostility that bespeaks the patient's grasp of how his ego is diminished through the lost love-object's impositions. Working-through fails, then, in the patient's inability to move from repetition to memory.

The second point has to do with how Freud is asking us to consider the mourning/memory—melancholia/repetition distinction in terms of *Hamlet*. If, as I have noted, "Mourning and Melancholia" reads at times as an extended gloss on his 1896 dream, his interpretive reconstruction of 1914 was also, I would suggest, mediated by his rereading and rethinking of *Hamlet*. Freud explicitly mentions Hamlet as a prime instance of this melancholic temperament (XIV, 246): such a temperament, in Freud's view, might explain everything from Hamlet's self-reproaches to his brutal honesty to his suicidal tendencies to his sense of possessing an interior space we can never fully access even to his desire and inability to sleep.[26] Furthermore, although Freud makes no reference to Hamlet's Oedipal crisis, Shakespeare's character still serves as Freud's test-subject for his new theories of a son's resentment toward the father. Hamlet's status in Freud's revisionary work also helps explain more fully Greenblatt's unpacked assertion that Hamlet experiences a "crisis of memory and mourning." If, as Freud remarked in 1897, "remembering is never a motive, but only a method—a mode" (*Origins*, 208), a crisis of mourning is expressed through a crisis of memory, a failure to remember in the right way. In other words, the patient repeats. And this pathological way of connecting to the past manifests a crisis of the impoverished ego that cannot sever its attachment to the deceased. In *Hamlet*, that crisis is represented in a son's relationship to a beloved father whose ghost demands to be remembered in an act of vengeance. But that way of remembering is indistinguishable from identification, which, as Freud notes, is one of the chief manifestations of pathological mourning. The haunting in the play is thus an instance of the shadow of the lost love-object falling upon the ego, and the plot recounts Hamlet's efforts to refuse melancholy, to refuse the father, in an attempt to find his way back to mourning through memory.[27] But what can that process possibly mean in a story in which the very locus of pathological mourning laments from the outset that he can do nothing but remember ("Heaven and earth, / Must I remember?" [1.2.142–43])?

As a sort of preface to that more detailed consideration of this question, I note here that the play self-consciously thematizes the very Freudian distinction between something we might call simple memory and some other relation to the past characterized by repetition. Since this issue will be examined subsequently from other angles, one example can suffice, a small but significant segment of the exchange between Hamlet and Horatio just before Horatio tells Hamlet of the sighting of the Ghost on the battlements:

HAMLET: My father—methinks I see my father.

HORATIO: Where, my lord?

HAMLET: In my mind's eye, Horatio.

HORATIO: I saw him once, 'a was a goodly king.

HAMLET: 'A was a man, take him for all in all,
I shall not look upon his like again.

HORATIO: My lord, I think I saw him yesternight.

HAMLET: Saw, who?

HORATIO: My lord, the King your father.

HAMLET: The King my father? (1.2.184–91)

I shall return to consider in more detail the significance of the repetitive phrasing that concludes this exchange ("King/father"). For now, I wish merely to call attention to the fact of the repetition rather than to its content. Whatever pathologies we may have already observed in Hamlet's conduct, at this moment he clearly articulates his father's death as a great felt absence but in a way that even Freud might have considered normal as opposed to pathological. And that loss points explicitly to a past Hamlet knows will not return, a past that only exists in memory: he "*was* a goodly king" / he "*was* a man." But as Hamlet's curiosity is piqued by Horatio's cryptic remarks, the form of his thinking about his father shifts from a kind of narrative past tense—"was"/"was"—to a temporally unmarked repetition (the lack of verbs in line 191 marks a subtle shift away from the past tense). At the outset of the exchange, that is, Hamlet is working precisely within the bounds of memory ("working through," we might say): his father is dead and buried; he will return no more. But even as Horatio barely hints that the past may not be behind them, that indeed, a living voice may speak from beyond the grave, Hamlet's remembering undoes itself in repetition: "the King your Father. / The King my father?"

In short, a passage that begins with a son in the act of remembering his deceased father concludes with a moment of repetition that will initiate the action of the rest of the play. That action will be shaped by a tension between repetition that cannot surrender the past—indeed that is pathologically compelled to reenact it—and something else in Hamlet (call it "conscience") that must insist on that surrender, an insistence marked by the refusal of revenge. This exchange between Hamlet and Horatio is thus an early conceptual turning point in the play: it marks a moment at which therapeutic memory becomes pathological repetition.

Such repetition itself speaks to a repressed hostility toward the deceased that might manifest itself in a variety of ways. In 1897 Freud writes that hostile impulses toward our parents "are repressed at periods in which pity for one's parents is active, at times of their illness or death. One of the manifestations of grief is then to reproach oneself for their death . . . or to punish oneself . . . by putting oneself into their position with an idea of retribution" ("identification"). Hamlet feels the stings of reproach because of his failure to avenge his father, and these feelings, just as in Freud's dream, evince a son's guilt over not showing proper filial piety. But Hamlet also, and perhaps more significantly, punishes himself, via identification-as-defense, by putting himself into his father's position: in an act of suicidal madness, he stakes out his father's "position with an idea of [self-]retribution," all but guaranteeing that he too will die at the hands of Claudius.[28] Like Freud in 1896, then, Hamlet (who over-idealizes his father at a conscious level) shows signs that he is actually repressing hostile feelings. Freud, as we have seen, saw identification as an especially important mode of repetition, one marked by a failure to distinguish between past and present and between self and other. Hamlet anticipates this insight in struggling throughout the rest of the play to draw a distinction between himself and his father. In his drive to individuate himself as the son whose very name repeats the father's, Hamlet discovers that remembering the father in the right way is a tragic business indeed.

IV

As we have noted, Shakespeare radically altered the trajectory of the story he inherited by establishing as the new central conflict the need for his hero to decouple memory and its attendant mourning from vengeance. In short, Hamlet struggles to accomplish the work of mourning because vengeance functions in terms of repetition (specifically as identification) rather than as memory. As this section will consider in more detail, in identifying with his father rather than remembering him, Hamlet cannot distinguish where or when he is from a past that he has forgotten precisely *as* the past, a past that literally haunts him.

Watson and Stanley Cavell (among others) are right to suggest that, whether coming from the true ghost of his father or from his own needs and longings, revenge is represented in the plot as a way by which the Ghost imposes—or Hamlet imposes upon himself—the necessity of sustaining his father's memory by acting as his father's surrogate. This is not just the fantasy that, as Watson notes of Fortinbras's quest, "the living child can repair the losses of the dead parent." Beyond that, the child comes to identify so completely with the dead parent—over-identify with the dead parent—that he loses all capacity for self-definition. Thus Hamlet's stirring proclamation, "this is I, Hamlet the Dane!" (5.1.257–58) (a naming that conflates or even confuses Hamlet with his dead father) is immediately followed by an even more powerful act of "sympathetic identification with a past life"—Hamlet's leaping into a grave—an act of identification that, as Watson argues, reveals itself as a kind of "demonic possession of the present."[29]

Hamlet thus attempts to remember/avenge his father by playing out in the scene of Ophelia's burial precisely what his father both did and failed to do while alive. Just as the dumb-show and play-within-the-play had earlier allegorized the major characters and events in the play (or in the backstory), so, jumping into the grave, Hamlet stands in for King Hamlet while the role of the brother who would steal or block a legitimate love-relationship, and substitute an incestuous one, is taken by Laertes, and the role of the beloved woman battled over by rivals is taken by Ophelia. (It is worth noting that in 5.2.244 Hamlet refers to Laertes as his "brother."[30]) Hamlet both identifies with his father and tries to correct his father's failings by asserting how his love for Ophelia surpasses that of Laertes and by attempting to back up that assertion by not allowing himself to be defeated by a mere brother (if, here, only by victory in an adolescent scuffle). Hamlet, in that sense, shows us just how haunted he is in this simultaneous act of identification and refusal of identification. In trying to live the life his father could not, Hamlet is, like his father, already in the grave.[31]

More broadly, the burial scene as a whole fixes our attention on one of the play's central preoccupations: how the issue of ceremony—what Greenblatt aptly terms "damaged rituals"—is linked to the vexed way in which a son needs to remember his father.[32] This arc is initiated in 1.2 by Hamlet's grisly joke that "the funeral bak'd meats / Did coldly furnish forth the marriage tables" (1.2.180–81), which not only suggests that we have entered into a world in which the living have not done their ceremonial duty to the dead but also may make us wonder, somewhat more fancifully, if perhaps the court dispensed with King Hamlet's funeral altogether. The conspicuously absent funeral with which, in a sense, the play symbolically begins is finally (re)staged in 5.1, King Hamlet and Ophelia sharing both suspect deaths and devalued ceremony.[33]

The play completes this arc in 5.2, which stages a symbolic recuperation of the proper burial lacking at the outset of the play:

> FORTINBRAS: Let four captains
> Bear Hamlet like a soldier to the stage,
> . . .
>   and for his passage
> The soldier's music and the rite of war
> Speak loudly for him.
> Take up the bodies. . . .
> . . .
> Go bid the soldiers shoot. (5.2.395–403)

What Fortinbras restores is precisely the concept of proper ceremony that was missing at the play's outset and that, as noted above, Shakespeare must have first noticed in his sources. But this restoration of proper ceremony in some ways merely continues the identification with his father that Hamlet is struggling to overcome. Hamlet is here identified precisely with his warrior-father to the extent that Fortinbras's eulogy seems more appropriate for the martial King Hamlet (precisely the figure that Shakespeare found in Saxo Grammaticus) than for the intellectual Prince Hamlet. And, once again, we don't actually see the funeral of a royal Hamlet: Prince Hamlet's funeral, Fortinbras notes, will take place offstage, on some "stage" toward which Fortinbras can only gesture.

But even as this ending asserts identification, it also refutes it. For the very context in which Hamlet's death appears to repeat his father's situation—the Norwegian Fortinbras's impending ascension to the throne of Denmark—has the effect of undoing his father's great legacy (King Hamlet's victory over Fortinbras the elder). Moreover, in his own death, Hamlet powerfully expresses hostility to his father in that the murder that is at the center of the play's action is, by the final scene, completely forgotten. This final rejection of (over)identification is part of what Watson means in arguing in relation to the burial scene of 5.1 that Hamlet's identification with his father "violat[es] a boundary between death and life that should be respected, for all our impulses to cross it."[34] The distinction, however, between the living and the dead (such as occurs at the funeral of a parent) is, in Shakespeare's presentation, also the occasion in which an even more foundational, and more problematic, boundary between one's own life and the life of another is made manifest. Hamlet must come to recognize, as does Gertrude, that the ghost of the dead father cannot be seen, cannot be heard, that in the wake of such a death there is "nothing but ourselves" (3.4.133). To discover this for himself (something he is not yet able to do even as late as 5.1), Hamlet must lose his father; indeed, he must, as we shall see, lose the very word "father."

V

To appreciate the full symbolic weight the play gives to this issue, I want to reconsider how the bold proclamation made at Ophelia's burial—"This is I, Hamlet the Dane!"—at once pulls together earlier passages and sets the conceptual stage for a transformative conceptual revision at play's end. Let us start by returning to Watson's observation that "This is I, Hamlet the Dane" is part of 5.1's broader representation of Hamlet's "sympathetic identification" with his father. In other words, Shakespeare seems to go out of his way here to raise a question in our minds: can the son distinguish himself from his father even at a moment that appears to mark emphatic self-assertion?

The ambiguity as to which Hamlet stands before us in 5.1 harkens back to a strange moment in 1.4. Unsure during his initial encounter just what the spectral apparition is, Hamlet yet decides to treat the "questionable shape" not just as an image of his dead father but as his actual father: "I'll call thee Hamlet, / King, father, royal Dane" (1.4.43–45). This proclamation, troubling given Hamlet's suspicions that the apparition may be a condemned spirit "bring[ing] . . . blasts from hell" (1.4.41), in turn looks back to that concluding repetition from Hamlet's initial exchange with Horatio:

> HORATIO: My lord, I think I saw him yesternight.
>
> HAMLET: Saw, who?
>
> HORATIO: My lord, the King your father.
>
> HAMLET: The King my father? (1.2.189–91)

Much more could, and should, be made of Hamlet's statement "I shall not look upon his like again" since Prince Hamlet, as son and namesake, is precisely *like* (if not identical to) King Hamlet. And indeed, this scene, and the play as a whole, is fascinated with the ways in which doubles of almost any kind may or may not be identical.[35] For my purposes here it suffices to note that the particular way of identifying Hamlet the elder (King/father) is repeated in line 191 and again in 1.4, this second time quite literally at the center of Hamlet's identification of the otherwise unintelligible apparition ("I'll call thee Hamlet, *King, father*, royal Dane"). Of course, the framing elements of the 1.4 identification—*I, Hamlet, Dane*—are precisely the elements that Prince Hamlet will employ for *self*-identification in 5.1: "This is *I, Hamlet* the *Dane*." The roles of king (the royal Dane) and father are thereby condensed into the name that Hamlet only appears to be claiming for himself. These roles, that is, along with the name of the nation that gives this king-father his primary authority, are precisely what young Hamlet collapses into a sympathetic identification that makes us wonder if he can truly answer the question with which Shakespeare chooses to begin this most maddening of plays: "Who's there?"

We should recognize, then, that the "I" in "This is I, Hamlet the Dane" is, at best, fluid. That this "I" refers not simply or exclusively to Prince Hamlet but is rather some uncanny intermingling of two identities is borne out by a strange aspect of the initial exchange between the Prince and the Ghost[36]:

> GHOST: Revenge his foul and most unnatural murder.
>
> HAMLET: Murder!
>
> GHOST: Murder most foul, as in the best it is,
> But this most foul, strange, and unnatural.
>
> HAMLET: Haste, haste me to know it, that with wings as swift
> As meditation or the thoughts of love
> May sweep to my revenge. (1.5.25–31)

Greenblatt astutely observes of the final three lines that, in "urgently demand[ing] the information that will enable him immediately to heed" the call for revenge, Hamlet expresses a "desire for haste . . . so intense that it erases the very person who does the desiring: the subject of the wish has literally vanished from the sentence."[37] That is, faced with the command of the dead father, the compulsion of filial duty is so powerful that it is grammatically registered in the very elision of the subject. This erasure of the "I," moreover, occurs not only in a context where vengeance comes to define and displace memory but also at a moment where Shakespeare again thematizes repetition ("murder / murder / murder"; "Revenge . . . revenge"). That erased "I" of 1.5 is, of course, what rematerializes in the assertion, "This is I, Hamlet the Dane!" But, as I have already argued, Hamlet's "I" in 5.1 appears not as self-assertion but rather as a kind of "demonic possession." The Ghost haunts him still.

It is all the more fascinating, then, when, given the opportunity both to identify and to identify with Hamlet the elder in the play's final scene, Prince Hamlet inexplicably does not employ the phrasing previously used to such powerful effect. Summarizing the events preceding the play for a bewildered Horatio, Hamlet says that Claudius "hath kill'd my king and whor'd my mother" (5.2.64). Conspicuously contrasted as it is with the reference to Gertrude as "my mother," the reference to Hamlet the elder as "my king" suggests that Hamlet is at last disentangling his identity from full paternal authority. It is crucial to note how different the 5.2 phrasing is from a very similar sentiment expressed in the previous act. There, as part of a soliloquy in which he berates himself for his inaction—and especially in contrast to the conduct of the faithful son, Fortinbras—Hamlet asks, "How stand I then, / *That have a father kill'd, a mother stain'd* . . ." (4.4.56–57; my emphasis). The most obvious difference, of course, is that, in the earlier passage, it is precisely the "father" and not the "king" who has been killed. More to the point, the earlier phrasing rather ambiguously suggests that Hamlet sees himself as his father's murderer ("I . . . that have a father kill'd"), whereas the 5.2 passage makes it clear that the murderer is Claudius. The 4.4 phrasing is consistent with Freud's statement in the draft of the 1897 letter that "one of the manifestations of grief is then to reproach oneself *for their death*"—that is, the child accepting both the responsibility and the "reproach" for killing the parents, however symbolically that is meant. Freud will become more explicit on this point in "Mourning and Melancholia," observing there that the "struggle of ambivalence" that is at the heart of melancholia manifests itself in the subject's "disparaging . . . , denigrating . . . , and even as it were *killing*" the lost love-object (XIV, 257; my emphasis). To the extent that, for Freud, this reproach manifests the repression that governs our attitudes toward deceased parents, Hamlet's self-liberation from that reproach in 5.2 (he clearly recognizes that it is Claudius who is responsible) suggests that he is also beyond what he has previously repressed: the hostility he has felt for his father. In asserting that

Claudius has killed his king rather than his father, Hamlet prepares us for the play's ending in which both the protagonist and the audience come to see that this story has from the start been about the necessity of leaving the father behind.

The play's drive toward this moment is powerfully marked in its fullest expression of tragic *anagnorisis*:

> HORATIO: If your mind dislike anything, obey it. I will forestall your repair hither, and say you are not fit.
>
> HAMLET: Not a whit, we defy augury. There is special providence in the fall of a sparrow. If it be now, 'tis not to come; if it be not to come, it will be now; if it be not now, yet it will come—the readiness is all. Since no man, of aught he leaves, knows what is't to leave betimes, let be. (5.2.217–24)

The rhetorical design of the passage forces us to conclude against our expectations that the "readiness" Hamlet's speaks of here refers to his own intimations of mortality rather than to his readiness to kill Claudius.[38] We are almost led to imagine that what he wants to "let be"—leave alone, untouched, unfulfilled—is precisely what we expect he should now, finally, be ready to do: avenge his father's murder. There is a paradox here. If, as Freud might have observed, Hamlet's suicidal drive for self-retribution was a way of identifying with the dead father (and so a way of repressing his hostility), at the very moment he registers just how close to death he is Hamlet completely forgets that his readiness should serve the first duty imposed upon him by the Ghost—*avenge* me.

This forgetting of the father's business is marked in the subtle deletion Shakespeare makes from the biblical source-text of this passage: "Are not two sparrows sold for a penny? Yet not one of them will fall to the ground apart from your father. And even the hairs of your head are all counted. So do not be afraid; you are of more value than many sparrows" (Matthew 10:26–31). Shakespeare here retains Matthew's core sentiment that every person, every moment, is uniquely special in the working out of God's inscrutable will. But even as this viewpoint depends on the comfort of faith in a beneficent God who loves us, Shakespeare chooses to leave out the very word Matthew employs to underwrite that faith: "father," or he in whose eyes and because of whom we have worth, even as his "providence" assigns us existence and a destiny. Without surrendering the notion that he might have a fate or destiny, Hamlet surrenders the presence of the father (whether divine or human) as the source and purpose of that destiny. Perhaps Hamlet just forgot to say "father," or perhaps Shakespeare just forgot to write it. But that sort of forgetting in which the father disappears can be read as a true remembering, the kind that permits a Hamlet or a Shakespeare or a Freud to move past the trauma of loss, to move from grief to mourning, from repetition to a memory, a process that makes the past past and keeps the dead where they belong.

VI

Ambivalence, resistance, resentment, and, at times, outright hostility move as powerful undercurrents in many of Freud's meditations on his father. Perhaps the most poignant of these occurs in the *Interpretation of Dreams*:

> At that point I was brought up against the event in my youth whose power was still being shown in all these emotions and dreams. I may have been ten or twelve years old, when my father began to take me with him on his walks and reveal to me in his talk his views upon things in the world we live in. Thus it was, on one such occasion, that he told me a story to show me how much better things were now than they had been in his days. "When I was a young man," he said, "I went for a walk one Saturday in the streets of your birthplace; I was well dressed, and had a new fur cap on my head. A Christian came up to me and with a single blow knocked off my cap into the mud and shouted, 'Jew! get off the pavement!'" "And what did you do," I asked. "I went into the roadway and picked up my cap," was his quiet reply. This struck me as unheroic conduct on the part of the big, strong man who was holding the little boy by the hand. I contrasted the situation with another which fitted my feelings better: the scene in which Hannibal's father, Hamilcar Barca [in the 1900 edition, Freud had written, "Hasdrubal," a point to which we shall return] made his boy swear before the household altar to take vengeance on the Romans. Ever since that time Hannibal had had a place in my phantasies. (IV, 197)

When he revisited this incident the following year in chapter 10 of the *Psychopathology of Everyday Life*, Freud noted almost in passing his youthful "phantasies of how different things would have been *if I had been born the son not of my father* but of my brother" (VI, 219–20; emphasis added).

The opening of that chapter deals in a very broad way with filial resentment toward the father (at least the lack of proper "filial piety" [VI, 220]). Freud describes, for example, the mythical incidents of Kronos and Zeus emasculating their respective fathers and afterward dethroning them (VI, 218 and 218n1). Freud there also reflects on "errors of memory" that—as in *Hamlet*—could just as easily be called, following Greenblatt, failing to remember "in the right way," or what Freud simply terms "remembering wrongly" (VI, 217). Furthermore, when Freud gives as a prime example of remembering wrongly the fact that in the *Interpretation of Dreams* he had mistakenly substituted Hannibal's brother's name (Hasdrubal) for Hannibal's father's name (Hamilcar), one might conclude that, for Freud as for Hamlet, remembering wrongly is inseparable from an ambivalence or hostility that is registered in the act of leaving out the father.

Freud had earlier noted that such errors of memory are "not the results of defective memory but displacements, symptoms" (*Origins*, 303), and these are "ultimately rooted in repressed material" (*Psychopathology of Everyday Life*, VI, 218).[39] In that sense, however, remembering wrongly might be understood as remembering correctly. Freud's own misremembering of the name of the father (remembering wrongly) may, in fact, be an example of *properly* remembering the dead, if proper remembrance, in the context of grief, is part of the process by which the grieving son distances himself from an over-idealized paternal figure. What Freud ventures in regard to his father's death—and what I am explicitly arguing in relation to *Hamlet*—is that the psychic distance gained by remembering rather than repeating helps the one grieving to address, if only half consciously, repressed hostility toward the deceased, hostility whose full motive force is coincident with the very tortured plot of Shakespeare's play.

That plot, as I have argued, anticipates Freud by staging the complex relation between memory and mourning. *Hamlet*, in a sense, ends by accepting the verdict of the gravedigger: both that the dead should be well buried and that a proper burial is inseparable from our ability to remember them, as the gravedigger can recall many things about those who have passed away and whose skulls he unearths. Watson's avowedly atheistic reading of *Hamlet* makes something of this same point in noting almost in passing that the play's "stage action reflects a psychological truth: that rising to the business of a new dawn means leaving behind . . . the memories of the dead."[40] Cavell develops this point in observing that the play finally marks "the work of mourning . . . [as] the severing of investment, the detaching of one's interests, strand by strand, memory by memory, from their binding with an object that has passed." Of course, as I have argued, the play's central psychological claim is precisely not that, in severing our investment in the dead, we should leave behind or unbind our memories of them, for it is only *through* memory that the dead can be left behind.[41]

There is thus a distinction to be made here between merely forgetting the dead and remembering them in the right way, a distinction that is powerfully on display at the close of *Hamlet*. Indeed, if, as I have suggested, the play's final scene marks how the father must be forgotten, it simultaneously aims to restore the father as memory and through memory. Thus, even as 5.2 twice "forgets" the father in the way I have already considered, in this same scene Hamlet invokes King Hamlet as his father one last time. Recounting his miraculous escape from his death sentence while in route to England, Hamlet tells Horatio, "I had my father's signet ring in my purse" (5.2.49). For all its importance as a marker of royal status, the father's ring is also a memento or keepsake. At play's end, then, the son's relationship to the deceased father is represented precisely as a thing to be remembered and not re-lived, an objectified memory, we might say, a memory that marks the past as distant and different from the son's present. This memento returns us to Hamlet's original conversation with Horatio in which, up until the moment when Horatio hints at the presence of the Ghost, Hamlet had viewed his father as a thing of the past ("*was* goodly king" / "*was* a man"). In those lines in 1.2 and now again in his recollection of the signet ring, Hamlet relates to his father as someone to be remembered and not repeated, a father who does not haunt the son.

What we witness between 1.2 and 5.2 is the son's psychic struggle. When the Ghost visits Hamlet for the second time, Hamlet's response acknowledges that he has failed to honor his promise to remember by obediently carrying out the command to revenge:

> Do you not come your tardy son to chide,
> That, laps'd in time and passion, lets go by
> Th' important acting of your dread command? (3.4.106–08)

There is, no doubt, self-reproach in Hamlet's rhetorical question. But there is also a note of defiance in the simple fact of a son's announcing that he has refused to submit to the duty to set right his father's life, a duty that would prevent the son from remembering his father by mourning him. This "tardy son," ever belated in relation to his father (the father *after* whom he was named), wants to rebel without ceasing to love. In 1896, when he came late to his father's funeral, Freud was also the tardy son, an act of defiance that yet made him feel like a tree "torn up by the roots." But the reason Freud came late to his father's funeral was because it was his time and no longer that of his father. His coming late—a belatedness that might have marked a submission to his father's priority—was yet the origin, the taking up the burden of existence and the origin of psychoanalysis. For in coming late to his father's funeral Freud had sought, like Hamlet, to father himself.

VII

We might get a clearer sense both of what self-fathering might have meant to Freud in 1900 and how he struggled to acknowledge his need for it by examining his pairing of two dreams from October 1898; following Freud's treatment of them in the *Interpretation of Dreams*, I will treat them as a single dream[42]:

> I had a very clear dream. I had gone to Brücke's laboratory at night, and, in response to a gentle knock on the door, I opened it to (the late) Professor Fleischl, who came in with a number of strangers and, after exchanging a few words, sat down at his table. This was followed by a second dream. My friend Fl. [Fliess] had come to Vienna unobtrusively in July. I met him in the street in conversation with my (deceased) friend P., and went with them to some place where they sat opposite each other as though they were at a small table. I sat in front at its narrow end. Fl. spoke about his sister and said that in three-quarters of an hour she was dead, and added some such words as 'that was the threshold.' As P. failed to understand him, Fl. turned to me and asked how much I had told P. about his affairs. Whereupon, overcome by strange emotions, I tried to explain to Fl. that P. (could not understand anything at all, of course, because he) was not alive. But what I actually said—and I myself noticed the mistake—was, 'NON VIXIT.' I then gave P. a piercing look. Under my gaze, he turned pale; his form grew indistinct and his eyes a sickly blue—and finally he melted away. I was highly delighted at this and I now realized that Ernst Fleischel, too, had been no more than an apparition, a 'revenant' [ghost—literally, one who returns]; and it seemed to me quite possible that people of that kind only existed as long as one liked and

could be got rid of if someone else wished it. (V, 421; original emphases deleted)

Although Freud will offer two separate, lengthy explications, he acknowledges that, out of deference to certain persons he "greatly value[s]," he must "content himself . . . with selecting only a few of [the dream's] elements for interpretation" (V, 422). But even as his explications reveal an almost chronic state of ambivalence toward friends and respected colleagues, his very selectivity seems to cover over the obvious fact that what he interprets as the dream's latent content is itself a screen for the subject he refuses to address, his much deeper and abiding ambivalence toward his father.[43]

Marthe Robert is no doubt correct in her assertion that the various named persons in the dream-work—Ernst Brücke, Ernst Fleischl von Marxow, Josef Paneth, and Wilhelm Fliess, friends and/or close professional colleagues of his early medical training—all function as father-substitutes.[44] Although he does make a passing reference to his father in each of his two explications, in neither does he use his father's name. More significantly as an instance of the very sort of screening mechanism he alludes to several times in his analysis, on both occasions he refers to Jacob Freud as his own nephew John's grandfather (on the second occasion he only subsequently clarifies that this person is therefore his own father [V, 424, 483–84]).[45] Even to the extent he acknowledges the friends and colleagues as substitutive figures, he explicitly states that these persons stand in for his nephew (V, 424–25, 483, 485–86), and he concludes that all the feelings of ambivalence experienced in the dream—"a convergence of a hostile and an affectionate current" (V, 423)—can be traced to this particular relationship. We shall have reason to revisit this particular misdirection, but for now we might simply note that when Freud says his relationship with John Freud that "had a determining influence on all [his] subsequent relations with contemporaries" (V, 424), we should suspect that he does protest too much. In short, he is doing everything he can to avoid acknowledging that the dream concerns his father and that, therefore, his own primary role in the dream's latent content is that of (ambivalent) son rather than of companionate uncle.

But Jacob Freud's centrality to the dream is marked in many other ways. For example, Freud portrays his relationship with John through the lens of a theatrical piece involving Julius Caesar and Brutus: "I was fourteen years old . . . and was acting with a nephew who was a year my senior" (V, 424); "my nephew himself re-appeared in my boyhood, and at that time we acted the parts of Caesar and Brutus" (V, 483). (It is clear that Freud, one year younger, took the part of Brutus [V, 424].⁴⁶) Although Freud was not performing the part from Shakespeare's *Julius Caesar*, the first reference to his acting with his nephew comes immediately after a citation from that play; Brutus is speaking: "As Caesar loved me, I weep for him; as he was fortunate, I rejoice at it; as he was valiant, I honor him; but, as he was ambitious, I slew him" (V, 424; *Julius Caesar* 3.2.24–27). Freud cites the line as a subtext of the dream precisely because of the way Shakespeare's Brutus's expression of ambivalence ("two opposite reactions towards a single person") serves as an analogy for his own feelings ("I had been playing the part of Brutus in the dream" [V, 424]). And while Freud does not mention Shakespeare's own speculation that Brutus was Caesar's son, when in his second explication he returns both to his Brutus-Caesar performance and to the lines from Shakespeare's play, he recollects another Shakespearean pairing in which the father-son tension is dramatically explicit: "Wherever there is rank and promotion the way lies open for wishes that call for suppression. Shakespeare's Prince Hal could not, even at his father's sick-bed, resist the temptation of trying on the crown [*2 Henry IV*, 4.5]. But, as was to be expected, the dream punished my friend, and not me, for this callous wish." Freud refuses to interpret his "callous wish" (for "rank and promotion") as anything other than his desire for advancement in Brücke's laboratory (V, 484). But it is precisely at this stage that Freud mentions the scene from *2 Henry IV*, and that play's depiction of a son's premature usurpation of his father's authority combined with the associative recollections of his playing the assassin Brutus to John's Caesar suggests that Freud's locating of a key element of the dream's latent content in his desire for "rank and promotion" is more properly analogical. In other words, the paired links to Shakespeare mark what Freud refuses to acknowledge: his filial drive to eliminate the father or at least to lay claim to his authority. Even as it is this figure whose precedence (both ontologically and temporally) stands in the way of the son's own ascension, the very fact that Freud shifts attention away from that relationship to the much less significant one with his nephew shows just how reluctant he is to address directly the real source of his ambivalence.

There are yet other ways in which the dream and its analysis call special attention to the very figure whom Freud so aggressively excludes. Deeply aware of the complex associative pattern involved in dream-making, Freud points to a Latin inscription on a memorial to the late Kaiser Josef in Vienna's Imperial Palace, a monument from which the dream draws some important details. The actual text of the memorial reads:

Saluti publicae vixit
non diu sed totus
[For the well-being of his people he lived not long but wholly].

But Freud (mis)quotes it as

Saluti patriae vixit
non diu sed totus
[For the well-being of his country he lived not long but wholly].

If both the Latin of the inscription and the imperial setting of the monument itself might reasonably be associated with Freud's recollection of his youthful Brutus-Caesar scene and, beyond that, to Shakespeare's *Julius Caesar*, it is noteworthy that Freud defines his native land, an empire ruled by a Kaiser/Caesar, not in terms of the people (*publica*) so much as in terms of the very place of the father (*patria*/*pater*). The misquotation reminds us once again that, Freud's explications notwithstanding, the "non vixit" dream memorializes precisely what it so conspicuously excludes, what has been passed down to him by his own (dead) father (*pater*/patrimony).[47]

We might go further down this interpretive path by linking the misquotation to another notable "mistake," though this one made in the dream itself and one that Freud actually registers there: "I tried to explain to Fl. that P. (could not understand anything at all, of course, because he) was not alive. But what I actually said—and I myself noticed the mistake—was, 'NON VIXIT.'" If, as Robert is no doubt correct to infer, Freud's substitution of *patriae* for *publicae* marks his unconscious effort "to bring back the father-phantom he had wanted to exorcise," we should also note that this restoration is marked with the very ambivalence that is so central to the dream as a whole.[48] Registering how, through the intermediary recollection of the Kaiser Josef monument, the phrase he should have said in the dream—"non vivit"—is replaced with "non vixit" (V, 421–22), Freud himself acknowledges that an expression of hostile affect here substitutes for a simple statement of fact: that is, "he is not alive" (whether applied to Kaiser Josef or, as in the dream's manifest content, to Josef Paneth) becomes a wish to utterly destroy ("get rid of," "annihilate," later "reduce to nothing") a person who, in an act of proper commemoration, should still have been accorded respect or even love. Freud's reconstruction shows, in other words, that the very monument he is creating to perpetuate the memory of his own Kaiser/Caesar is founded on the ambivalence that inheres in the "non vixit." Thus, he concludes, "hostile and distressing feelings—'overcome by strange emotions' were the words used in the dream itself—were piled up at the point at which I annihilated my opponent . . . with two words" (V, 480).

Just as important, in both explications the analysis of the "non vixit" substitution is linked to the use of the French *"revenant"* (ghost [V, 421, 480]), a word Freud will subsequently gloss as "those we have lost [who] come back" [V, 486] and whose resonances extend deep into the dream-analysis. As we have noted, Freud will assert that the ghost from the past now reincarnated in the figures in the dream and dream-thoughts is his nephew John. But John played Caesar (the father) to Freud's Brutus (the son), and as we recall that in Shakespeare's play Caesar's ghost (*revenant*) visits Brutus on the eve of the battle of Philippi (*Julius Caesar* 4.3) we might reasonably surmise that one *revenant*, John, is simply standing in for another one, Jacob.

Even if we dismissed as irrelevant to Freud's dream-thoughts Shakespeare's own belief that Caesar was Brutus's father, the complex nephew-father-son dynamic Freud constructs calls attention to the triangulated relationships at the heart of the Shakespearean play that follows, *Hamlet*. In that play, of course, the *revenant* as the one who comes back is most definitely the father. Moreover, unlike in *Julius Caesar*, in *Hamlet* the son's relation to the ghost-father is defined explicitly in the context of mourning and proper commemoration, and this subtext leads us to understand why in the "non vixit" dream the sense of something coming back is strongly associated with various acts of memorialization for people who have died (but John Freud was still alive in 1900). In short, the ghost as the one who comes back through the ambivalence-laden monument that is the "non vixit" dream and indeed the *Interpretation of Dreams* as a whole is undoubtedly the person who *can* come back from the dead some four years later, the person Freud was still struggling to mourn properly: his father. It is in response to the death of this figure that the son—Hamlet or Freud—is "overcome by strange emotions." The contradictory nature of these emotions (variously hostility, distress, anxiety, anger, self-reproach, satisfaction) is aptly understood through Freud's notion of ambivalence.

To the extent ambivalence itself comes back into Freud's thought along with the (dead) father, we might say that the "non vixit" dream symbolically reenacts his initial memorial to Jacob Freud, the 1896 dream on the night after his father's funeral. The 1898 dream(s) as well as what Freud calls its "exciting cause" (V, 480) are, of course, also heavily entangled in the work of mourning. The reference to "my friend Fl." (Fliess) who in the dream spoke about his own dead sister marks Freud's concern about Fliess's own failing health.[49] Freud's anticipation of his own mourning for Fliess is linked generally to others mentioned in the dream: by the time of the dream Brücke, Fleischl, and Paneth had all already died, and even inside the dream Freud is strangely aware of his "dealings with people who were dead" (V, 422). But Freud is even more concerned with how recognition of the dead might be ritually expressed and how one personally experiences the loss of another, issues, we might also observe, that link the dream directly to *Hamlet* through the play's own interests in both mourning and the ceremony of funeral rites. Immediately after his mention of the Kaiser Josef monument, Freud writes that "this train of ideas . . . reminded me that I had the dream only a few days after the unveiling of the memorial to Fleischl in the cloisters of the University. At that time I had seen the Brücke memorial once again and must have reflected . . . with regret on the fact that the premature death of my brilliant friend P. . . . had robbed him of a well-merited claim to a memorial in these same precincts. Accordingly, I gave him this memorial in my dream" (V, 423). And in his second explication, Freud recollects that

> at my friend's [P's] funeral, a young man had made what seemed to be an inopportune remark to the effect that the speaker who had just delivered the funeral oration had implied that without this one man the world would come to an end. He was expressing the honest feelings of someone whose pain was being interfered with by an exaggeration. But this remark of his was the starting-point of the following dream-thoughts: 'It is quite true that no one is irreplaceable. How many people I've followed to the grave already! But I'm still alive. I've survived them all; I'm left in possession of the field.' A thought of this kind, occurring to me at a moment at which I was afraid I might not find my friend [Fl.] alive if I made the journey to him, could only be construed as meaning that I was delighted because I had once more survived someone, because it was he and not I who had died, because I was left in possession of the field . . . This satisfaction, infantile in origin, at being in possession of the field constituted the major part of the affect that appeared in the dream. (V, 485)

In part because this latter reflection comes right after the reference to Prince Hal's taking of his father's crown—and Hal, we should note, similarly muses on the nature of his own impending mourning (*2 Henry IV* 4.5.20–47)—we are surely right to associate Freud's reflections on his feelings for Fliess as repeating something of his response to Jacob Freud's death. In 1896, he had followed his father to the grave but only to bury him, not to die himself; he was still alive and, like Prince Hal (soon to be Henry V), was now in "possession of the field" once possessed by his father. Perhaps most crucially, just as they had been for his father, his feelings for Fliess are nothing if not ambivalent: he is afraid Fliess might die, but he knows he will take satisfaction, delight even, in his own survival.

That said, if this feeling of ambivalence generally connects the experience of mourning in the dream to his father's death almost exactly two years earlier, the "non vixit" dream returns to that ambivalence precisely through the repetition of several critical details of the 1896 dream. For example, even as proper commemoration of—a doing of one's duty toward—the dead and thus the nature of mourning itself are key concepts in both dreams (as also in *Hamlet*), the particular expression of Freud's concern with mourning and commemoration hinges on his tardiness. As we saw earlier, he feels both reproaches from others and self-reproach on account of his arriving late to his father's funeral: "On the day of the funeral I . . . arrived at the house of mourning rather late. The family . . . took my lateness in rather bad part." And the consequences of late arrival clearly play a similarly crucial role in the "non vixit" dream.

Thus, Freud offers two different descriptions to cover over some of the real backstory underlying the dream and how that reality figures both into the dream and into his own final interpretation:

> The central feature of the dream was a scene in which I annihilated P. with a look. His eyes changed to a strange and uncanny blue and he melted away. This scene was unmistakably copied from one which I had actually experienced. At the time I have in mind I had been a demonstrator at the Physiological Institute and was due to start work in the morning. It came to Brücke's ears that I sometimes reached the students' laboratory late. One morning he turned up punctually at the hour of opening and awaited my arrival. His words were brief and to the point. But it was not they that mattered. What overwhelmed me were the terrible blue eyes with which he looked at me and by which I was reduced to nothing—just as P. was in the dream, where, to my relief, the roles were reversed. No one who can remember the great man's eyes, which retained their striking beauty even

in his old age, and who has ever seen him in anger, will find it difficult to picture the young sinner's emotions. (V, 422)

***

The dream-thoughts informed me that I feared for my friend's [Fliess'] life. . . . (In the dream Fl. spoke about his sister and said that in three-quarters of an hour she was dead.) I must have imagined that his constitution was not much more resistant than his sister's and that, after getting some much worse news of him, I should make the journey after all—and arrive too late, for which I might never cease to reproach myself. This reproach for coming too late became the central point of the dream but was represented by a scene in which Brücke, the honored teacher of my student years, levelled this reproach at me with a terrible look from his blue eyes. It will soon appear what it was that caused the situation [in regard to Fl.] to be switched to these lines. The scene [with Brücke] itself could not be reproduced by the dream in the form in which I experienced it. The other figure in the dream was allowed to keep the blue eyes, but the annihilating role was allotted to me . . . My anxiety about my friend's recovery, my self-reproaches for not going to see him, the shame I felt about this[,] . . . the need I felt to consider I was excused by my illness—all this combined to produce the emotional storm which was clearly perceived in my sleep and which raged in this region of the dream-thoughts. (V, 481)

Virtually everything in the dream and/or the dream-thoughts described here points back to Freud's dream on the night after his father's funeral. Indeed, his own observation that "reproach for coming too late became the central point of the ['non vixit'] dream"—he will make this point again two paragraphs later: "the reproach against me for coming too late" (482)—should have alerted Freud to how the later dream revisited the earlier one.[50] In the first place, the "non vixit" dream places the causal relation between coming late and reproach in a chain of associations that links a scene of mourning to the authority of an older man who chastises Freud for shirking his duty. Second, Freud's citing of Brücke's "terrible . . . eyes" as the key symbol of reproach (and thus also of his own acknowledgement that he had failed to perform his job properly) recalls the shop-notice from the 1896 dream:

I found myself in a shop where there was a notice up saying:

> You are requested
> to close your eyes. . . .

The phrase on the notice-board has a double meaning. It means "one should do one's duty toward the dead" in two senses—an apology, as though I had not done my duty and my conduct needed overlooking, and the actual duty itself.⁵¹

But Freud all too conspicuously does not draw the connection between the earlier and later dreams and so closes his eyes in a different sense: he refuses to see that what haunted the "non vixit" dream—its "apparition" or *"revenant"*—was Jacob Freud himself. In short, Freud effectively refuses to trace back to its origin and so to understand how and why the 1896 dream comes back in the "non vixit" dream's combination of two powerful, guilt-laden experiences: the earlier one, with his mentor (old man) Brücke's "terrible blue eyes" reproaching Freud for arriving late for work; the latter one, his inexplicable refusal to go see his ailing friend Fliess and his sense that, should he "arrive *too late*" at the place of death, he would "never cease to reproach [him]self." Anticipating his mourning for Fliess, Freud might have returned to the unfinished business of 1896. Indeed, the "emotional storm" that he tells us "raged" in the "non vixit" dream might have prompted him to reflect on an earlier feeling about a death that had left him "torn up by the roots." But, for now, Freud will not or simply cannot grasp that connection consciously.

If the "non vixit" dream as analyzed in 1900 effectively marks Freud's refusal to fully acknowledge his father's ghost, it is no doubt because he was still uncertain about the feelings set loose by Jacob Freud's death four years earlier. At the end of his original analysis of 1896 dream, Freud had concluded that "the dream was . . . an outlet for the feeling of self-reproach which a death generally leaves among the survivors." But if such self-reproach might arise because survivors shirked their duty toward the dead by failing to mourn properly, it also masks, even as it reveals, other feelings.

Thus, as we have saw earlier, in "Remembering, Repeating, and Working-Through" and, in more developed form, in "Mourning and Melancholia," Freud would come to understand how self-reproach in the face of the loss of a loved one functions as a way of denying the ambivalence felt for that person (especially, for Freud, where the context is a son's loss of his cherished father). If love, respect, admiration, and identification sit on one side of that feeling, defiance, hostility, and even hatred sit on the other. Thus it is that, even in the "non vixit" dream, the feeling of being "reduced to nothing" by the force of Brücke's "terrible blue eyes with which he looked at me" is turned around to express the opposite, Freud's own power and superiority over others. He explicitly notes that, with regard to the withering power of the old man's gaze, in the dream itself "the roles were reversed" (that is, it was Freud who "annihilated P. with a look" [V, 422]). Later, he writes that "the other figure in the dream [P.] was allowed to keep the blue eyes [which in reality had belonged to fatherly Brücke], but the annihilating role was allotted to me" (V, 481). And this is Freud's full recounting of the situation from the dream itself: "I then gave P. a piercing look. Under my gaze he turned pale; his form grew indistinct and his eyes a sickly blue—and finally he melted away. I was highly delighted at this . . . and it seemed to be quite possible that people of that kind only existed as long as one liked and could be got rid of if someone else wished it." In sum, if in 1896 closing one's eyes had symbolized Freud's guilt in the face of the father's imagined chastisement for failing to mourn properly, the reversal in the 1898 dream (the son now keeps his eyes open) grants to Freud the power to cause death, to render others "non vivit" ("he is not alive") or even worse "non vixit" ("he did not live"). The failure to do one's duty to the dead (to build a proper memorial) thereby appears less an act for which Freud might deserve censure and more a form of self-assertion, the claim to the power to annihilate anyone who would dare reduce him to nothing.

But what would Freud's own fear of being reduced to nothing mean in the context of mourning a ghost, a father already four years dead? We might find a hint of an answer in an observation he makes almost in passing about his youthful rivalry with his companion-nephew. Freud's formulation of the focus of that rivalry—at least the specific reason provided for why he and John "came to blows" at one point—is instructive: "Each of [us] claimed to have *got there before the other*" (V, 483; emphasis in original). If throughout the account of the "non vixit" dream John is always a substitute for Jacob, the fight to claim precedence—to get there *before* the other—points to Freud's desperate attempt to precede his true *revenant*, his father, the lost one who keeps coming back. He is the figure about whom it could be reasonably said that he was the "determining influence on all [his] subsequent relations with contemporaries." And so the figure who got there before Freud (and precisely for that reason can keep coming back to determine his relations with others) is the one who in his role as a father can reduce a son to nothing. Unless, of course, as Freud dreams in fantasy, the roles might be reversed. Freud writes of his conflict with John, "from this point the dream-thoughts proceeded along some such line as these: 'It serves you right if you had to make way for me. Why did you try to push *me* out of the way? I don't need you" (V, 484). Of course, in the crisis of belatedness that is at the heart of filial ambivalence, not needing this "you" means not needing the father or perhaps even doing away with the need for any father. Then, the son might truly be able to say "non vivit," or even more radically, "non vixit": he did not live. And to come before the father would thus also mean that the son could not have arrived too late.

All this Freud sees and doesn't see in 1900, for he both opens his eyes and closes them. Even four years after his father's death, he is not ready to complete Hamlet's task: to distance himself from his father by mourning instead of identifying with his father in melancholy. In other words, he has not yet reached the stage where he can overcome his ambivalence. In fact, he will not succeed in this task until, like Hamlet, he is about to die. With the publication of the full text of *Moses and Monotheism*, which will take place in the year of his death (1939) and which itself, perhaps not coincidentally, will take place in Shakespeare's own *patria*, Freud will, because he must, find a way to claim his life as his own, something other than what was bequeathed to him by his father, something other than a mere patrimony.

Toward the close of *Moses and Monotheism*, Freud will reflect that his account of Moses, the figure he considers the great father of the Jews and thus the father of Jewish sons like Freud himself, had "haunted him like an unlaid ghost" (*Moses and Monotheism*, 132). Freud's story of Moses (the subject of chapter 6) will thus also trace out Freud's account of no longer being haunted. And to the extent his completion of the book ended this haunting, it also permitted him to annihilate the opponent who had always filled him with strange emotions. But this opponent is not Moses himself so much as the father-imago that continued to live in Moses. In short, the *revenant* of *Moses and Monotheism* is not Moses but Jacob Freud, the figure that had haunted Freud, the figure who had died in 1896 and then kept coming back. Of the "father imago," Freud writes in 1939 that "longing for the father . . . lives in each of us from his childhood days," but he adds immediately that in legend this is "the same father whom the hero . . . boasts of having overcome" (*Moses and Monotheism*, 140). And the hero of *Moses and Monotheism*, also, paradoxically, represented in Moses, is thus the son who could overcome the father. As the conclusion and culmination of his career, becoming the hero of his own life by overcoming the very father he longed for was what finally was at stake in

Moses and Monotheism. In short, his last major work shows what it meant for Freud to work through and finally, like Hamlet, to father himself. But before we turn to that text we must further consider Freud's theorization of filial ambivalence and his continuing attempts to evade its true psychical origins in the problem of the origin itself. Chapter 4 will take up these issues primarily in relation to his 1919 essay, "The Uncanny."

Afterword

Against what he calls "the bafflement of psychoanalytic interpretation" before the complexities of early-modern notions of identity, Greenblatt champions an historically inflected critical practice that, at its best, evokes a "disconcerting recognition" that the force of the past "lies not in an absolute otherness that compels us to suspend all our values in the face of an entirely different system of consciousness, but rather in the intimations of an obscure link between those distant events and the way we are." He thus insists that a conceptually productive application of psychoanalysis to a text like *Hamlet* requires that psychoanalysis's own historical situatedness be taken into account.[52]

I shall return in a moment to reconsider Greenblatt's particular understanding of the dialogic possibilities between early-modern and psychoanalytic notions of identity. But I will note here that, while they do not always conform to Greenblatt's own strictures, scholars of early-modernity whose work is informed by psychoanalysis have made a variety of efforts to return Freudian and post-Freudian theory and practice to history. Reflecting on psychoanalytic responses to *Hamlet*, for example, Julia Reinhard Lupton and Kenneth Reinhard aptly remark that the "reductive allegoresis" typically associated with strict Oedipal readings has in large measure given way to an understanding of the central role that mourning serves in the play. They note, moreover, that the "mournful Hamlet is already at play throughout Freud's texts," a recognition paired with the historically minded observation that "Freud's autobiographically enunciated theories of the Oedipus complex and mourning" are tied together "within a legacy of melancholic self-reflection."[53]

That said, while my general argument is in obvious accord with the notion that we are dealing here with "a legacy of melancholic self-reflection," I do not accept Lupton and Reinhard's critical assumption that the Oedipus complex is central to what mourning entails. For even to extent they register how mourning involves antagonism toward the deceased (the son's toward the dead father in case of both Hamlet and Freud), they are, in my view, too accepting of Freud's own verdict: that the son's antagonism derives from his *sexual* rivalry with the father. Historicizing the trajectory of Freud's thought in a different way, I would like to venture against this understanding that Freud's move toward his Oedipal theory (on display as early as 1897 and firmly in place by 1900) was, in effect, his attempt to *explain* the ambivalence he felt toward his father as registered in the 1896 letter to Fliess.[54] But even accepting that antagonism or, more accurately, ambivalence toward the dead is a very real part of mourning, is the Oedipus complex a sound explanation of the motive force of such ambivalence? Or is it possible that the Oedipal theory actually represents Freud's swerving away from, even a disavowal of, what his ambivalence meant? More generally, what is the precise psychical situation in response to which ambivalence toward the dead forms as a symptom?[55]

Although he also relies overmuch on the notion of Oedipal opposition, Cavell's reading of *Hamlet* envisions an alternative explanation for Hamlet's ambivalent response to his father's death. When at the close of "Mourning and Melancholia" he discusses what it means for the ego to sever its "attachment to the lost object," Freud observes that "mourning impels the ego to give up the object by declaring the object to be dead and *offering the ego the inducement of continuing to live*" (XIV, 257; my emphasis). Cavell at once echoes and builds on Freud's claim in arguing that the "condition of this work [of mourning] is that you want to live." Or, as he later ventures, mourning entails finally the "burden of proving that [one] exists . . . finding how to say, 'I am, I exist'; not . . . to say it just once, but at every moment of your existence; to preserve your existence, *to originate it*."[56] Following Cavell, I would like to suggest that, by explaining filial ambivalence in terms of Oedipal hostility, Freud lost contact with his own deepest intuition: that something primal in the constitution of identity—something more primal even than sexual rivalry—is at stake when the son confronts what Freud called "the most poignant loss of a man's life," the death of his father. In melancholy, in short, the son "cannot consciously perceive what he has lost" in his father because, torn up by the roots as he is, the son is confused precisely about where his origin truly lies.

The experience of the tardy son, Hamlet, is reenacted in 1896 in the experience of the grieving son who arrived late. Such tardiness is not simply descriptive of the son's perception of one moment in time (Hamlet's in relation to the command to vengeance or Freud's in relation to his father's funeral). Rather, filial tardiness speaks to a temporal priority (the father's) that is also an ontological priority. Or, to look at this notion from the opposite point of view, the son's tardiness speaks to an existential belatedness that forces him to confront his father's identity in him. In the context of mourning for his father, then, the grieving son must stake a claim to an identity in relation to a father whose life the son is otherwise doomed to repeat.

Greenblatt argues that the psychoanalytically conceived notion of selfhood is itself historically constituted in the early-modern period: "it is only when proprietary rights to the self have been secured—rights made most visible . . . in moments of self-estrangement or external threat—that the subject of psychoanalysis, both its methods and the materials upon which it operates, is made possible."[57] It is also conceivable, then, that in creating the discursive possibility of "proprietary rights to the self" the early-modern period simultaneously created an anxiety that the self might not truly own its own origin. If prior to the emergence of such proprietary rights Western European religious discourse made it virtually impossible to register this sort of anxiety, surely the weakening or at least the transformation of religious claims (theological, ethical, ecclesiastical) at once permitted and compelled a novel nonreligious discourse of selfhood that made the problems of the self's origin visible for the first time.[58] Moreover, if the early-modern subject encountered itself (or its self) in the radically new experience of what Greenblatt terms "inalienable self-possession," precisely where did the self originate if not in God? Greenblatt argues that the early-modern period articulated a new discourse of "identity *as* property," where "the crucial consideration is ownership."[59] To own is one sort of act; to be one's own more complex still: "nothing but ourselves" as the undervalued Gertrude puts it. How did we get there to begin with?

In *Love and its Place in Nature*, Jonathan Lear notes that "psychic health, Freud discovered, depends on abandoning the fantasy that one can be one's own child"; psychoanalytically speaking, that is, the most difficult recognition is precisely that we are not our own point of origin.[60] Hamlet almost casually articulates the play's broader anxiety in this matter when he laments that while "in their birth . . . they are not guilty" yet "since *Nature cannot choose his origin*" men still "take corruption" (1.4.25–26, 35; my emphasis). Tinged with the Augustinian melancholy of original sin, Hamlet's strange reflection here seems poised on the edge of modern existential angst. For the full weight of this "corruption" is not the mere fact of birth but the possessing or being possessed by an origin we did not choose for ourselves. Yet, as the experiences of both Hamlet and Freud bear out, mourning appears to demand precisely that we create the fantasy that identity can be bounded off, that we are self-possessed to the point of being able to claim that we are our own point of origin. Thus Cavell finds both in *Hamlet* and in Freud (is this *Hamlet* read through Freud or Freud through *Hamlet*?) the lesson that in mourning we "find . . . how to say, 'I am, I exist'; . . . to preserve . . . existence, to originate it." When at play's end Hamlet asks Horatio to tell his story—and *not* the story of his murdered father—we recognize that the son has taken up the burden: he wants to preserve *his* existence (if perhaps only as a memory or as a story), to be the author of his own life. At the end, Hamlet finally realizes that his dramatic existence has been encompassed by the "tragedy of Hamlet," the Prince, not the King, of Denmark.

If Greenblatt is right to argue that the early-modern period invented the notion that, in some mysterious way, we own our identities, then it might be that the Freudian subject of mourning takes its cue from Hamlet's powerful vision of what it means to be one's own even where Freud himself explained away mourning's existential longing in a sexual rivalry he then "discovered" in *Hamlet*. Greenblatt refers to Freud's sense of "primary creatural individuation" as more burden than blessing, "the tragic inescapability of continuous selfhood."[61] The paradox of *Hamlet* is that its protagonist's full recognition of this selfhood comes only at the moment of tragic *anagnorisis*: he can only lay claim to his origin when he reaches his end.

If as tardy sons Hamlet and Freud both assert a claim to self-ownership, Freud will subsequently fail to register how another such son is ultimately defeated by a paternal authority and priority he can never overcome. Composed in between "Remembering, Repeating, and Working-Through" and *Beyond the Pleasure Principle*, Freud's "The Uncanny" attempts to reconstruct E. T. A. Hoffmann's story "The Sandman" so as to argue that Hoffmann's protagonist Nathanael's sense of impoverishment in relation to multiple father-figures is merely an expression of his castration anxiety. Freud, in short, reads Hoffmann's story as a manifestation of filial ambivalence as it is embedded within and metonymically representative of the full Oedipal economy. But rereading Freud's essay in conjunction both with Hoffmann's full narrative (much of which Freud ignores) and with the essay that first gave rise to Freud's speculations (Ernst Jentsch's "On the Psychology of the Uncanny"), we will see more clearly in chapter 4 that as an expression of the uncanny Hoffmann's Nathanael struggles to come to terms with an origin that always lies elsewhere, in an act of fathering from which he is necessarily if impossibly absent. The act that concludes Hoffmann's story, Nathanael's suicide, is thus completely unlike Hamlet's death in that Hoffmann there represents the fully disabling effects of the ego's impoverishment as that is best understood as a symptom of the traumatic encounter with belatedness.

And if Hoffman and Jentsch in certain key ways anticipate Freud's grappling with these issues, like Shakespeare in *Hamlet* they also offer anticipatory corrections to what Freud refused to see: that the feeling of the uncanny lies not in castration anxiety experienced as the return of the repressed but in an experience of existential anxiety in the face of the Emersonian Fall, a discovery "too late to be helped" that is, at the same time, a recognition of what is means to always already come too late.

4

The Afterwards of the Uncanny

> For Man to tell how human Life began
> Is hard: for who himself beginning knew?
>
> —Milton, *Paradise Lost*

I

As we observed in the study's introduction, his 1918 case-history of the Wolf Man is the text in which Freud first fully described his concept of the primal scene. Reflecting on that concept toward the end of the piece, Freud includes the following as part of a long footnote:

> I admit that this is the most delicate question in the whole domain of psycho-analysis. I did not require the contributions of Adler and Jung to induce me to consider the matter with a critical eye, and to bear in mind the possibility that what analysis puts forward as being forgotten experiences of childhood (and of an improbably early childhood) may on the contrary be based upon phantasies created on occasions occurring late in life. . . . On the contrary, no doubt has troubled me more; no other uncertainty has been more decisive in holding me back from publishing my conclusions. I was the first—a point to which none of my opponents have referred—to recognize both the part played by phantasies in symptom-formation and also the "retrospective phantasying" of late impressions into childhood and their sexualization after the event. (XVII, 103n1)

Elsewhere, Freud claimed to have completed the case-history by November 1914, but even if this is true one must ask why he chose to delay publication. Or, conversely, we might speculate on the later developments in his thought that might have prompted him to return to work that for whatever reason he had set aside. Reading the footnote in relation to Freud's "The Uncanny" (1919) and, to a lesser degree, *Beyond the Pleasure Principle* (1920), Neil Hertz has argued that in the footnote "Freud again is engaged with questions of origins and their subsequent rehearsals."[1] As Hertz observes, moreover, these questions are bound up with concerns over priority and originality (e.g., "*I was the first* . . . to recognize"), concerns that, set in the context of his rivalry with Adler and Jung, suggest how much Freud's professional interests were intertwined with vexed personal ones.

We might extend Hertz's suggestion to note more broadly that his phrase "subsequent rehearsals" should be taken to include the many ways in which, within psychoanalytic interpretation, later moments in our experience are understood not just as deriving from but also, in some inexplicable way, as pathologically drawn back to earlier ones (the "origins"), whether those earlier moments actually happened or are rather the product of what Freud here calls "retrospective phantasying." However that looking back is to be conceptualized (and, among other possibilities, we might include the notions of repetition compulsion, *Nachträglichkeit* or deferred action, and the return of the repressed), Freud imagines a sequence unfolding in time in which the impact of an original event is deferred and, only thereafter, experienced backwards (for example, as something repeated). Read in relation to the sequence of writings that includes "The Uncanny" and *Beyond the Pleasure Principle* (where the concept of repetition-compulsion is fully articulated), the 1918 footnote and indeed the whole of the case-history can be seen as caught up in Freud's evolving concern with how the past is problematically retrieved in the present, in the anxiety over what it means to come before or after (and thus including questions of origins, originality, and priority), and in the struggle to distinguish actual experiences from what is imagined after-the-fact.

While it is not clear that he is endorsing this concept, it is yet worth noting that Hertz places all of these issues under the broader heading of "Freud's Oedipal model."[2] We should give some special consideration to that phrase because in the 1918 footnote Freud reluctantly acknowledges that the "sexualization" that appears so central to "symptom-formation" might itself come late(r) and thus not belong to the original experience. In other words, the sexual motive that is so fundamental to his theorizing (and opposed, of course, by both Adler and Jung) might have very little to do with "the experiences of childhood" and mark instead what is imposed upon those experiences only belatedly. And does this retrospective imposition of the sexual belong only to the patient or is Freud here calling into question the work of the analyst as well? In other words, is Freud expressing a concern that the sexualization of the experiences of childhood may simply be part of psychoanalytic discourse and thus a perspective produced and imposed "after the event" on something that may not have happened in the patient's life at all?

We might go even further here. Hertz is certainly correct that the footnote powerfully expresses Freud's anxiety over priority and originality in the context of a deepening rivalry with his two former disciples (we might almost think of Adler and Jung as unruly sons). And, as I have been suggesting throughout this study, we might speculate that the Freudian inclination to sexualize psychical experience (the "Oedipal model" itself) actually serves to displace or even deny an intense preoccupation with those other concerns, which, though still grounded in some filial-paternal conflict, could conceivably derive from another motive-force entirely.[3] Might it be then that Freud retrospectively imposes a sexual meaning upon a patient's past experience to explain or even explain away the more intractable problem of what priority and originality mean within human relationships? We might wonder, in short, if Freud's footnote unwittingly calls attention to how the obsessive need to look back, to refer the present to the past (for Freud, at least, especially within the context of the father-son relationship), marks the human psyche's even more primal struggle with what it means to come after.

What the remainder of this chapter will explore is how, in dialogue with his own conceptual precursors on the topic, E. T. A. Hoffmann and Ernst Jentsch, and despite his efforts to offer a sexualized account, Freud will most provocatively if unintentionally locate the uncanny in the vexed experience of having an origin in relation to which one is always and necessarily belated. Especially pronounced for Freud in the son's ambivalent relationship to his father, this experience is registered, as we shall see, in the obsessive revisiting of the past that is itself marked simultaneously by a desire to know, a revulsion at knowing, and the impossibility of knowledge. Admittedly trying to use Freud's own ruminations to articulate a meaning of the uncanny that he would have rejected, I offer what follows as a way of addressing the question that Derrida, in the passage I use as the second epigraph of my study's introduction, sees as already marked by belatedness ("it is *too late* to deny"), "what happens . . . when a son is *after* his father?"

II

The most well-known part of Freud's reading of the uncanny deals with Hoffmann's 1816 short story "The Sandman," which we will look at in detail in section III. Freud's interest in this story was no doubt prompted by Jentsch's passing reference to Hoffmann's writings in his 1906 essay, "On the Psychology of the Uncanny," an essay Freud cites and that itself must have spurred his initial attention to the psychological aspects of the broader topic. Freud famously dismisses Jentsch's interpretation, suggesting that Jentsch's primary locating of the uncanny in "intellectual uncertainty" misstates its true cause, at least in terms of its application to Hoffmann's story:

> Jentsch writes: "In telling a story, one of the most successful devices for easily creating uncanny effects is to leave the reader in uncertainty whether a particular figure in the story is a human being or an automaton, and to do it in such a way that his attention is not focused directly upon his uncertainty, so that he may not be led to go into the matter and clear it up immediately" [Jentsch, "On the Psychology of the Uncanny," 13]. . . . This observation . . . refers primarily to the story of "The Sand-Man" in Hoffmann's *Nachstücken*, which contains the origins of Olimpia, the doll . . . But I cannot think—and I hope most readers of the story will agree with me—that the theme of the doll Olimpia, who is to all appearances a living being, is by any means the only, or indeed the most important, element that must be held responsible for the quite unparalleled atmosphere of uncanniness evoked by the story.
>
> ***
>
> There is no question . . . of any intellectual uncertainty [in Hoffmann's story] . . . The theory of intellectual uncertainty is thus incapable of explaining that impression. (XVII, 227; 230–31)[4]

Freud is playing a bit loose here in that Jentsch's brief mention of Hoffmann (he never even explicitly references "The Sandman") and even his broader interest in the confusion as to whether a figure is "a human being or an automaton" are only parts of his "*theory* of intellectual uncertainty" as that idea shapes his understanding of the uncanny. And Freud will later complicate matters even more in asking, though without recalling Jentsch, whether "we are after all justified in entirely ignoring intellectual uncertainty as a factor" in the evocation of uncanny feelings (XVII, 247).[5] But at the point in the argument where he is explicitly addressing Jentsch's essay, Freud makes an extended reference to Hoffmann's story in which he substitutes for Jentsch's intellectual uncertainty Hoffmann's "theme of the 'Sand-Man' who tears out children's eyes" (227); at least in the context of "The Sandman," it is this "theme" (in the figure of the Sandman) to which, according to Freud, "the feeling of something uncanny is directly attached" (230; ". . . daß das Gefühl des Unheimlichen direkt an der Gestalt des Sandmannes . . . haftet" [*Gesammelte Werke*, XII, 242]). "*Directly* attached" is somewhat misleading in that "the idea of being robbed of one's eyes" is itself a replacement based on the "substitutive relation between the eye and the male organ"; hence, what is really at stake in the uncanny, at least as Freud reads Hoffmann's story, is not the fear caused by intellectual uncertainty about a figure's status as animated or lifeless but rather "the dread of being castrated" (231), which in its deferred form—via the return of the repressed—becomes the chief instance and a synecdochic emblem of Freud's new interpretation.

We might observe here that the main reason Freud needs to reject Jentsch's notion of intellectual uncertainty is that, psychically speaking, repressed material is *not* uncertain. It is, rather, psychically forgotten or lost sight of. Or, we might say, it is because this material is all too certain—too close, too familiar—that the mind must hide it away in the unconscious as what cannot be faced. Thus, clarifying his earlier remark, Freud will state that "the uncanny is something which is *secretly familiar*, which has undergone repression and then returned from it" (XVII, 245).[6] Still, by dismissing Jentsch's reading so quickly, Freud not only avoids any real confrontation with the idea that doubt as to whether a figure is alive or not is central to the experience of the uncanny but also misses the opportunity to explore the relation of that idea to his own notion that the uncanny is primarily enacted through the recurrence of the secretly familiar.

Those remarks require some qualification. Although he does rightly observe Jentsch's interest in automata as a prime example of how the uncanny is grounded in uncertainty over a figure's status (alive or lifeless), Freud misses Jentsch's broader point: the deeper, more troubling questions as to what actually constitutes aliveness, how we respond to our own confusion regarding that issue, and, even for something that is unquestionably alive, what it means to be externally determined (by natural laws, or by something or someone else) as opposed to being free, autonomous, and self-determined. Still, it would be misleading to suggest that Freud completely fails to register these matters. He does note, for example, that Jentsch's interest in a diverse range of particular objects and experiences links them all to the animate-inanimate question in the special way they "excite in the spectator the impression of automatic, mechanical processes at work behind the ordinary appearance of mental activity" (XVII, 226). And later, though without reference to Jentsch, he will link uncanny effects to other material that is "offensive to the ego" in the way it undermines those "acts of volition which nourish in us the illusion of Free Will" (236).

That said, Jentsch's point is more developed and much more central to his argument than even these comments register. Jentsch's linking of the uncanny to "the impression of automatic, mechanical processes at work behind the ordinary appearance of mental activity" is founded on how certain objects and situations give their spectators the eerie impression that human consciousness itself is but a mechanical process. (This impression is less uncertain than it is disorienting.) Indeed, going well beyond Freud's almost passing reference to the "illusion of Free Will," Jentsch's "psychology of the uncanny" enters into the realm of existential speculation. For Jentsch, that is, the uncanny is not about intellectual uncertainty simply or even that more specific uncertainty over a figure's status as alive or lifeless; the uncertainty at the heart of the uncanny is not, that is, about the simple "what" of the figure (person or object). If a faith in what Jentsch variously calls "man's individuality," "a unified psyche," and "psychical freedom" (what we might call self-possessed volitional autonomy) and a belief that this human condition might be traced ultimately to our "transcendental origin" are central to our normal impressions of existence, the uncanny marks the unnerving evocation that such impressions might be wrong. As Jentsch puts it, in the experience of the uncanny we are confronted with the possibility of "hidden psychological" or "mechanical processes" in the mind that "undermine one's hasty and careless conviction of the animatedness of the individual" (14–15).[7] Within the context of Jentsch's own argument, the word translated here as "animatedness" ("Beseelung" [205]) does not point to the simple difference between alive or not alive (a person vs. a doll, for example). Rather it calls our attention, problematically, to our assumptions as to what constitutes life—*human* life—at all.

Elaborating on the animate-inanimate problematic, Jentsch observes how one can be disoriented by something that, having "at first seemed completely lifeless[,] suddenly reveals an inherent energy." He adds that "this energy," which might "have a psychical or a mechanical origin," is capable of generating a "feeling of terror" precisely because of "the obscurity of its cause" (11). He doesn't make the connection himself, but we might associate the phrase "obscurity of its cause" with an earlier part of his discussion in which he relates the uncertainty-uncanny link to "processes . . . whose *conditions of origin* are unknown." While at this point in his argument he hasn't yet delved into the richer existential implications of the uncanny, he goes on to observe that "a slight nuance of the uncanny effect . . . can be explained psychologically in terms of *one's bafflement regarding how the conditions of origin . . . were brought about*" (10; my emphases). I would like to suggest that such "bafflement" ("Rathlosigkeit" ["Zur Psychologie des Unheimlichen," 197]) can and should be associated with the anxiety over whether what we thought possessed "psychical freedom" might actually be determined by mere mechanical processes. In other words, the phrase "bafflement regarding how the conditions of origin . . . were brought about" might be applied to Jentsch's later discussion of the confusion over "the animatedness of the individual." For the existential question at the heart of this confusion is not simply how one is to distinguish what is alive from what is lifeless but in what sense a living thing (something undoubtedly "animated") might not be able to call its life its own. And this question arises because the *cause* of one's animate condition is obscure. In the experience of the uncanny, Jentsch remarks, "dark knowledge dawns" (14), and if this darkness is yet more bafflement than knowledge it is because what we once thought we could take for granted about existence is, at best, uncertain. The uncanny unnerves, in short, by reminding us that we exist—we are conscious, we think, we are *animate*—without knowing how or why.

But how exactly do the conditions of origin become a problem of knowledge? As we already noted, one of the points Freud picks up on from Jentsch is the notion that the experience of the uncanny is often grounded in a certain temporal lag: "In story-telling, one of the most reliable artistic devices for producing uncanny effects is to leave the reader in uncertainty as to whether he has a human person or rather an automaton before him in the case of a particular character. This is done *in such a way that the uncertainty does not appear directly at the focal point of his attention, so that he is not given the occasion to investigate and clarify the matter straight away*" (Jentsch, 13; my emphasis; Freud, XVII, 226–27). Jentsch is more obviously addressing an aspect of narrative technique—how to build fictional suspense—but he hints more broadly that the experience of the uncanny is typically grounded in a similar temporal lag: that between an original moment where an event or situation's meaning is not fully registered and a later moment at which intellectual uncertainty gives way to clarity, but clarity about an idea or state of affairs one finds repulsive or horrifying. Although he is rather more implicit than explicit on this point, we might say that, for Jentsch, one of the keys to the uncanny is a process of discovery we would avoid if we knew what was coming. But because we fail to focus our attention directly upon this scene of uncertainty when we first encounter it—we don't recognize it or, perhaps, we simply miss it—we are set in motion toward a later epiphany we do not want and whose full force produces feelings of dread, horror, shock, and revulsion.

In dealing with definitions of the uncanny in the first section of his essay, Freud makes a similar point in linking his notion of the "secretly familiar" back to his earlier philological analysis of the two words *heimlich* and *unheimlich* and in particular to his finding "that among its different shades of meaning the word '*heimlich*' exhibits one which is identical with its opposite, '*unheimlich*.' What is *heimlich* thus comes to be *unheimlich*" (XVII, 224). Although Freud does not acknowledge it here, this sense of the uncanny as involving a reversal of meaning—what is familiar suddenly being perceived as containing within itself something unfamiliar—appears in Jentsch's formulation as well:

> That which has long been familiar appears not only as welcome, but also . . . as straightforwardly self-evident. . . . It is only when one deliberately removes [an idea] from the usual way of looking at it . . . that a particular feeling of uncertainty quite often presents itself. . . . It is thus comprehensible if a correlation "new/foreign/hostile" corresponds to the psychical association of "old/known/familiar." . . . [T]he emergence of sensations of uncertainty is quite natural, and one's lack of orientation will then easily be able to take on the shading of the uncanny. ("On the Psychology of the Uncanny," 8–9)

Freud alters Jentsch's formulation by offering a different way of understanding the correspondence between "new/foreign/hostile" and "old/known/familiar." For Freud, what appears new, unfamiliar, and thus uncertain is actually something we already know without for all that recognizing that we do. Of course, the unfamiliar can be something we already know (the secretly familiar) because of repression. But, by itself, repression is not enough to cause uncanny feelings. The emergence of such feelings also requires that what has been repressed returns in an unfamiliar way, a process in which our normal forward movement in time (from past to present) turns back on itself: if "the *heimlich* . . . comes to be *unheimlich*," it is because the uncanny "*leads us back* to what is known of old and long familiar" (XVII, 220; my emphasis).[8] For Freud, the uncanny is thus precisely a belated revelation of something the mind has kept a secret from itself: the "secret and hidden" is somehow familiar (we've experienced it before in some form) and so it is *heimlich*; but because it has come to light unexpectedly and in some deferred way it also has the quality of the *unheimlich*.[9]

What Freud recognizes, in short, is that what is *unheimlich* is hidden away precisely in the *heimlich*. In that context, what is repulsive or horrifying in the experience is not just something frightening in itself. Rather, we are unnerved by the experience of coming to see *subsequently* that some other reality—something uncertain or unexpected—is concealed within what is most familiar, personal, and intimate. In other words, the experience of the uncanny is a moment of reversal, the point at which our sense of reality as what is comforting, safe, or friendly (*heimlich*) is suddenly exposed as unfamiliar, obscure, or self-estranging. We might even say that the experience of the uncanny resides in this disorienting duality: what is at once insufficiently and too secretive, insufficiently and too concealed, insufficiently and too familiar. And to the extent that, as I have already suggested, a *deferred* coming-to-know (a temporal lag) defines this experience, the uncanny also, typically, refers to a past that we cannot fully grasp, conceptualize, or remember, a past we did not or could not know directly at the time even though, in some inexplicable way, we must have been present for it.

But there is another crucial factor to consider. For if, as Freud notes, the uncanny compels us to revisit (and also revise) "what is known of old and long familiar" (XVII, 220), what it means to be "known of old and long familiar" is precisely what is at stake: known by and familiar to whom? I would like to suggest that what is most frightening in the uncanny is that its deferred coming-to-know marks a recognition of something "known of old" only *not by us*. In other words, a key part of the uncanny is experienced through our slowly dawning awareness that others do not share our ignorance. At one stage Freud notes as an aspect of the shared definition of *un/heimlich* the notion that it can mean "concealed . . . so that others do not get to know about it, withheld from others" (223). But it is more likely that behind this sense of a *knowledge withheld* is the terrifying prospect of knowledge being withheld from us *by* others: it is as if part of what we discover is that others have known this secret all along (known of old and long familiar *to them*). Summarizing Jentsch, Freud notes that the notion of "intellectual uncertainty" means that "the uncanny would always, as it were, be something one does not know one's way about in" (221; see Jentsch, 8). But this disorientation exists in relation to intimate and forbidden knowledge that is not denied to others, who, by contrast, know *their* way about in it.

The image Freud himself offers of being lost in the red-light district of a certain "provincial town in Italy" perfectly captures this feeling. Freud's "feeling of helplessness" in inadvertently returning "again and again to one and the same spot" is exacerbated by the fact that the onlooking "painted women" seem perfectly at home in the situation and thus have an easy and familiar knowledge of what is unfamiliar to him. In other words, they already know precisely what baffles Freud, and the fact that others know what he doesn't makes the situation worse. Indeed, their knowledge as against his ignorance, along with the fact that Freud keeps returning to where he began (his origin), is central to making the experience uncanny and not just frustrating (XVII, 237). The secret unearthed in the experience of the uncanny is something that has been known to others who appear to know more about us than we do ourselves and who therefore appear to have direct access to a past—*our* past—that we do not share. And if, then, we experience the uncanny when we feel a sudden exposing of what we would prefer would stay hidden, part of its terror is the fact that the secret has been known by others whose strange power over us is defined by their prior knowledge.

To sum up this part of the discussion, although on one level Freud explicitly rejects Jentsch's notion of intellectual uncertainty as a central feature of the uncanny, he effectively reinstates that notion in psychoanalytic terms by positing an *un/heimlich* duality. More specifically, he revises Jentsch's idea of a temporal lag through which certainty replaces uncertainty so that the uncanny comes to be experienced expressly in terms of delayed recognition: what had only seemed normal and so comforting is defamiliarized; or, the *unheimlich* comes to be seen as residing within the *heimlich* (what Freud calls the secretly familiar is thus also the strangely unfamiliar). Without perhaps being fully aware of the reworking, Freud also adds to Jentsch's theory of the uncanny the sense that what is uncertain is not simply what isn't known. For beyond what is obscure to us—*what* we cannot see or understand—is the sense that we may not truly want to see, that we refuse a knowledge offered. But against Freud's position that such refusal is a mark of repression (and the knowledge that returns from that state), I am suggesting that in the uncanny what we seek to disavow is knowledge at once there and not there, available yet inaccessible, something we actually missed and did not simply psychically forget. Returning from Freud to Jentsch, we might observe, finally, that, in linking intellectual-psychical processes to the very question of our animate condition, Jentsch more so than Freud situates the uncanny at a moment of existential anxiety, a dawning awareness of our own previously unrecognized bafflement regarding the conditions of our very origins as conscious and self-conscious creatures. And what is most discomforting in the uncanny is the self-estranging experience of coming to see how the origin that defines us is our own and not our own simultaneously.

In what remains of this chapter, I would like to combine Jentsch's and Freud's theories of the uncanny, adapted as I have thus far suggested, and read them in relation to Hoffmann's "The Sandman." I would like to suggest that the narrative structure of the story plays on the interconnected issues I have just described: the uncanny as a moment we cannot fully understand as it happens (and which, inexplicably, we have missed despite having been present); a truth of our past denied to us but not to others; knowledge that comes to us only belatedly and even then without full certainty. Borrowing from Jentsch, I want to suggest, further, that "The Sandman" can and should be read precisely as dealing with the existential question *par excellence*: how do we understand the animatedness of the individual? As we shall see, in the tale of young Nathanael who must confront the very possibility that he is but an automaton, Hoffmann treats the question of animatedness metaphorically to raise a series of broader questions. How are we to understand our animate/d condition? What does it mean to have had an origin we seem not to remember? Why is the secret of our origin known only by others? And how does this origin mark our present as forever belated?

III

Before we take up specific plot-details, it is worth observing how Hoffmann's play with point-of-view offers a kind of oblique commentary on the issues we have been addressing.[10] While the story's basic chronology moves through four major temporal episodes starting with the childhood of the protagonist, Nathanael, its narrative structure is divided between an initial epistolary section (three letters comprising roughly one-third of the whole) and a larger section narrated by an anonymous friend of one of the minor characters (Lothar). The latter section begins as follows: "No invention could be stranger or more extraordinary than the fate which befell my poor friend, the young student Nathanael, and which I have undertaken to recount to you, dear reader" (97). The origins of this statement are obscure: it is unclear who is speaking or how this person is connected to Lothar or Nathanael (both termed friends)[11]; it is unclear why the story begins with the letters rather than with the narrator's deferred observation (why is that observation only now being related?); and it is unclear just what motivates the telling in the first place ("I must confess, kind reader, that nobody has actually asked me to tell the story" [98]). Moreover, as Hertz astutely notes, the narrative intrusion calls to mind "the classic problem of the Romantic writer: how to begin."[12] Our narrator (female or male?) thus tells us that s/he has "laboured in vain to find words with which to begin," that s/he has "racked [her/his] brains to find a portentous, original, and arresting way of beginning," and that, finally, "unable to find words . . . to reflect . . . [her/his] "inner vision, [s/he] decided *not to begin at all*" (97–98; my emphasis). That last statement is, of course, contradicted both by its very writing and by the inclusion of the letters, which, the narrator tells us, were "communicated" by Lothar and which provide a suitable introductory "sketch" of the full story (98). In short, even as s/he actually does begin or perhaps begins again (are the letters the beginning or not?), our narrator marks her/his (re)beginning by disavowing it: "I resolved not to begin." But after s/he has already begun, what is such a resolution worth?

For the narrator, then, the story begins with a beginning that, as Freud might say, has lost its way. On the one hand, identifying the origin is difficult because it is unavailable for some reason (no words with which to begin; a resolution not to begin); on the other hand, it is not so much missing as displaced: either it is not to be found where we expected it or it is present where we did not expect it. It is as though the story's origin must always lie elsewhere even as we are left to wonder how we missed it. The problematic nature of the origin is marked in a particularly telling way in the narrator's claims regarding her/his own representational practice: "[A]s I tell the story, . . . I may, like a good portraitist, succeed in depicting some figures so well that you find them good likenesses *even without knowing the originals*" (98; my emphasis). Where the origin(al)s are missing, how can we even begin to assess the quality of the representation? Indeed, what would representation (*re*-presentation/repetition) even mean in this context? In short, the story's narrative structure thematizes as problematic the very notion of what it means to begin, to have an origin, or to see the present in relation to some beginning we cannot access. Read in conjunction with Jentsch's phrase—"bafflement regarding how the conditions of the origin were brought about"—the narrator's (non)beginning might be taken as a warning that any origin is always already uncanny.

If this missing or misplaced beginning is the situation of the tale's telling, it is also, and more importantly, a major element of Nathanael's situation. Although, as we have seen, Freud dismisses its relevance to the production of uncanny feelings, most readers no doubt see Nathanael's discovery of what Olimpia really is (a mechanical doll created by the joint efforts of Spalanzani and Coppola) as the central event of the story. But while her status becomes clear as the story proceeds, the revelation also forces

Nathanael (or at least the reader) to look back, retrospectively, to redefine what *he* is. We thus get the following two passages, the first describing Nathanael's recognition of what Olimpia is, the second Nathanael's earlier and rather more cryptic description of an incident from his youth while he was in his father's study:

> Nathanael stood stock still. He had perceived only too clearly that Olimpia's deathly pale wax face had no eyes, just black caverns where eyes should be; she was a lifeless doll. Spalanzani was writhing on the floor . . . [b]ut he summoned all his strength and cried: "After him, after him! Why are you standing there? Coppelius—he's stolen my best automaton—twenty years work . . . the clockwork—language—walk—all mine—the eyes—he stole your eyes . . . !" (114)

***

> . . . the two of them [Nathanael's father and Coppelius, the Sandman] donned long black smocks. I did not notice where these came from. My father opened the folding doors of a cupboard; but I saw that what I had so long taken for a cupboard was instead a dark recess containing a small fireplace. Coppelius walked over to it, and a blue flame crackled up from the hearth. . . . [B]randishing a pair of red-hot tongs, [he] was lifting gleaming lumps from the thick smoke and then hammering at them industriously. It seemed to me that human faces were visible on all sides, but without eyes, and with ghastly, deep black cavities instead.
> "Bring the eyes! Bring the eyes!" cried Coppelius in a hollow rumbling voice. . . . [The hidden Nathanael is then discovered by Coppelius.] With a piercing laugh, Coppelius cried: "All right the boy may keep his eyes . . . ; but let's examine the mechanism of his hands and feet." And with these words he seized me so hard that my joints made a cracking noise, dislocated my hands and feet, and put them back in various sockets. (90–91)

Although Freud himself can do no better than to link the paired disassembling of Nathanael and Olimpia as a "new castration equivalent," the general connection between the two scenes is clear enough: the image of what even Freud recognizes as Coppelius "screw[ing] off [Nathanael's] arms and legs as an experiment" (XVII, 232n1) is linked to the discovery that Olimpia is a "lifeless doll." In short, the second scene in some sense reenacts (without simply repeating) the first so as to reveal what is not clear initially. Perhaps more accurately, what Nathanael finds in Olimpia is, inexplicably, himself or at least what he experienced of himself, though unknowingly, in that earlier episode.[13]

Though without reference to Jentsch, Stefani Engelstein has recently shown that Hoffmann's own interests anticipate Jentsch's interpretation of the uncanny in certain key respects. Writing explicitly in response to late eighteenth- and early nineteenth-century developments in biological science and natural history, especially those studies with an emphasis on procreative and regenerative processes, Hoffmann is attuned to how the body might be said to govern itself; or, with a more philosophical bent, he creatively engages the period's conceptual interlacing of an emerging view of the mechanistic-materialist "instrumentality of the body" with a "wider confusion in the boundaries of the self." This confusion, Engelstein notes, could "elicit with urgency the question of the final purpose of human existence, and whether it proceeds in a determinate fashion from our physical structure."[14] In other words, Hoffman aims to represent the terrifying possibility of the human body functioning through purely natural or material processes without any reference to a higher spiritual purpose and without any capacity to express self-motivating agency (intellectual, moral, or spiritual).

That said, despite registering the deeper issues at stake in Hoffmann's writings, Engelstein yet has a fairly narrow sense of how these are played out in "The Sandman." For the most part Engelstein focuses on the limited question of what exactly Nathanael is, even as she completely literalizes the answer: like Olimpia, Nathanael turns out to be a machine of some kind.[15] The problem with this view is that it gives to Hoffmann's telling more clarity than it actually has and so imagines the story's *denouement* as a simple question of fact. Even more to the point, at least when Hoffmann's story is read in relation to Jentsch and Freud, the focus on what Nathanael "is" has almost nothing to say about how his situation evokes the uncanny.

I would like to suggest that Engelstein is closer to the heart of "The Sandman"—and thus also closer to the uncanny—in noting in relation to another story in *Nachtstücken* ("Die Automate") that Hoffmann "sets up the puzzle of human consciousness *through* the automaton."[16] And so too for "The Sandman": the final aim of the story isn't simply to reveal that Nathanael isn't human (or even, as Jentsch might put it, to leave us in doubt for as long as possible whether an apparently living being is animate). Rather, it aims to puzzle us, even, in Jentsch's words, to "undermine our hasty and careless convictions" about consciousness, what it means to be animate, and how the simple fact of being alive can become uncanny. I would venture further that Hoffmann's puzzle anticipates Jentsch's under-theorized intuition that the uncanny is connected to our bafflement regarding how the conditions of origin come about.

Let us return, then, to Nathanael's special connection to Olimpia. Clearly, for a time Spalanzani and Coppola (or is this Coppelius?) alone know what Olimpia is, a secret identity that only later comes to light. But, cryptic as it is, Spalanzani's wording in his final meeting with Nathanael strongly suggests that he and Coppola (and perhaps also Nathanael's father) possess a similar secret about Nathanael himself: "[Spalanzani] summoned all his strength and cried: '. . . *he stole your eyes*'" (my emphasis). It isn't just that Spalanzani is here revealing some secret knowledge about Nathanael (although that may also be true). Rather, Spalanzani's revelation is marked precisely as delayed, knowledge that, for some reason, could not be recognized earlier. Clearly, the discovery that Olimpia is a machine—and in particular Spalanzani's association between her eyes and Nathanael's—is intended to draw us back to the earlier scene in Nathanael's father's study. The relation between the two scenes highlights what was so strangely missing in the first: at the very moment where Coppelius is shown dismantling the young Nathanael, Nathanael remains strangely oblivious. What thus gets revealed as the latter scene *leads us back* isn't simply that Nathanael is an automaton but rather that he cannot recognize himself in the first instance. Faced with how the conditions of his origin were brought about, Nathanael can only (re)discover himself, as Freud might say, after the event.

But why must this (self-)knowledge be deferred? I would venture that this belated structure of knowing is at once linked to the temporal lag Jentsch associates with fictional representations of the uncanny and points to the uncanny's most fundamental characteristic: it is an experience of always already coming after, of having an origin that, inexplicably, remains obscure (inaccessible to us, at least, though perhaps known to others) and in relation to which we *always* come too late. Aptly referring to how Hoffmann's story represents "an *unheimlich* episode in the history of the subject," Françoise Meltzer argues that Hoffmann's Nathanael marks such an episode precisely in how he is caught up in "the preordained order into which the subject is situated *before* he acquires knowledge of his relation to 'others.'"[17] I place special stress on that "before" because it is defines the history of the subject as the history of one who has a *before* in his relation to others but who acquires knowledge of it only later (after the event). It is this vexed contrast, I argue, that makes a situation uncanny.

That said, Meltzer's otherwise provocative reading is marred by her strange insistence that Nathanael's belated self-knowledge yet leads him back to something eminently knowable. Building on her notion that, in his final encounter with Olimpia (seeing her as but a mechanical doll), Nathanael is "only repeating the trauma of the conceptual primal scene which he witnessed from the closet [in his father's study]," Meltzer argues that this primal scene offers Nathanael (and the reader) the clear if unnerving revelation "that he is the other incarnate: the automaton."[18] As we saw at the outset, Freud himself openly pondered whether the primal scene could be understood as an actual event and accessible to the observing child. But Meltzer has no such qualms; she thus uses the verb "witness" four times to suggest that, once he conceptually returns from the Olimpia episode to the scene in the father's study—once, that is, he understands the latter as a repetition of the former—Nathanael has recovered the actual origin in the form of stable knowledge, available even to direct sense-experience.[19] But if there is a sense that the story's key plot development hinges on Nathanael's deferred knowledge of his very identity (rendered visible only in the mediating figure of Olimpia), that self-knowledge is precisely not something accessible in this way.

This limitation—the fundamental inaccessibility of the origin—is powerfully, if subtly, on display in Coppelius's most cryptic remark in the scene in the father's study: "And with these words he seized me so hard that my joints made a cracking noise, dislocated my hands and feet, and put them back in various sockets. *'They don't fit properly! It was alright as it was! The Old Man knew what he was doing!'* hissed and muttered Coppelius" (my emphasis). We have no idea who the "Old Man" is (German: *Der Alte* ["Der Sandmann," 10]), but Coppelius's reassembling of Nathanael's joints (". . . put them back in various sockets . . .") appears to be repeating the moment at which Nathanael was first assembled. In other words, what both Nathanael and the reader encounter in the father's study is the very inaccessibility of that earlier scene. Conceptualizing the incident in the study as the story's primal scene, Meltzer refers to it by its French term: *la scène originaire*. But she fails to register that Nathanael's true origin is what the story is at pains *not* to give us. Indeed, in relation to Meltzer's "before"—the subject's situatedness within relationships prior to a knowledge of them—Nathanael's present can but gesture toward a time existing prior to the scene in his father's study. And that before-time can thus only be known through a repetition that belatedly marks the original as missing. For Nathanael as for the reader, the knowledge of how our very identities are caught up in the conditions of our origin remains, in some fundamental sense, at once belated and obscure.

In his first mention of primal scenes in a May 1897 letter to Fliess, Freud links them to "phantasies [that] arise from things *heard* but only understood *later*"; he adds in his notes that such "phantasies serve the purpose of refining the memories, of sublimating them. They are built up out of things that have been heard about and then *subsequently* turned to account" (*Origins*, 196–97). In his first formulation, then, the Freudian primal scene appears to have something in common with the temporal lag that Jentsch will associate with the experience of the uncanny. Just as important, what is "understood *later*" or "*subsequently*" typically leads us back to an event that is not immediately available to the mind, something we may have "heard about" without our having an actual memory. In this context Freud notes that these "psychical structures . . . are not properly speaking memories" (*Origins*, 196) because we may not in fact have experienced them except as reconstructions after the fact.

Hoffmann offers his own version of a not quite being there in Nathanael's almost passing description of how his repeated attempts at knowledge could never quite catch up with their object: "I would slip out of my bedroom into the corridor, but I never managed to discover anything; for the Sandman had always entered the room before I reached the spot at which he would have been visible" (88). As Freud himself did (XVII, 232n1), we might recognize how Hoffmann doubles the father-image in Coppelius (the Sandman) and Nathanael's actual father (significantly, always referred to as "father" even by his wife). In the context of this doubling it is as though the situation of always arriving late at the scene of knowing cannot escape the existential urgency of the question posed by Derrida: "What happens . . . when a son is *after* his father?" For both Hoffmann and Freud, we might say, the uncanny is precisely that psychical response of the son who, when confronted with the question, discovers that he cannot answer it.

It is both as an attempt and a failure to answer that impossible question that we should we read Nathanael's suicidal leap from atop the town hall at story's end:

> [H]e uttered a horrible bellow, like a tormented animal; then he sprang aloft and cried in a piercing voice, interspersed with hideous laughter: "Spin, wooden dolly! Spin, wooden dolly!" . . . Nathanael was raving . . . , leaping into the air and

shrieking: "Fiery circle, spin! Fiery circle, spin!" . . . Suddenly Nathanael paused and stood stock still; he bent down, perceived Coppelius, and, with a piercing shriek of "Beautiful eyes-a! Beautiful eyes-a!" he jumped over the parapet. By the time Nathanael was lying on the pavement, his head shattered, Coppelius had vanished. (117–18)

This scene leads us back to the final incident at Spalanzani's house where Nathanael goes mad after he is hit by the "pair of bloody eyes" taken from Olimpia: "Spalanzani picked them up . . . and threw them at Nathanael, so that they struck him in the chest. Madness seized him . . . , tearing his mind to pieces. 'Hey, hey, hey! Fiery circle, fiery circle! Spin, spin, fiery circle! Come on! Spin, wooden dolly, spin, pretty woman dolly . . .' and with these words he flung himself on the Professor and clutched him by the throat" (114). But, more impressionistically, the shared image of the "fiery circle" (German: *Feuerkreis* ["Der Sandmann," 38, 43]) leads us back to the scene in Nathanael's father's study and the "small fireplace" with crackling "blue flame" (90) onto which Coppelius hurls Nathanael. If, as I have suggested against Meltzer's reading, the scene in the father's study marks a repetition of precisely what *cannot* be witnessed (an earlier scene figured in the unidentified "Old Man"), we might interpret Nathanael's suicide as another kind of repetition of that scene, an attempt to force what is missing into the open. In other words, if the missing scene must have shown the Old Man first assembling Nathanael, Nathanael's disassembling of his body ("his head shattered") returns him to the lost origin by undoing it.

Of course, the very self-destructiveness of this act reveals the essential helplessness that one feels in the uncanny. Like Shakespeare's Hamlet in relation to King Hamlet, in killing himself Nathanael undoes the work of his creator—the "father" who exists in the son's "before." But whereas Shakespeare presents the tragic protagonist in a heroic light—Hamlet does, in some meaningful way, claim himself, even father himself—Hoffmann's Nathanael can only reclaim in fantasy (and thus futilely) what was never his, the choice to exist. For in the wake of that inaccessible origin—*la scène originaire*—what Nathanael experiences or, more accurately, what he is forced to experience against his will is his absence precisely where he should have been present. If, whatever Freud might have thought, the primal scene is best understood as the belated discovery that we were, inexplicably, absent from the scene of our own creation, the uncanny registers that the choice of our existence belongs to another, someone mysteriously residing at the origin in relation to which we necessarily come forever after.

IV

Meltzer and Sarah Kofman both interpret the scene in Nathanael's father's study as a prolepetic representation of Freud's concept of the primal scene as that will be formulated in the case-history of the Wolf Man. Implicitly reminding us that Freud was simultaneously at work on the case-history and "The Uncanny," they suggest thereby that uncanny feelings are akin—perhaps even identical—to what is experienced in the primal scene. But where we earlier observed Hertz's effort to align the case-history (1918), "The Uncanny" (1919), and, to some extent, *Beyond the Pleasure Principle* (1920) in terms of their shared concern with origins, originality, and priority, Meltzer and Kofman, despite some attention to these issues, understand Freud moving toward the concept of endings and in particular toward the death drive as that notion gets its full articulation in *Beyond the Pleasure Principle*. In other words, Meltzer and Kofman both view the place of the primal scene in "The Uncanny" (the link established by the role Hoffmann's story plays in Freud's essay) as bound up with what is perhaps the key post-Oedipal insight in Freud's metapsychological thinking.

Meltzer and Kofman both argue that, in the experience of the uncanny (in Hoffmann's story most powerfully expressed through a proto-Freudian representation of the primal scene and its subsequent repetition), the subject encounters the ultimate incomprehensibility: how our being-in-the-world is always our being-toward-death. To put this idea most simply, they both read the uncanny as the sudden, inexplicable awareness (perhaps best understood as a drive or instinct in the Freudian sense) of how death shadows life as its *unheimlich* double.[20]

Although a full engagement with Meltzer's and Kofman's arguments is beyond the scope of this chapter, I would like to suggest by way of conclusion that a link between "The Uncanny" and *Beyond the Pleasure Principle* does exist and that this link is itself associated with Freud's earlier effort to theorize the primal scene. That said, although he doesn't trace the full development, I would also venture that Hertz's understanding of what is at stake in these texts more accurately captures the particular trajectory of Freud's thought. In short, Freud's notion of the death drive as formulated in *Beyond the Pleasure Principle* conceptually points toward a crisis of origins and not, as Meltzer and Kofman would have it, the other way around. So how should we understand the relationship between "The Uncanny" and *Beyond the Pleasure Principle*?

Let us return to Freud's reworking of Jentsch's "psychological theory of the uncanny." Because he knows in advance what he is looking for, Freud fails to grasp what Jentsch's theory really entails: intellectual uncertainty over the disturbing border between the animate and the inanimate—exactly what is on display in Hoffmann's story. But what does it mean to be animate? In what we might call a kind of anticipatory gloss on Jentsch's essay, Hoffmann clearly imagines that "animate" does not simply mean being alive, that which has life as opposed to what is lifeless (a human being, for example, as opposed to a mechanical doll). After all, a central issue of "The Sandman" is that the apparently human Nathanael shares something with the inanimate Olimpia without for all that actually being a doll: he is too much like her without being identical to her in any literal sense. In other words, there is something potentially inanimate—some latent inanimateness we might say—within the animate. So perhaps the better question would be what does it mean to move from one state to the other; what, in short, does it mean to become animate/d? There are two words here, or two parts of the same concept, and I give both to stress that, at least as far as *Hoffmann's* uncanny is concerned, the condition of being animate is precisely a condition registered in the passive voice: something imposed upon one by someone else.

If in "The Uncanny" Freud turns away from Jentsch's animate-inanimate problematic to reassert a central element of the Oedipal model (castration anxiety), in an important sense he returns to it in *Beyond the Pleasure Principle*. More specifically, as we saw in chapter 1, Freud there describes the origin of the death drive as a crisis of the ending that is, in reality, a crisis of the beginning: "The attributes of life were at some time evoked [*erweckt*/awoken] in animate matter by the action of a force of whose nature we can form no conception. . . . The tension which then arose in what had hitherto been an inanimate substance endeavored to cancel itself out. In this way the first instinct came into being: the instinct to return to the inanimate state" (XVIII, 38). This sudden and unwelcome awakening into life from an inanimate state marks consciousness itself as originating in a kind of trauma but a wound registered by the incomprehensibility of its cause.[21]

In his typically cryptic fashion, Hoffmann provides a symbolic mini-narrative of precisely the moment at which something inanimate first becomes animate/d:

> With a piercing laugh, Coppelius cried: "All right the boy may keep his eyes . . . ; but let's examine the mechanism of his hands and feet." And with these words he seized me so hard that my joints made a cracking noise, dislocated my hands and feet, and put them back in various sockets. "They don't fit properly! It was alright as it was! The Old Man knew what he was doing!" hissed

and muttered Coppelius; but everything went black and dim before my eyes, a sudden convulsion shot through my nerves and my frame, and I felt nothing more. A warm, gentle breath passed over my face, and *I awoke from a death-like sleep*; my mother was bending over me . . . her darling boy who was thus restored to life. (90–91; my emphasis)

Nathanael's recovery from the unnerving experience of seeing himself as a constructed, perhaps even inanimate object is re-presented in this passage as a naturalized event: his birth, with a real mother "bending over . . . her darling boy," replaces the work of fathering that, within the confines of Hoffmann's story, actually created ("animated") him.[22] The full movement of the passage, in short, marks the coming into existence we know as birth as an awakening out of some state we might call inanimate. Significantly, while Nathanael's recovery seems like birth, it is yet only a "*re*storation to life"; that is, his quasi-birth is marked as a return, a secondary event that, at best, looks back to an unrepresentable earlier one. What we thus get is an image of birth as both a movement from inanimate to "animate matter" and a repetition of an origin that remains inaccessible, the experience of missing what necessarily came before.

Just what all this might mean for an understanding of the uncanny in its relation to the death drive more generally is hinted at in one of Nathanael's more obscure ruminations. Although it largely stands apart from the main action, this passage seems, in retrospect, to address the existential threat at the heart of Hoffmann's story:

> He fell into gloomy reveries . . . To him, all life consisted of dreams and premonitions; he kept saying that each individual, fancying himself to be free, only served as a plaything for the cruelty of dark forces; that it was in vain to resist, and one must acquiesce humbly in the decrees of destiny. He went so far as to assert that artists and scholars were under a delusion when they believed that their creative endeavors were governed by the autonomy of their will: "for," said he, "*the inspired state which is indispensable for creation does not arise from ourselves*; it is due to the influence of a higher principle that lies outside ourselves." (100; my emphasis)

At the commonsense level, the sentence I have italicized is simply a statement about artistic inspiration. But the "inspired state" is, literally, the condition of having been breathed into (*in* + *spirare*); it means *to have received* breath, "anima," life. Understood in those terms, the sentence provides a cryptic gloss on the "gloomy reveries" of the uncanny itself: we lack freedom and autonomy of will, we are subject to the decrees of destiny, because what is "indispensable for creation"—*our* creation—"does not arise from ourselves."[23] To be animate/d, in other words, is precisely the condition of having been brought into existence by that which inspires or animates, a "principle that lies outside ourselves" and "of whose nature we can form no conception." We earlier noted Jentsch's observation that a "slight nuance of the uncanny effect . . . come[s] to light now and then . . . and can be explained psychologically in terms of one's bafflement regarding how the conditions of origin . . . were brought about." In *Beyond the Pleasure Principle* Freud will assert that this bafflement marks the beginning of the death drive ("the instinct to return to the inanimate state"), but the drive toward that ending becomes a solution to living only because the "conditions of origin" are so problematic. For, as Jentsch intuited but could not fully articulate, to be animate/d is precisely the condition of having been brought into existence by an "influence . . . that lies outside ourselves."[24]

One final perspective on the relationship between Jentsch's theory and Hoffmann's story can help us see why Jentsch's understanding of the uncanny, unfinished as it is, is superior to Freud's (at least as a reading of "The Sandman"). In addressing the notion that part of what generates the uncanny is the impression that a living human being is a mere automaton, Freud offers this summary of Jentsch's view:

> Jentsch has taken as a very good instance "doubts whether an apparently animate being is really alive; or conversely, whether a lifeless object might not in fact be animate"; and he refers in this connection to the impression made by wax-work figures, ingeniously constructed dolls and automata. To these he adds the uncanny effect of epileptic fits, and of manifestations of insanity, because these excite in the spectator the impression of automatic, mechanical processes at work behind the ordinary appearance of mental activity. (XVII, 226)

He returns to this point subsequently: "The uncanny effect of epilepsy and madness has the same origin. The layman sees in them the working of forces hitherto unsuspected in his fellow-men, but at the same time he is dimly aware of them in remote corners of his being" (243). It is interesting to note that, even as Freud will later dismiss this aspect of Jentsch's theory, he doesn't even report it accurately. Jentsch does indeed take up the paired topics of epilepsy and insanity (or at least mental instability) but precisely to distinguish them as sources of uncanny impressions in onlookers. And, for our purposes, the reason Jentsch distinguishes them is particularly instructive.

Jentsch begins the section Freud summarizes with the following: "Another confirmation of the fact that the emotion being discussed is caused in particular by a doubt as to the animate or inanimate nature of things—or, expressed more precisely, as to their animatedness as understood by man's traditional view—lies in the way in which the lay public is generally affected by a sight of the articulation of most mental and many nervous illnesses. Several patients afflicted with such troubles make a decidedly uncanny impression on most people" (14). As Jentsch proceeds, he does address what Freud calls "the impression of automatic, mechanical processes at work behind the ordinary appearance of mental activity"; however, he does so in order not only to emphasize the appearance of mere mechanicality on display but also to stress how such an appearance raises anxiety about the lack of a "unified psyche":

> [P]eculiarities become apparent when strong affects make themselves felt, whereby it can suddenly become evident that not everything in the human psyche is of transcendental origin, and that much that is elementary is still present within it even for our direct perception. . . . [I]f this relative psychical harmony happens markedly to be disturbed in the spectator, . . . then the dark knowledge dawns . . . that mechanical processes are taking place in that which he was previously used to regard as a unified psyche. (14)

Significantly, in the case of bouts of hysteria (the one case of mental disorder he addresses explicitly), Jentsch is at pains to note that its appearance is *less* likely to evoke uncanny impressions than is an epileptic fit (so Freud is wrong to conflate the two) precisely because the onlooker's assumption of a normal human consciousness operating behind hysterical symptoms does not disappear:

> It is not unjustly that epilepsy is therefore spoken of . . . as an illness deriving not from the human world but from foreign and enigmatic spheres, for the epileptic attack of spasms reveals the human body to the viewer—the body that under normal conditions is so meaningful, expedient, and unitary,

> functioning according to the directions of his consciousness—as
> an immensely complicated and delicate mechanism. . . . On the
> other hand, the hysterical attack of spasms generally has a limited
> alienating effect . . . since hysterics usually retain consciousness,
> falling over and hitting out so that they do not . . . harm them-
> selves—whereby they reveal precisely their latent consciousness.
> Then their type of movement again frequently reminds one of
> hidden psychical processes, in that here the muscular distur-
> bances follow a certain higher ordering principle. (14)

Reading this distinction between consciousness (a unified human psyche) and what lacks or appears to lack consciousness back into his discussion of the uncanny, we realize that, for Jentsch, the "doubt as to the animate or inanimate nature of things" is an instance of the mind-body problem. Inanimation—the material existence of the body, its mere mechanistic aspect—isn't so much a source of the terror of the uncanny because a bodily object is perceived to lack life. Rather inanimation causes terror where it is accompanied by a perception of the lack of human-defining consciousness. Jentsch's earlier statement—the chief source of the uncanny is "doubt whether an apparently living being is animate"—can be taken, then, to mean doubt whether what appears to be human has the kind of consciousness that would distinguish it from something that, while alive, does not operate on the basis of "a certain higher ordering principle." This anxiety that what appears to be living and human is merely a functioning body, one without the "latent consciousness" that grounds and orders it and that therefore distinguishes human from merely animate life, stands in opposition to the faith in what Jentsch calls the "transcendental origin" of that life. Jentsch does not appear to mean *divine* origin here, but he does seem to be imagining animation in terms of belief in a unifying human consciousness that precedes (both temporally and ontologically, in the sense of taking precedence over) a mere "living body."

It is of special significance, then, that Jentsch immediately continues by addressing a concern that, as we have seen in Nathanael's "gloomy reveries" (Jentsch's "dark knowledge"?), Hoffmann similarly takes up for its special contribution to the terror that inheres in the uncanny. "The uncanny effect," Jentsch writes, is "based on the fact that a more or less clear idea of the presence of a certain . . . mechanism . . . appears in man which, standing in contradiction to the usual view of psychical freedom, begins to undermine one's hasty and careless conviction of the animatedness of the individual." Jentsch here links the "conviction of the animatedness of the individual" to our belief in the possibilities of freedom. But such conviction, he notes, may be "careless," undermined by our inability to distinguish our animation from lack of animation, an inability that generates the uncanny sense that the inanimate lurks within the animate, the intuition of which is the origin of the Freudian death drive (to return to some inanimate state from which one was inexplicably awakened). But more precisely than Freud, both Jentsch and Hoffmann understand the experience of the uncanny as grounded in our suspicion that what we think of a human life—human animation as embodied in a consciousness that appears both to emanate from and to grant us freedom—is in reality simply the marker of our very lack of autonomy. As Nathanael puts it, we lack this animating autonomy not because we are not alive but because our existence has been imposed from "outside ourselves."

These conditions are uncanny because they whisper of what we cannot fully know about ourselves: "dark knowledge dawns" as Jentsch aptly puts it. But the paradox is that such knowledge—about the conditions of our origins—is precisely what baffles us. The incomprehensibility of this situation resides both in our impossible absence from the scene of our own creation and, more pointedly, in the temporal lag between our creation and our retrospective understanding, the condition of "afterwardsness" that Jean Laplanche puts at the center of traumatic experience.[25] Following Laplanche, Cathy Caruth observes, as we noted in chapter 1, that "the peculiar temporality of trauma" resides in "the sense that *the past it foists upon one is not one's own*," a "perspective," she adds, that may "be understood in terms of a temporality of the other." In a related context Laplanche himself adds that in trauma there is always "*something that comes before* . . . the [other's] implantation of [an] enigmatic message."[26] Coming after our origin does not simply mean then that we can never know it; it means, more precisely, that a true knowledge of this moment always resides elsewhere and that, in relation to which, our knowing always comes too late.

The problematic, perhaps insurmountable distance to one's very beginning is figured in Hoffmann's story by the spyglass through which Nathanael observes Olimpia: "He picked up a small, beautifully made pocket spyglass and tested it by looking out of the window. Never before in his life had he come across a spyglass that brought objects before one's eyes with such clarity, sharpness, and distinctness. He involuntarily looked into Spalanzani's room; Olimpia was sitting as usual at the little table . . . Only now did Nathanael behold Olimpia's wondrously beautiful face" (106). Seeing through the spyglass is represented here as a revelation of something that is necessarily viewed over a distance and, as the story recounts it, not properly viewed before. The spatial distance overcome by Nathanael's use of the spyglass thus also figures the temporal distance to his own origin. Of course, the fact that Nathanael needs the spyglass at all—when he first sees Olimpia without the spyglass he cannot see her clearly—suggests that his vision of his own past is always mediated: he cannot see his origin directly but only as represented and so as repetition.

In "The Uncanny," Freud will make a brief, anticipatory comment on his forthcoming elaboration on the theory of repetition in *Beyond the Pleasure Principle*. We might give special attention to the odd phrasing Freud employs there: "all these considerations prepare us for the discovery that whatever reminds us of this inner 'compulsion to repeat' is perceived as uncanny" (XVII, 238). To the extent the experience of the uncanny "leads us back" (220), we are expecting Freud to tell us that we revisit some experience from the past (or at least the mental residue of an earlier event). But Freud's phrasing makes the actual content of the earlier event seem curiously beside the point. For what is "perceived as uncanny" is not the recollection of the past itself but the reminder of our own compulsion to repeat.[27] That is, what is most at stake in the uncanny is our *awareness* of the compelling force of repetition and not the repetition *per se*. To put this another way, for Freud the uncanny resides, in part at least, in the unexpected reminder of the simultaneous inescapability and necessity of what comes before and our belated relationship to an origin(al) that constantly draws us back.

That said, even with the spyglass Nathanael does not fully understand what he is seeing in Olimpia. At the literal level, he doesn't yet know that she is a mechanical doll; at the figurative level, he doesn't yet grasp that he is looking at a version of himself. And so, within the full design of the narrative, Nathanael's awareness of his origin as revealed in the mediating figure of Olimpia is not just deferred until the incident in which Spalanzani throws Olimpia's eyes at him. That revelation must also point backwards to an earlier time at which, inexplicably, understanding was not truly available. The revelation at the heart of the story thus points to something lost or at least lost sight of, just as the earlier scene in Nathanael's father's study can but point backwards in time to the unidentified Old Man who, mysteriously, must have been present from the beginning. As a synecdoche of the entire story, the knowledge that comes through his use of the spyglass suggests, in short, that Nathanael never achieves full access to his own originary moment. Read in terms of Laplanche's *afterwardsness*, Nathanael's seeing is always after the event. *Pace* Freud, then, there is much intellectual uncertainty both in Hoffmann's story and in the experience of the uncanny because, in paradoxically being absent from the scene of its own origin, the subject is always belated in relation to what the origin at once reveals and conceals: what is most intimately oneself.

V

I conclude this chapter with a brief reflection on its epigraph, three lines from Milton's *Paradise Lost* in which Adam, in a conversation with the angel Raphael, struggles to find the words to describe his own beginning. Unlike Hoffman's Nathanael, Milton's Adam is not unduly troubled by his lack of knowledge of the origin and even imagines that lack as a universal condition ("for who himself beginning knew?" [8.251]). Yet, like Nathanael, Adam comes to witness something akin to his own origin in the creation of another, a female version of himself:

> Mine eyes he [God] clos'd, but op'n left the Cell
> Of Fancie my internal sight, by which
> Abstract as in a transe methought I saw,
> Still glorious before whom awake I stood;
> Who stooping op'nd my left side, and took
> From thence a Rib, with cordial spirits warme,
> And Life-blood streaming fresh; wide was the wound,
> But suddenly with flesh fill'd up and heal'd:
> The Rib he formd and fashond with his hands;
> Under his forming hands a Creature grew. . . . (8.460–70)

Like Nathanael, Adam will fall in love with this father-made "Creature" and indeed for much the same reason: where, as we previously noted, Nathanael says that Olimpia "reflect[s]" back to him his "whole existence" so Adam sees in Eve an image of himself ("I now see . . . my Self / Before me" [8.494–96]).

Of course, Nathanael becomes horrified precisely when he comes to understand the createdness of Olimpia, an epiphany that, as I have suggested, comes to him in the uncanny awareness that she reflects back to him his own status as a made-thing. In other words, the uncanny is the delayed discovery that we have an origin and that, while we are necessarily present for it, we are also inexplicably absent from it; it is our origin yet the power to make it so belongs to someone else. For his part, Adam might not feel revulsion at having to witness Eve's creation (though "wide was the wound," he feels no trauma) in part because he sees that she, and therefore he himself, is flesh and blood rather than a machine: "cordial spirits warme" / "Life-blood streaming fresh." Moreover, Milton's theodicy is premised on God's rational creatures (angels and humans if perhaps not animals) having precisely that "unified psyche" that is at once the sign and cause of freedom (and for Milton the "transcendental origin" of that psyche is most assuredly a testament to humankind's divine potential). In short, for Milton, free will, at least in its prelapsarian form, can never be reduced to what Jentsch and Freud both call mere "mechanical processes." This may be why Adam can intuitively grasp that he has been created (animated) by another without feeling horror (which may be another reason that his subsequent witnessing of Eve's creation has nothing of the uncanny about it):

> My self I then perus'd, and Limb by Limb
> Survey'd, . . .
> . . .
> But who I was, or where, or from what cause,
> Knew not; . . .
> . . .
> Not of my self; by some great Maker then,
> In goodness and in power præeminent. (8.267–79)

Adam is, in a sense, an inversion of Nathanael, one happy to know that he is constructed and animated by another.

That said, as we shall see in chapter 5, the uncanny as I have tried to describe it still haunts Milton's poem. Even the submissive Adam will, by the epic's next book, demonstrate a deep ambivalence toward the father-god. Of course, the full representation of filial rebellion, and indeed its psychological basis, are made available to us in Milton's Satan who, much like Hoffmann's Nathanael, experiences the burden of his belatedness in almost physical terms: in this character especially, the father-as-origin is imagined as a literal truth and not simply as an idea. And if Adam, at first, seems to glory in not being able to claim his origin as his own—he can't even remember it—Satan by contrast will use all of his considerable imaginative powers to try to sustain the paradox of creaturely existence: that to "know no time when we were not as now"—that is, *not* to remember "while the Maker gave [us] being"—must mean that we were not created but "self-begot, self-rais'd / By our own quick'ng power" (5.858–61). But, *pace* Freud, Satan has not so much repressed his origin (that God, through the Son, created him). Rather, Milton's poem represents both the temporal lag that is part of the primal scene and the primal scene itself, the moment of discovery at which Satan and the other angels are confronted with the origin they never knew precisely because they were mysteriously absent from it. In response to Satan's claim that the angels are "self-begot," Hoffman might reply, as his Nathanael theorizes, that we do "not arise from ourselves." The uncanny marks for Satan an existential crisis in which the created son discovers that he cannot escape the burden of an imposition of an origin, an origin imposed by the father's priority.

Milton's Adam and Milton's angels are all sons without mothers and so driven by something other than Oedipal rivalry. They are driven precisely by the uncanny, but the uncanny understood in Jentsch's terms rather than in Freudian terms. We might also say that, even as Milton helps to invent Freud by imagining the psychological basis of the uncanny, he does not create it out of whole cloth. One of the reasons Satan's rebellion is so caught up in the Genesis stories of creation is not simply because, in Christian terms, Satan, in the guise of the Serpent, is the immediate cause of the fall of Adam and Eve. More crucially, as Milton rightly intuits, the creation-stories themselves are heavily invested in, even to the point of needing to disavow, ancient Judaism's own anxiety of origins. In part III, we shall consider how Judeo-Christian concepts—in biblical, Miltonic, and, finally, Freudian versions—all grapple with the afterwards that lurks in the uncanny. In ways that it cannot openly acknowledge, in short, the Judeo-Christian tradition at once reveals and conceals what it means to come too late.

Appendix: Synopsis of Hoffmann's "Der Sandmann"[28]

The story can be broken down into four major temporal episodes. The first of these, narrated in the opening letter from the protagonist, Nathanael, to his fiancé's brother, Lothar (the friend of the anonymous narrator), describes scenes from Nathanael's childhood. These scenes feature the mysterious Coppelius—the Sandman (so-called because Nathanael takes him to be the living embodiment of a fictional bogey-man described by the family nurse). They include an initial episode in which Coppelius first captures the young Nathanael, who has been spying on his father and Coppelius at work on some strange project, and then threatens to burn Nathanael's eyes with hot coals only to be dissuaded from the act by Nathanael's father.[29] And they culminate in the death of Nathanael's father in an unexplained chemical explosion, one associated with Coppelius's presence and suggesting either the completion or the failure of their project.

The second episode recounts the increasing strain in the adult Nathanael's relation with his fiancé, Clara, over his morbid obsessions and in particular over his belief that an optician he has met while away at university, Giuseppe Coppola, is none other than Coppelius, who had disappeared at the time of the explosion. The centerpiece of this episode is the narration of a poem that Nathanael writes for Clara.

The third and longest episode is a third-person account of Nathanael's meeting and falling in love with Professor Spalanzani's daughter, Olimpia, while back at university. This episode concludes with Nathanael's shocked discovery that Olimpia is actually a mechanical doll, the shared creation of the mechanician Spalanzani and the eye-maker/optician Coppola. Nathanael's discovery and, more particularly, Spalanzani's action in throwing at him Olimpia's "bloody eyes," inexplicably left behind by Coppola who escapes with the mechanized body, send Nathanael into a temporary madness: he begins to chant words that appear to have some association both with the initial episode with Coppelius and with the poem he had composed for Clara. He then tries to strangle Spalanzani, who is saved by others but who is then banished from the town for his deceit.

Finally, after Nathanael has recovered from his madness and has returned home and to Clara's love, there is a second incident in which he is drawn into murderous insanity. Clara and Nathanael together climb to the top of the town hall while Lothar remains on the street. Taking out the spyglass that he had received from Coppola and first used to observe Olimpia from afar, Nathanael sees something through its lens (Freud says it is Coppelius, but, although Coppelius has in fact returned, Hoffmann doesn't make it clear just what Nathanael has seen[30]). In a fit of madness, Nathanael begins to repeat certain words and actions from previous scenes; these culminate in his attempt to kill Clara. Lothar races to the top of the town hall and manages to free Clara from Nathanael's clutches; all the while Nathanael continues to rave. Before the townspeople can get to him, Nathanael throws himself off the building to his death.

Part III

"Is not He the Father who created you?"

*Belatedness and the Judeo-Christian Tradition
(the Bible, Milton, Freud)*

Shame on him who argues with his Maker,
Though naught but a potsherd of earth!
Shall the clay say to the potter, "What are you doing?
Your work has no handles"?
Shame on him who asks his father, "What are you begetting?"

—Isaiah 45:9–10

I would thou hadst told me of another father.

—Shakespeare, *As You Like It*

Introduction to Part III

Gazing on God

It is quite clear that the Father alone is a self-existent God; clear, too, that a being who is not self-existent cannot be a God.

—Milton, *De Doctrina Christiana*

[W]e find that the ambivalence implicit in the father-complex persists in totemism and in religions generally. Totemic religion not only comprised expressions of remorse and attempts at atonement, it also served as a remembrance of the triumph over the father. . . . We shall not be surprised to find that the element of filial rebelliousness also emerges . . . in the *later* products of religion.

—Freud, *Totem and Taboo*

In imitation of its very subject, this introduction to part III looks back to much of what has gone before. And so I start by revisiting the existential crises of my two children as I briefly discussed those at the opening of part I. More to the point, I do so with special attention both to how my children's experiences match up with a series of biblical passages and to how those passages themselves articulate a crisis of belatedness. That crisis, I will argue, is a central, if largely unrecognized, aspect of the religious vision of the ancient Israelites at least as recorded in biblical accounts. Just as important, as we shall see here as well as in chapters 5 and 6, over the long historical trajectory of the Judeo-Christian tradition, that vision and its attendant crisis are sustained as part of what we might call the tradition's heretical undercurrent, a disruption of orthodoxy that will emerge in everything from early Christian writings (the Gospel of John, for example), in Milton's *Paradise Lost*, and, finally, in Freud's strange attempt to reconstruct the hidden history of the Israelites in his last major work, *Moses and Monotheism*.

So back to my children, and first to the crisis of my daughter, Emma. Her encounter with mortality at age five, I would like to suggest, has a particular conceptual affinity with the story of the Fall as recounted in Genesis 3. In an episode of the Bill Moyers's series, *Genesis: A Living Conversation*, Biblical scholar, Robyn Darling Young, claimed that she saw "no analogy" between this story and anything in our own lives, but I have to disagree. This is the one story that everyone has to tell. And by "has to" I mean both as possession (we possess the story to tell) and as obligation (the story we each must tell).[1] For what the so-called J-writer has so brilliantly rendered is a parable of growing up, maturing, moving away from the garden of innocence—childhood, our parents' home and protection—and taking on the fears and possibilities, the new limits and promises, of adult life.[2] In Dostoevsky's *The Brothers Karamazov*, Ivan Karamazov effectively points this out when, in the preface to the Grand Inquisitor episode, he distinguishes the suffering of children from that of adults, who have, he says, already tasted the fruit.[3] Such a perspective might even enable us to see the rule-making Yahweh of Genesis 3 as sympathetic: as a parent, he desires at once to protect his children (to keep them ignorant and thereby innocent) and to guide them toward the burdens of adult life he can at best forestall. Adam and Eve cannot stay children forever, just as we cannot live forever under the shadow of our own parents. And so they must be disciplined for the reality of this world, prepared to be free and responsible, capable of understanding that choices have consequences.

Consequences suggest limits, and among the limits Genesis 3 imagines we must certainly include death. Initially, however, the story is a bit vague on what death is and even when or how it will happen. God tells the human couple that "as soon as [they] eat of [the tree of the knowledge of good and bad, they] shall die" (Genesis 2:17). The serpent certainly tells some part of truth here: Adam and Eve do not die upon eating the fruit, and their eyes are opened and they do become "like divine beings who know good and bad" (3:5). This latter point is confirmed by God himself at the end of the story: "Now that the man has become like one of us, knowing good and bad" (3:22). But if the divine threat of immediate death isn't meant literally, how then does the J-writer want us to understand its place in the story?

The key to J's presentation comes in two subtle verses toward the end of the chapter. The first of these is verse 19:

> By the sweat of your brow
> Shall you get bread to eat,
> Until you return to the ground—
> For from it you were taken.

We should take special note of what the verse does not say. We tend to assume that Adam and Eve are cursed to mortality because of the Fall, in part, no doubt, because the pun *'adam/'adamah* resonates through the full story: "the LORD God formed man [*'adam*] from the dust of the earth [*'adamah*]"; "Cursed be the ground because of you / . . . For dust you are, / And to dust you shall return" (2:7; 3:17, 19). But the curse does not include death: the acknowledgment of death only sets the temporal term of the curse ("*Until* you return to the ground"). In other words, death was inevitable, something that was going to happen anyway, "natural" rather than "voluntary" as the Pelagian Julian of Eclanum argued in his famous debate with Saint Augustine.[4] This point is confirmed in 3:22: "And the LORD God said, 'Now that the man has become like one of us, knowing good and bad, what if he should stretch out his hand and take also from the tree of life and eat, and live forever!'" Yahweh makes it clear that, without eating from the tree of life, the human couple won't become like gods, at least in one critical respect: they won't live forever. For even in their unfallen condition Adam and Eve were not immortal.

That same Julian argued against Augustine that the story presented death as something figurative rather than literal: a spiritual death rather than a physical one, a death experienced as alienation from God and from one's own moral purpose.[5] But that view refuses the keener edge of the story that Augustine, for all his perversity as an interpreter, comes closer to recognizing. For within the context the J-writer provides (a story of growing up), it makes more sense to accept that the loss of innocence includes the *recognition* of death's inevitability—that is, recognition of a literal physical death and not merely, as Julian would have it, the spiritual death attendant upon alienation from God. The story of the Fall, then, registers the fact of human mortality but not because Adam and Eve *become* mortal when they were not so before. Rather, in their case, as also in my daughter's, the Fall coincides with the emergence of adult wisdom, and central to that wisdom—that loss of innocence—is the *discovery* of a mortality that was always there. Because, as Julian properly understood, death is natural to human beings, whether pleasant or unpleasant, sooner or later it must come for all.

By contrast, as I suggested in the discussion in the introduction to part I, what was troubling my son Ian had nothing to do with death and everything to do with being born. And that crisis just before his fifth birthday finds its proper biblical analogue in the story that precedes the Fall: Genesis 2, the second or J story of creation.[6] In marked distinction to the first creation-account in Genesis 1, the version in Genesis 2 makes explicit humankind's inferior status in relation to God (now Yahweh). Moreover, right from the start, Genesis 2 defines that inferiority in terms of humankind's (*'adam's*) secondariness in relation to God's creative power. The second creation-story's opening image, for example, insists on this relation:

> When the LORD God made heaven and earth—when no shrub of the field was yet on earth and no grasses of the field had yet sprouted, because the LORD God had not sent rain upon the earth and there was no man to till the soil, but a flow would well up from the ground and water the whole surface of the earth—the LORD God formed man from the dust of the earth. He blew into his nostrils the breath of life, and man became a living being. (Genesis 2:4–7)

Humankind comes to be (acquires life) in a situation of belatedness. Yahweh, of course, exists before "man" does (we must always remember that, even acknowledging the sexism of the formulation, "man"—*'adam*—is meant to be humankind as a whole, an individual as synecdoche for the species), but the land itself—a land in the first fragile hints of a Judean spring—is already there as well. We cannot tell for how long the land has existed: has it only just been created in anticipation of a human tiller? But the fact that the time before humans existed is registered so clearly in a place from which they are absent is a reminder that there was a before-time and that, therefore, humans were not even present at, perhaps not even necessary for, the first stirrings of creation.

The most striking reminder of humankind's status as a product of God's creative power—perhaps even a mere afterthought in creation—is its close connection to, even derivation from, the ground (earth, the dust): *'adam* from *'adamah*. Initially, at least, it is not even correct to think of what God creates as "man" because what God first forms doesn't possess life. The gross materiality of human existence is thus given special treatment, a materiality that, as we have noted, will be echoed after the Fall: "For dust you are, / And to dust you shall return." Even the way the narrative presents God finally giving life to the clay figure—blowing the breath of life into its nostrils—is heavy with sensuous physicality, an image that also makes unmistakable not just how God creates us but *that* he creates us. In other words, not only does God create in the sense of giving us a shape or form, but he also animates us, *authors* us, in the sense given by Giorgio Agamben in the passage we considered in the introduction: as *auctor*, God alone sets into being, he alone grants life, a life we do not and could not possess on our own. We might say that the creation of *'adam* at the opening of Genesis 2 sets out in narrative terms the answer to the rhetorical question that will be posed subsequently in Deuteronomy 32:6, the passage from which I draw the title of part III: "Is not He the Father who created you, / Fashioned you and made you endure?" Clearly, the biblical answer is yes.

Harold Bloom makes the apt observation that "the preferred biblical way of representing an object is to explain *how it was made*." Bloom is thinking here of such objects as the Ark of the Covenant, the Tabernacle, the Temple, and Solomon's Palace—"stories of how they were built constitute depiction."[7] But it makes sense to include *'adam* in this list of objects since a story of how (and that) he was made is precisely the J-writer's way of depicting him.[8] Adam's secondariness thereby becomes doubly evident: even after the earth exists, he is fashioned by God, initially, as a sort of figurine (perhaps anticipating the Decalogue's idea of a "sculptured image" [Exodus 20:4], the making of which, as we shall see, will be prohibited to the Israelites themselves); and only after that first making does God create "a living being" by adding the "breath of life." It is God who makes and it is God who grants life, and these tasks are his alone in his role as creator. In short, Genesis 2:4–7 shows us that we are not our own authors because we are ever belated in relation to an origin that derives uniquely from God's creative power.

Though not immediately obvious, this discovery is also one of the crucial lessons of Genesis 3, at least if Genesis 3 is read as part of a single continuous story with Genesis 2 (together comprising the opening of the J-narrative). Genesis 3, of course, focuses on death. The human couple's (and thus also the reader's) discovery of mortality is linked to their (and our) discovery that we are not God/gods; we are not like them and that is why we die. But what is here registered as the problem of having an end shows itself as inseparable from the problem of having a beginning: the recognition recorded in Genesis 2 that we are first created. In other words, the discovery of both necessities—a beginning and an end—includes the recognition that we are not, as Milton puts it in *De Doctrina Christiana*, "self-existent" (VI, 218, 263). As we saw in the study's introduction, Emerson states that our "discovery we have made that we exist"—the Fall itself—"comes too late to be helped." But, as we also saw, the "when" of that discovery is inextricably bound up with its "what" because the discovery we make is precisely of our inescapable belatedness. We must die because we have been brought into being afterwards. And the single story running through Genesis 2–3 teaches us that this is so because, whatever we might have thought, we were never gods.

Just in case we might have missed it, this point is consistently stressed in the so-called Primeval History (Genesis 1–11, up to the call of Abraham). Made in the image and likeness of God in Genesis 1:26–28, humankind might appear almost too godlike, too much like the creator. So the repetition of Genesis 1:26–28 in Genesis 9:6–7 provides some necessary clarification:

> For in his image
> Did God make man.
> Be fertile, then, and increase; abound on the earth and increase on it.[9]

The latter verses come at the conclusion of the flood-story, which is itself conceived as another version (perhaps even a revision) of the first creation-story. Now, in the wake of God's destruction of the world, the reminder that humankind is made in God's image stands as a corrective assertion that to be made in the image of God is not the same thing as being (a) God.

The biblical emphasis on the human-divine gap is perhaps why the J-narrative, which doesn't otherwise make any reference to humankind being made in the image of God, frames its version of the flood with two brief stories that, taken together, suggest just how problematic this gap is. There is, first, the image the "sons of God" who took for themselves human wives ("daughters of men") and so begat "the heroes of old, the men of renown" (Genesis 6:1–4). After the flood, we get the story of Babel with its central image of the human-made tower, "its top in the sky" (11:4). Recontextualized within the fully redacted (post-Captivity) text, the two stories of what we might call boundary-violators call special attention to what is at stake in the flood-story: to clarify, even correct, the first creation-story by establishing beyond doubt that the human claim to have been made in the image of God must yet sustain the awareness that the gap between human and divine is unbridgeable.

Nevertheless, those two framing stories suggest a real concern on the part at least of the J-writer and perhaps of the entire Hebrew biblical tradition that human beings might imagine themselves as quasi-divine.[10] If the line of demarcation between the human and divine is precisely what the story of the Tower of Babel aims to reaffirm, the threat of violating that boundary yet provides the narrative center of the story: "The LORD came down to look at . . . the tower that man had built, and the LORD said, 'If, as one people with one language for all, this is how they have begun to act, then nothing that they may propose to do will be out of their reach'" (Genesis 11:5–6); in his *The Book of J*, David Rosenberg translates the last part of Yahweh's speaking here as, "'They conceive this between them, and it leads up *until no boundary exists* to what they will touch.'"[11] However translated, God's warning in Genesis 11 points forward to part of the Mount Sinai sequence in Exodus (both passages are from the J-narrative):

> So Yahweh descended to Mount Sinai, to the summit. He called Moses to ascend to the top. Moses climbed up and Yahweh spoke to him, "Descend, hold the people's attention: *they must not be drawn to Yahweh, to destroy boundaries.* Bursting through to see [or, "break through to the LORD to gaze"], they will fall . . . The priests and the people shall not come up, *as boundaries destroyed will be their destruction.*" (Exodus 19:21–24 in Rosenberg, 159–60; my emphases)

At once echoing the account of the building of Babel and suggesting that much more is at stake, Exodus 19 shows Yahweh as particularly obsessed with maintaining a definitive boundary between himself and, now, even his own chosen people; paradoxically, the very people he has invited to his presence cannot truly come to him. The passage in Exodus 19 hints, moreover, that the boundary might be violated by an act of seeing ("bursting through to see" or "breaking through to gaze"). We presume that this forbidden act would derive from the simple desire to see Yahweh himself, and we might then wonder if that was originally the point of the Tower in Genesis 11, to ascend to a point where human beings could *see* God. But what is the problem with seeing God?[12]

To begin to understand how and why this question is fundamental, let us briefly consider how the emerging monotheism of the ancient Israelites articulated itself against the surrounding pagan world. In regard to the latter, Karen Armstrong summarizes a key moment in the Babylonian creation epic, the *Enuma Elish,* and speculates on its broader implications:

> Finally, . . . Marduk created humanity. . . . The first man [was] . . . created from the substance of a god [Kingu, the consort of Tiamat]; he therefore shared the divine nature, in however limited a way. There was no gulf between human beings and the gods. The natural world, men and women and the gods

themselves all shared the same nature and derived from the same divine substance. The pagan vision was holistic. The gods were not shut off from the human race in a separate ontological sphere: divinity was not essentially different from humanity.[13]

The corollary to this argument is that Hebrew monotheism, slowly developing as it was and, in its earliest phases, not always distinct from paganism, was not holistic in this sense. Hebrew monotheism, that is, *did* see a gulf between human beings and God (or even the gods—Yahweh and El or, the plural, *Elohim*) and so viewed divinity as "essentially different from humanity." Robert Alter argues for this very different vision as central to what he calls the "monotheistic revolution" in observing that "the whole spectrum of biblical thought presupposes an absolute cleavage between man and God, man cannot become God and God (in contrast to later Christian development) does not become man."[14] We shall have reason to return to this issue several times in what follows. But for now we might simply challenge part of Alter's assertion. For it is not clear at all that the "*whole spectrum* of biblical thought presupposes" such an "absolute cleavage." Looking forward in history, Alter makes reference to "later Christian development" as attempting to overcome the human-divine divide, an issue we will consider in more detail in chapter 5. But much earlier Hebrew thought, perhaps more bound to its pagan roots than Alter wants to admit, could, like its child Christianity, imagine that divide somewhat more ambivalently.

Indeed, like the word "uncanny," the verb "to cleave" links together two opposed meanings in one concept: to separate and to cling together. Keeping that duality in mind, we might better understand the Hebrew-monotheistic "cleavage between man and God" as a border-event at once marking human separation from God and hinting at a certain permeability at the boundary-point. To suggest, as Alter does, that Jesus as the Christ challenges a discursive division previously established in Hebrew monotheism (and in that sense Christianity would mark a partial return to paganism) might be only to acknowledge that the Christ-figure embodies the paradox inherent in cleaving, a paradox that, in subtle ways, had always been part, even if only a repudiated part, of Hebrew monotheism. In the gospel tradition, of course, Jesus is the *son* of God and, in John's gospel at least, was "with God" from "the beginning," mysteriously co-eternal with this father-god or even, as later Christian tradition would put it, of one substance with him. That said, the brief account in Genesis 6 of the "sons of God" siring children at once anticipates the Christ-figure (including the shared notion of "daughters of men" acting as divine receptacles) and reveals a remnant of the early Israelites' more openly pagan orientation. And both 2 Samuel 7 and Psalm 2 (to take two obvious later examples) imagine David as Yahweh's son. Finally, the post-captivity Book of Job portrays Satan (actually *the* Satan) as among the "sons of God" (Job 1:6) whatever the human Job's own very radical distance from his creator. Those who are God's sons may not be precisely gods themselves (though John is clearly wavering on this point as would later Gnostics), but such sons are yet *affiliated* (*filius/filial*) with God: they cleave to (with or against) God as sons to their father. We might argue against Alter, then, that the "cleavage between man and God" is a site of ambivalence or, conversely, that an "*absolute* cleavage" in this relationship (full distinction or separation) is precisely what Hebrew-monotheistic discourse must both invent and invest with authority. And it must do so because the Hebrew God's status as father to his creature-sons means that some part of creation is, mysteriously, at once god and not-god, at once separate and inseparable from what, in John's terms at least, is there from "the beginning."

What forms does such invention take? Two examples will have to suffice: the first, the continuation of the Exodus 19 passage we have just considered, and the second from the Priestly tradition as recorded in the following book, Leviticus. Both examples, I suggest, need to be understood as at once expressions of and compensations for an ambivalence concerning the human relationship to God and in particular an ambivalence concerning the nature of origins themselves.

Consider, then, the opening of the first account of the giving of the Decalogue at Sinai (Exodus 20:2–6):

> ²I the LORD am your God who brought you out of the land of Egypt, the house of bondage: ³You shall have no other gods besides Me. ⁴You shall not make for yourself a sculptured image, or any likeness of what is in the heavens above, or on the earth below, or in the waters under the earth. ⁵ᵃYou shall not bow down to them or serve them. ⁵ᵇFor I the LORD your God am an impassioned God, visiting the guilt of the fathers upon the children, upon the third and upon the fourth generations of those who reject Me, ⁶but showing kindness to the thousandth generation to those who love Me and keep My commandments.[15]

Verses 4–6, the statement of and commentary on the second commandment, are especially curious.[16] How should we understand the connection they make between the commandment itself (vv. 4–5a) and everything that comes after the explanatory or contextualizing "For"—Hebrew *Ki* (vv. 5b–6). The commandment itself makes some sense both because it follows the first commandment's more general prohibition against worshipping other gods besides Yahweh (more literally, having other gods before his face) and because it lays the conceptual framework for the Golden Calf story later in the Sinai sequence (Exodus 32): freed for a short time from Moses's leadership, the Israelites immediately violate the second commandment by offering sacrifices to the molten calf that Aaron had cast for them. (The calf is an example of precisely the sort of idol or sculptured image Exodus 20:4–5 prohibits.[17]) The NRSV's translation of the Hebrew *pessel* as "idol" (translated above as "sculptured image" but more famously in the King James Version as "graven image") makes the point unmistakable: we are dealing here with the threat of idolatry, a violation that over time will come to rouse the Israelite imagination to fits of indignation and loathing more typically reserved in the signifying universes of other cultures for instances of sexual deviance.

We might at first think that the commentary on the commandment (vv. 5b–6) makes sense precisely in that context, or rather, that the commentary supplies the clarifying context. Why should the Israelites not bow down before images that they have themselves "sculpted" (before the idols they have made)? *Because* Yahweh is an "impassioned God," or, as the King James Version has it, a "jealous God." But why then do verses 5b–6 not appear after verse 3 ("You shall have no other gods besides Me"), where Yahweh's jealousy would make at least as much if not more sense? After all, he has more reason to be jealous of the worship of actual other gods than to be jealous of mere images. In what sense should he be jealous of a fabricated golden calf rather than of, say, Baal or Dagon or Astarte?

The more implicit concern of the second commandment appears to be something other than idolatry itself. Indeed, the prohibition against making any "sculptured image (*pessel*) or any likeness (*temounah*) of what is in the heavens above, or on the earth below, or in the waters under the earth" appears to give special (negative) emphasis to the human capacity to make images. One might wonder if the phrase "what is in the heavens above" refers not just to birds or clouds or the sun but even, if not especially, to Yahweh himself. Although the commandment does not explicitly forbid the making of an image of the one true God, that prohibition is certainly implied even though such an act would not technically be idolatry in the sense articulated in the first commandment (v. 3). And if depictions of Yahweh himself are forbidden as surely they are, we might then imagine that the deeper concern of the second commandment is less that we might make an image of God than that we might be led thereby to understand God *as* an image.

There are several corollaries to this concern. The first might simply be that to represent Yahweh as an image is tantamount to restricting him, to understand him as something fixed in space and locatable at a specific time and so bounded or limited by space and time.[18] In that context, it is possible that the real purpose of verses 5b–6 is less to warn that God is jealous or mark how God might respond in his jealous state (visiting guilt over many generations) than to distinguish how he is *not* to be encountered (in an image/as an image) from how he *is* to be encountered. Alter is no doubt correct in saying that the "God of Israel . . . is above all the God of history," and Bloom similarly reminds us, somewhat more pessimistically, that "the Hebrew Bible commands the Jews to remember, because its God is primarily 'the God of your fathers, the God of Abraham, Isaac, and Jacob,' known only through his historical self-revelations."[19] We shall return to this insight in a moment, but for now we might note that, especially with the recognition that the Temple could be destroyed—but undoubtedly something of this understanding existed in the very beginnings of Israelite religion—Judaism came to privilege memory and time over seeing and space, and so also privileged corresponding modes of temporal representation: history, genealogy, prose narrative, and interpretation, modes that were appropriately open to change, debate, evolution, non-fixity. In that context, God's self-proclaimed jealousy in Exodus 20:5 might simply be a reminder that the divine presence can only be experienced as it unfolds in and through time, something that is to be registered not spatially but temporally, not with the eye but with the memory, especially that communal memory that extends even to the thousandth generation.

But if Jewish culture and its corresponding consciousness eventually learned how to experience God in that temporally mediated form, in Exodus 20 the people of Israel must be warned not to attempt to encounter God in other ways, ways we might imagine as preferable or desirable, perhaps even dangerously so. Exodus 19:21 depicts God giving voice to that danger: not just a risk to the Israelites who might "burst through to see" him but some threat to himself, the risk of being seen by them. And the boundary God literally sets there (19:23) becomes, in the next chapter, codified in and as Law. That is, the Israelites are prohibited from making images even of the one true God because even an image of him might encourage them to believe that they could see him or, perhaps more to the point, that they could cross the separating gulf he had so carefully established. Part of the issue must be that to be able to make images of God—to see

Yahweh himself *as* an image—is to set up humankind as rival image-makers: if God makes *'adam* in his image and likeness (Genesis 1) or if God can fashion *'adam* as a kind of statue (Genesis 2), then *'adam's* ability to turn God into an image or statue (perhaps in *'adam's* own image and likeness) makes humankind "like" God. Becoming like god(s) is precisely what the closing verses of Genesis 3 worry about and why Adam and Eve must be expelled from the garden.

The prohibition, then, tells us very little about the worship of other gods—idolatry in the traditional sense—and much more about the fear that Israelites, like their pagan neighbors (and undoubtedly their own pagan ancestors) might worship themselves or at least view themselves as fundamentally inseparable from the gods. In its most primal sense, the making of images of God wouldn't just permit the people to see God but would also permit them to see themselves seeing God: in turning God into an idol, they would be able to witness the process by which their seeing of God became possible. What must be rejected at the very the beginning of the Law is the possibility that God's chosen people might put themselves in the place of God. Bursting through to see him, they would also see that they too were present at the beginning, perhaps before God himself and thus claiming a kind of temporal priority. The concern that is raised in Exodus 19—a reversal of the chronology of creation as recorded in Genesis 1–2—must then become subject to law-giving in Exodus 20, an act that will at once invent an "absolute cleavage between man and God" and invest it with an authority that places it beyond scrutiny.[20]

This notion of authority is precisely how Leon Wieseltier understands what comes after Exodus, the Book of the Law we know as Leviticus. But for Wieseltier, the determining feature of Leviticus is that Law becomes expressive, indeed the central symbolic enactment, of Jewish tradition itself. More to the point, the emergence of tradition must be understood as the culmination of the invention of Alter's human-divine cleavage but now as a concept that will take on an explicitly temporal form.

About tradition generally, Wieseltier argues that "for the Jew, the idea of tradition holds a consolation for the loss of immediacy, or at least the immediacy of the founding illumination."[21] There is in this sense of tradition a simultaneous acknowledgment of loss and a consolation for it, with "tradition" taking on both psychosocial functions simultaneously. Observing that Judaism "is based on a revelation that is over," Wieseltier goes on to describe how the loss of immediacy must confront what we might call the "past-ness" of the past: "[T]he faith of the Jew is premised upon the denial of contemporaneity with revelation. . . . Coming too late, the Jew detests time. He attempts to abolish it. Naturally, it is not abolished. . . . Coming too late, he has nothing but time. History is oxygen for Jews. It is the essential environment for a faith that calls itself a transmission" (28–29). In short, the loss of immediacy at the foundation of Judaism (Wieseltier calls Leviticus "the origin" of Judaism [38]) is inseparable from the experience of belatedness—a *coming too late*—it can never escape.[22]

As a mode of compensation, Wieseltier suggests that Jewish ritual practice in particular aims to counter the lost immediacy of revelation precisely through the "abolition of time," "planned disruption[s] within a highly organized commitment to temporality" (27–28). The extended example he offers is the climactic moment of the priestly anointing in Leviticus 8–9, where Moses's and Aaron's (and Aaron's sons') meticulous adherence to the prescribed rules for the burnt offering culminates in the immediacy of God's self-revelation in the consuming fire (9:22–24). But his example *par excellence* for what he calls the "re-creation of contemporaneity" is "that theater of the recovery of experience . . . known as the Passover seder" (27). Wieseltier consistently suggests that, in opposition to later rabbinical commentary which can at best offer a sort of record of a now lost simultaneity of God and his people, scripture itself enacts something akin to a full revelatory immediacy.[23] In that context, however, it is especially noteworthy that Wieseltier refers here to the actual *ritual* of the seder and not to the account of Passover provided in Exodus. For what we cannot help but notice in the text of Exodus 12 is just how much Jewish tradition carries the burden of its own afterwardsness even in what may be its most powerful attempt to reclaim its origin.

The actual story of the Passover is inseparable from the recounting of the construction of the very ritual that will later commemorate it. Exodus 12 does, of course, offer the basic narrative of the events of Passover, including the meal eaten in advance of the coming plague and the Israelites' subsequent departure from Egypt:

> This is how you shall eat it; your loins girded, your sandals on your feet, and your staff in your hand; and you shall eat hurriedly. It is the Passover of the LORD. For I will pass through the land of Egypt, and I will strike down every firstborn in the land of Egypt, both human beings and animals; on all the gods of Egypt I will execute judgments: I am the LORD. The blood shall be a sign for you on the houses where you live: when I see the blood, I will pass over you, and no plague shall destroy you when I strike the land of Egypt. . . . Then Moses called all

the elders of Israel and said to them, "Go, select lambs for your families, and slaughter the Passover lamb. Take a bunch of hyssop, dip it in the blood that is in the basin, and touch the lintel and the two doorposts with the blood of the basin. None of you shall go outside the door of your house until morning. For the LORD will pass through to strike down the Egyptians; when he sees the blood on the lintel and on the two doorposts, the LORD will pass over that door and will not allow the destroyer to enter houses to strike you down." . . . The Israelites went and did just as the LORD commanded Moses and Aaron. At midnight the LORD struck down all the firstborn in the land of Egypt . . . Pharaoh arose in the night . . . He summoned Moses and Aaron in the night and said, "Rise up, go away from my people, both you and the Israelites! Go, worship the LORD, as you said. Take your flocks and your herds, as you said, and begone!["] . . . The length of time that the Israelites had lived in Egypt was four hundred thirty years. At the end of four hundred thirty years, on that very day, all the companies of the LORD went out from the land of Egypt. (Exodus 12:11–13, 21–23, 28–32, 40–41)

Yet interspersed with and in many ways mediating that narrative are the instructions about what the account calls the "perpetual ordinance" to be observed *in the future*, even including how this new festival will come to mark the calendrical organization of time:

The LORD said to Moses and Aaron in the land of Egypt: This month shall mark for you the beginning of months; it shall be the first month of the year for you. Tell the whole congregation of Israel that on the tenth of this month they are to take a lamb for each family. . . . You shall keep it until the fourteenth day of this month; then the whole assembled congregation of Israel shall slaughter it at twilight. . . . This day shall be a day of remembrance for you. You shall celebrate it as a festival to the LORD; throughout your generations you shall receive it as a perpetual ordinance. Seven days you shall eat unleavened bread [etc.] . . . You shall observe this rite as a perpetual ordinance for you and your children. When you come to the land that the LORD will give you, as he promised, you shall keep this observance. And when your children ask you, "What do you mean by this observance?" you shall say, "It is the Passover sacrifice to the LORD, for he passed over the houses of the Israelites in Egypt, when he struck down the Egyptians but spared our houses." (12:1–6, 14–15, 24–27)

We earlier noted Bloom's observation that "the preferred biblical way of representing an object is to explain how it was made." Here, we might say, the account of the original Passover is shown simultaneously explaining the process by which Passover will be (re)made as a ritual. In other words, the biblical story of Passover doesn't recount the event so much as describe how immediacy can only be repeated as ritual reenactment. Biblical Passover, then, is the record of an immediacy that is mediated by time: it is no longer the original event of God's presence to the people of Israel but the record of the process by which a future people will only ever be able to commemorate an event in relation to which they will always come after. In this context, tradition emerges both as compensation and as a way of giving voice to nostalgia as the pained recognition of the elusiveness of "a past without end" (Wieseltier, 38).[24]

Celebrating normative Judaism as he does, Alter reads the "absolute cleavage between man and God" as a simple *recognition of* rather than as a *resignation to* that carries its own existential cost. What Wieseltier calls the "apotheosis of alterity" within normative Judaism—"separation [from God]" as "the condition of meaning"—is now also the "deeper objective of the Law" and, more broadly, of the tradition expressed through the Law. In this context, Wieseltier concludes, "the creation and the regulation of structure are how man imitates God" (36). Such spiritual imitation, *mere* imitation, is but a pale version of an original glory, humankind's creation in the image and likeness of God. But in the movement from paganism to monotheism, Jewish tradition first confronts and then invents as spiritual consolation what it cannot deny: "the gulf that separates that world from this world" (Wieseltier, 33). Law first in Exodus; Law becoming tradition in Leviticus: both are sites of ambivalence within Israelite-Jewish consciousness. And, as ambivalence, Law and tradition simultaneously articulate the desire to violate a boundary (one that can never truly be violated) and defend against that desire.

That said, the desire to violate still exists. In the Hebrew Bible this (under)current of hostility comes out, among other ways, in the desire to burst through to see God. That desire (Wieseltier calls it a "longing" [32]) still seeks ways to be where God is (to touch, to see: a primal seeing or scene), to overcome, even reverse, one's belatedness in relation to that "past without end." In his most optimistic mood, Wieseltier imagines that tradition might point the way, for "it ensures," he argues, "that those who come after are those who come before, that the inheritors are also the bequeathers." To the extent tradition, paradoxically, can look more to the future than to the past ("the future," Wieseltier observes, "not the past, is the term of Jewish desire") it also has the "ironic consequence of restoring the Jew to a position of priority, of coming before" (28). But such "coming before" is precisely desire or mere fantasy: Jewish consciousness can never be *restored* "to a position of priority" because it was never there to begin with. In relation to their own faith-experience, the people of Israel are ever belated in relation to their origin.

Of course, against the consolation of tradition in which "the sons are also the fathers," there yet stand other sons who refuse tradition and its consolation, the "impatient son" or the son who is not obedient (Wieseltier, 28, 37), the son who longs not merely to imitate but to stand with or perhaps even in the place of the father, at the origin. Even within Judeo-Christianity, there are thus less orthodox responses to loss, ones less given to spiritual subordination and its resignation to afterwardsness. Read in relation to the Tower of Babel and the theophany at Sinai, Christianity's complex (late) relation to normative Judaism might suggest that such heresy (the desire/the longing) goes underground only to resurface when conditions are right. The site, more temporal than spatial, that John's Gospel associates with the overcoming of human-divine cleavage is especially significant in this regard: it is precisely "in the beginning"—the point of origin itself—where a father-son (re)union is possible.

John tells us almost nothing about the son's/Son's status "in the beginning," though this is clearly a beginning that comes before the beginning recorded in Genesis 1:1. (Wieseltier calls this time "pre-Biblical," the " 'was' before the beginning," whereas the Hebrew Bible "begins 'in the beginning' " (31).] But John does suggest some things: for example, the divine son created the world ("Through him all things were made" [1:3]). Still, within most versions of what eventually will become orthodox Christianity (John both initiates and represents a rival tradition of sorts), even the "divine son" Jesus must acknowledge the father's priority and thus his own continuing subordination. But there will be other sons even more heretical within the tradition. Jesus performs the father's will, but that other son, Satan, rebels: the son's ambivalence toward the father breaks out as violence, a doomed act but all the more instructive for its very illogic.

In Milton's casting of such filial ambivalence in *Paradise Lost*, the focus of the next chapter, the son-problem (Satan's problem) is the mere existence of the father who creates, even as the poem's angel-prophet, Abdiel, mockingly asks that same question from Deuteronomy 32:6: "Is not He the Father who created you?" But Satan will not answer in the affirmative; instead, he rebels. And that violence is an expression, as Sartre rightly recognized, of "the refusal to be born." Satan's problem, that is, is the problem of the origin itself or, more precisely, the problem of having an origin from which, paradoxically, he was absent.

In creating Satan's story in *Paradise Lost*, Milton will accept the evangelist John's core idea of the "'was' before the beginning" and expand beyond it. In doing so, he will both draw on and freely invent within the broader Christian tradition as formulated by Augustine and others.[25] In that sense, Milton attempts to assume "a position of priority, to come before." But the true beginning he locates and by which he endeavors to place himself before tradition is the ambiguously presented begetting of the Son in Book 5, a moment that, in its very concealments, reveals that sons of God can never come to the place where God creates because that place resides in a past without end. As much as Milton will show the fantasy at the heart of Satan's rebellion, the hostility to the creator (to the true original whose authority/*auctoritas* is something we can never claim) is thus Milton's own. He too is the belated son who, even in imagination, can never quite catch up. It is to *Paradise Lost*'s depiction of that failure that we now turn.

5

Satan's Gnostic Fantasy

> [T]o Adam, formed out of the dust, God was creator rather than Father; but he was in real sense Father of the Son, whom he made of his own substance. It does not follow, however, that the Son is of the same essence as the Father. Indeed, if he were, it would be quite incorrect to call him Son. For a real son is not of the same age as his father . . . : otherwise, father and son would be one person.
>
> —Milton, *De Doctrina Christiana*

> We do not share the belief of some investigators that myths were read in the heavens and brought down to earth; we are more inclined to judge . . . that they were projected on to the heavens after have arisen elsewhere under purely human conditions. It is in this human content that our interest lies.
>
> —Freud, "Theme of the Three Caskets"

I

Although the focus of this chapter will be Milton's portrait of the great fallen angel, Satan, I begin with a brief reflection on *human* experience, a passage from St. Augustine's *On Free Choice of the Will*:

> The following question . . . troubles those who consider it: "Was it by folly that the first man departed from God, or was the first man made foolish by his departure from God?" This is troublesome, because if you answer that it was by his folly that

he departed from wisdom, it appears that he was subject to folly
before he departed from wisdom, so that his folly was the cause
of his departure. Likewise, if you reply that he became subject
to folly by departing from God, they will inquire whether it was
through folly or through wisdom that he departed.[1]

Brutally oversimplifying, we might say that Augustine is troubled by this paradox: humankind might have been fallen before it was fallen. Clearly the same question could be posed of angelic experience: were Satan and his cohort already fallen before their fall?

Augustine revisits the problem of the fallen angels many times over his writing career, and he has no single answer. At various points, he merely pleads tradition in attributing the cause of Satan's fall, as any sin, to pride:

> If, however, [a spirit] . . . is satisfied with itself, seeking to imitate God in a perverse way, so that it wills to delight in its own power—if the spirit takes this road, the more it desires to be greater, the less it becomes. Thus, "Pride is the root of all sin; and the root of pride is apostasy from God" [Ecclesiasticus 10:14–15]. (*On Free Choice of the Will*, III.25.262–63)

As Augustine himself recognizes at times, however, this position merely begs the question: was a preexisting inclination toward pride already a mark of Satan's fallenness, especially if the unfallen angels did not share this pride? Augustine's continuation of the passage just quoted—"but to the pride of the devil *was added* a most malevolent ill will and envy" (my emphasis)—and his references elsewhere to "defect[s]" and "flaw[s]" in the "nature" of the fallen angels force us to wonder at the cause of the fallen angels' "malevolent will" and of their desire "to be greater."[2] Were not their will and desire part of how they were created? And is God not responsible for creating that will and instilling that desire in the first place?

Augustine is clearly sensitive to the problems of his own argument. In *City of God*, for example, he will observe with some defensiveness that, exemplifying the ontological status of evil in general, the presence of evil will among the fallen angels simply has no cause, at least none that the human mind can grasp:

> No matter how thoroughly we examine the matter, . . . we can discover nothing which caused the particular will of one of them to be evil. . . . Let no one, then, seek an efficient cause for an

evil will. For its cause is not efficient, but deficient, because the evil will itself is not an effect of something . . . Now to seek for causes of these defections, which are, as I have said, not efficient causes, but deficient, is like wishing to see darkness or hear silence. . . . Let no one, then, seek to know from me what I know that I do not know; unless, perhaps, he wishes to learn how not to know that which he should know cannot be known. For those things which are known not by their appearance, but by their lack of it, are known . . . only by not knowing them. (XII.6–7)

The convoluted phrasing here bespeaks Augustine's frustration: he cannot come up with an argument to exonerate God from the charge that he is the true cause of the evil of his creatures. But it is clearly disingenuous to argue that "the evil will is not an effect of something" when, especially in the case of angels, that will seems precisely to be the effect of God's purposeful creative act.

Whether Milton the theologian might have found Augustine's abstract speculation persuasive, Milton the storyteller finds Augustine's paired notions—Satan's fall has no cause and/or we simply cannot grasp it intellectually—quite unacceptable.[3] In fact, Milton is so determined to dig out *the* cause of Satan's fall that, in terms of the narrative of *Paradise Lost*, he overdetermines it. More to the point, as we shall see in more detail, for Milton cause is virtually synonymous with motive, and, at the risk of sounding anachronistic here, I would suggest that the probing of motive for Milton (as indeed for Milton's great mentor in such matters, Shakespeare) necessarily entails a sort of proto-psychologizing—that is, exploring the interior state of consciousness prompting speech or conduct. Milton will thus effectively psychologize Satan's experience as later he will psychologize the experience of Adam and Eve, the latter portraits to a certain extent modeled on the former.

To the extent he would have recognized his own narrative tendencies, Milton undoubtedly would have imagined that psychological investigations of fallenness served the end of higher theological speculation and argument. But, following the Freudian logic of this chapter's second epigraph, I would like to reverse Milton's priorities—the privileging of the theological over the psychological—to suggest, as part III of my study aims to demonstrate more broadly, that Judeo-Christian thought often bears the mark of displaced psychological or psychoanalytic concepts.[4] In the case of Milton's Satan, one might, for example, view his fall through the lens of a psychoanalytically-conceived notion of trauma, with all that comes after the fall as a post-traumatic condition.⁵ Or, we might understand Satan's rebellion—a son's rebellion against an all-powerful father—as caught up in the same problem of filial ambivalence that, as we saw in part II, vexes Shakespeare's Hamlet and Freud himself. In that context, Satan's rebellion might be seen as at once an overt act of hostility, an expression of identification with a hated-and-beloved rival, and a defense mechanism against his own helplessness.

In the effort to align Milton and Freud, two of the previously quoted Augustinian statements about Satan's fall are particularly useful. First, caught up as he is in his own uncertainty (his "not knowing"), Augustine effectively argues that, when it comes to the question of the origins of evil, there is some fundamental lack or deficiency in the human mind's capacity to understand the very notion of a first cause: "Now to seek causes of these defections [toward evil] . . . is like wishing to see darkness or hear silence." In short, to seek to arrive at a knowledge of what is effectively the origin of human experience as we do know it is necessarily to come up against absence ("darkness," "silence," what "cannot be known," "lack," "not knowing"). But, as this chapter will try to demonstrate, the origin of Satanic evil as mysteriously immersed in absence becomes, in Milton's telling at least, less a problem of our not knowing what sets Satan against God than it is the problem of the origin itself as the site from which the act of knowing is always already absent. In other words, Milton (re)presents the Augustinian problem of uncertainty regarding the *cause of evil* as the problem of the knower's inescapable deficiency—seeing darkness, hearing silence—in regard to its own cause, the cause of its very existence. Following the logic of another son traumatized by "deficiency" with regard to his origin (Hoffmann's Nathanael), we might say that the cause of evil as depicted by Milton in *Paradise Lost* is the son's experience of the uncanny. For, like Nathanael, Milton's Satan belatedly encounters an unknowable origin, an origin in relation to which he necessarily comes too late.

The second Augustinian observation of special note involves what we might call a symptom of the uncanny (at least of the filial ambivalence that derives from the uncanny). While in quoting from Ecclesiasticus 10:15 he employs the tautology that "the root of pride is apostasy from God," Augustine prefaces that biblical quotation with the more subtle observation that, in its apostasy, the fallen consciousness more specifically "seek[s] to imitate God in a perverse way . . . so that it will delight in its own power." I would like to suggest that this effort to imitate God will be narrated in *Paradise Lost* as an enactment after-the-fact, an effect of that fallenness described in the passage from Emerson's "Experience" we have previously encountered: "It is very unhappy, but too late to be helped, the discovery we have made that we exist. That discovery is called the Fall of Man." As we shall see, what Augustine portrays as a creature's "delighting" in its "own power" becomes, in Milton's portrayal of Satan, a creaturely way of coping with the Emersonian "too late." Satan's divine imitation, in short, is at once a belated response (it comes *after* something else) and a response by which Satan (as symbol of all of God's disaffected sons) defends against the discovery, as Milton puts it in *De Doctrina Christiana*, that "a being who is not self-existent cannot be a God" (VI, 218). As a proto-psychoanalytic revision of Augustine's account of the unknowable origins of evil, Milton's poem portrays precisely what Augustine cannot conceptualize, the cause of Satan's fall. The poem offers this cause as what we might call the Ur-primal scene: the son's recognition that what is not God can only exist in the divine afterwards. Satan's "seeking to imitate God" may be as futile as it is perverse, but, as Milton imagines it, this failed effort is precisely Satan's fantasy of his own priority, the fantasy, that is, of putting himself in the very place of his creator. If this act is pathetic it is also tragic in the way Stanley Cavell understands that term: "tragedy is the result . . . of a burden of knowledge, of an attempt to deny the all but undeniable."[6] In what follows, I will try to demonstrate that, as a model for the human fall, the experience of Milton's Satan is at once an attempt to deny what cannot be denied—his own status as a creature—and the discovery of the inescapable condition of his own belatedness.

II

> say first what cause
> Mov'd our Grand Parents in that happy State,
> Favour'd of Heav'n so highly, to fall off
> From thir Creator, and transgress his Will
> . . .
> Who first seduc'd them to that foul revolt? (1.28–33)

The narrator of Milton's *Paradise Lost* asks this question at the opening of Book 1. The full answer, extended over the poem as a whole, will be developed in substantially greater and subtler detail. But here, there is a single, simple answer to the question: the "infernal Serpent" (1.34), Satan. As we saw earlier in regard to Augustine's reflections, however, that answer merely begs another question: if Satan is the cause of Adam and Eve's fall, who, or what, caused his?

There is certainly no shortage of motivation in Milton's account of Satan's fall. If we judged simply from Book 1, and if we accepted Satan's own claims on the matter, we might say that his fall was motivated by a political decision: his courageous, if doomed, determination to stand against the "Tyranny of Heav'n" (1.124). The poem, of course, will problematize the heroic, republican Satan in a number of ways. One of the most intriguing of these, if not the most obvious, comes in the only prelapsarian portrait we get of Satan, the unexpected image provided by Gabriel at the end of Book 4:

> And thou sly hypocrite, who now wouldst seem
> Patron of liberty, who more then thou
> Once fawn'd, and cring'd, and servilly ador'd
> Heav'ns awful Monarch? (4.957–60)

Brief as it is, Gabriel's account is certainly surprising, for it leads us to believe that, at some unspecified point in the past, Satan was not particularly bothered by God's tyranny. Even if, as we suspect, Satan is lying in Book 1 about his republican sentiments, we still need to ask what motivates his shift from cringing adorer of God to self-proclaimed rebel against a tyrant or, as Gabriel appears to believe, to one who wants to replace God and become the grand tyrant himself ("wherefore but in hope / To dispossess him [God], and thy self to reigne? [4.960–61]).

We might pause for a moment to notice the rhetorical design of Gabriel's lines. They are structured to achieve their chief effect by surprising us (that is, they surprise the reader rather than Satan). The lines generate an expectation that Gabriel's exposing of Satan's hypocritical self-representation as "Patron of liberty" will lead to a fuller examination of Satan's motive for rebellion: that it was actually motivated by his desire to rule the cosmos himself. The image of Satan the would-be sultan that opens Book 2 has already provided sufficient evidence of this possibility, and more will be provided in Books 5 and 6 in Raphael's account of the rebellion. Under the circumstances, we would not be shocked to discover that Satan had found it difficult to keep this desire hidden. That is, his ambition to reign in heaven might have been manifest in his prelapsarian conduct and perfectly obvious to such an astute angel as Gabriel. But if that is what the lines lead us to expect, they manage to create meaning by defying our expectation. For what we discover, instead, is that Satan is a hypocrite in rebelling against

God because, at that unspecified point in the past, not only did he accept but, apparently, he even endorsed divine despotism.

A similar rhetorical surprise has come earlier in Book 4 in the soliloquy in which Satan self-consciously reflects on his various motives for rebelling against God. Here is part of that soliloquy:

> Ah wherefore! he deservd no such return
> From me, whom he created what I was
> In that bright eminence, and with his good
> Upbraided none; nor was his service hard.
> What could be less then to afford him praise,
> The easiest recompence, and pay him thanks,
> How due! yet all his good prov'd ill in me,
> And wrought but malice; lifted up so high
> I sdeind [disdained] subjection, and thought one step higher
> Would set me highest.... (4.42–51)

Before looking more carefully at the rhetorical play of this passage, we might simply ask why one who previously had so obsequiously fawned over, cringed before, and adored God would *now* want to be placed above him ("set . . . highest"). If Satan is motivated primarily by his own tyrannical ambitions, the lines in the soliloquy make sense—deposing God is necessary to that end—but they would fail to explain Satan's earlier relationship to God, at least as that relationship is described by Gabriel later in Book 4.

The first part of the soliloquy offers one possible solution to this conundrum, that Satan's rebellion is motivated primarily by envy against the Son:

> Sometimes towards *Eden* which now in his view
> Lay pleasant, his grievd looks he fixes sad,
> Sometimes towards Heav'n and the full-blazing Sun,
> Which now sat high in his Meridian Towre:
> Then much revolving, thus in sighs began.
> O thou that with surpassing Glory crownd,
> Look'st from thy sole Dominion like the God
> Of this new World; at whose sight all the Starrs
> Hide thir diminisht heads: to thee I call,
> But with no friendly voice, and add thy name
> O Sun, to tell thee how I hate thy beams

> That bring to my remembrance from what state
> I fell, how glorious once above thy Spheare . . . (4.27–39)

As something akin to sibling rivalry, Satan's envy would largely be unconscious; hence, his cathexis is here transferred by a pun from the actual object of his feelings to a substitute: from Son to sun. The elevation of the Son to a position of special eminence in the heavenly court, what Milton understands as the begetting of the divine son described in Psalm 2, is narrated by Raphael to Adam as the first event in his celestial chronicle:

> Hear my decree, which unrevok't shall stand.
> This day I have begot whom I declare
> My onely Son, and on this holy Hill
> Him have anointed, whom ye now behold
> At my right hand; your Head I him appoint;
> And my Self have sworn to him shall bow
> All knees in Heav'n, and shall confess him Lord:
> Under his great Vice-gerent Reign abide
> United as one individual Soule
> Forever happie. . . . (5.602–11)

Satan, we are immediately told, although he "seemd well pleas'd" with this change in the structure of heavenly governance, was not pleased in fact. And his distaste for the Son's "Vice-gerent Reign" will prompt the first motions of rebellion (5.657–71). Read in the context of filial envy, the political motives of Satan's rebellion might appear as an afterthought. For in this new context, the attempt to depose God makes better sense as an act of vengeance: he wants to punish God for changing what was, to his mind, a perfectly adequate arrangement. Read along with Gabriel's account of Satan's earlier attitude toward God, then, the rebellion appears to have had a motive that was at once simpler and more complex. What Satan really wanted was to topple the Son from his preeminent position in the new divine hierarchy so that he might return to his servile adoration in the role of the favorite child.[7] But if that is the case we are certainly within our rights to ask another question: if the Son were suddenly out of the picture, would Satan then be satisfied with returning to his former role as fawner-and-cringer-in-chief?

I think we would instinctively say no to this possibility in part because it is difficult for us to imagine that the Satan in Gabriel's portrait is the same being who so roused us in Book 1 as the "Patron of liberty." I would also suggest, however, that, in the Book 4 soliloquy, Milton is showing us that Satan could never return to his old relationship with God, a truth Milton unveils by offering yet another motive for Satan's rebellion, but one that offers an even deeper, more traumatic prompting for it.

We can tell that Milton wants to call attention to this other motive because of the special rhetorical play he provides in the soliloquy. For just as in the Gabriel passage I quoted earlier, a key section of Satan's soliloquy generates meaning by defying our expectation of how the statement will be completed. Note how the passage I previously quoted from the soliloquy (ending in the phrase "one step higher / Would set me highest") raises certain expectations in our minds. We are expecting that Satan will either lay bare his own tyrannical ambitions or acknowledge his jealousy toward the Son. But as we see in the lines that immediately follow he does neither:

>   . . . lifted up so high
> I sdeind subjection, and thought one step higher
> Would set me highest, *and in a moment quit*
> *The debt immense of endless gratitude,*
> *So burthensome still paying, still to ow*;
> Forgetful what from him I still receivd,
> And understood not that a grateful mind
> By owing owes not, but still pays, at once
> Indebted and dischargd; *what burden then*? (4.49–57; my emphases)

To the extent Satan is here articulating a motive for rebellion, this motive is different from any we have previously seen, and it is not obviously consistent with what will come later in the poem. Indeed, I would go so far as to say that this motive is the most profound of all Satan's conscious or unconscious motives for rebelling against God. It is such a profound motive that it is difficult to be sure that Milton is himself fully aware of it and its implications. And it is certainly impossible to determine if, from Milton's view, this motive is intended to supersede and absorb the other motives, displace them, or simply mark the fact that, psychologically speaking, the rebellion is overdetermined.

Certainly, unless Gabriel's portrait of Satan is simply wrong, it is hard to figure out if the Satan who during the Book 4 soliloquy speaks of the burden of owing God can possibly have the same attitude toward God that the Satan depicted in Gabriel's scathing denunciation (toward the close of Book 4) might have had. That is, if Satan felt about God *then* (at the point in the past alluded to by Gabriel) the way Satan feels about God *now* (in the soliloquy), then how is it conceivable that he could he have fawned over, cringed before, and servilely adored this God? This shift in attitude would only make sense if something had fundamentally changed in his relationship to God or to himself, something that would now make him understand just how "burthensome" it is to worship this God. Given what Satan is saying at the opening of Book 4, one would think that in his earlier manifestation (what is being recalled by Gabriel) he would have been more like Gabriel himself, who, in his exchange with Satan, appears rather put off by the very necessity of worship (a point we shall take up in section V). How, then, should we understand this new motive for rebellion, this sudden recognition of and reaction against the "debt immense of endless gratitude," the burden of giving thanks to God? How and why are we being encouraged to view the worship of God as a burden for an angel or for a host of angels? In what sense does this particular motive displace, supersede, absorb, or conceptually compete with all the other motives for Satan's rebellion?

III

To understand just what is at stake in Milton's representation of Satan's predicament, we might take up Harold Bloom's almost casual observation that "Milton overtly assigns to Satan a Gnostic stance." Bloom is explicitly focused on how the Gnostic Satan functions in *Paradise Lost* as an "allegory of poetic origins."[8] But because the Gnostic stance encompasses more than just Milton's fashioning of his own poetic authority, we must go beyond Bloom's suggestive intuition to get a more complete understanding of the Gnostic vision at the heart of the poem.

At its core, Gnosticism is marked by its defiance of, even a hostility toward, the traditional Judeo-Christian notion of God.[9] Primarily understood as the Old Testament Yahweh or Jehovah, though also referred to by the Greek concept of the "Demiurge" or by other names, such as "Ialdabaoth," this god stands as a kind of dark caricature of the creator-god of Genesis. The Gnostic Demiurge is not just a lesser and flawed deity but is also, and variously, conceived as wicked, corrupt, cruel, jealous, punitive, and resentful, a tyrant who rules over the scattered sparks of divinity trapped in the botched, prison-like creation we know as the material universe. Against this tyrant and against the false world he has created, the Gnostic *heretic*—etymologically, the one who has the power of moral and spiritual choice—seeks freedom in a forbidden knowledge or *gnosis* that at once challenges the Demiurge's despotic imposition of false authority and (re)claims itself through a sort of mystical liberation theology. What we thus get in Gnostic writings is a general depiction of human existence as a cosmic counter-insurgency in which, if spiritual-ontological liberation is the ultimate goal, epiphanic awareness of our current oppression marks the first act of rebellion. The imagistic and narratological corollaries of this theology include: (1) a view of the world as a hostile place (the work of that flawed, small-minded, or in some accounts simply incompetent creator-god); (2) a revisionary stance toward Genesis 3—toward the meaning of the Fall generally, the value of disobedience, the nature of both the tree of knowledge and, most especially, the serpent, which is typically reimagined as the bearer of truth against what Milton's postlapsarian Eve will call "Our great Forbidder" (9.815); and, (3) a reconceptualization of the figure of the Son of God (the Christ), who is now viewed less as redeemer in a moral sense and more as a spiritual guide or teacher who opposes the law of the oppressive father and who is thus frequently associated or even equated with the serpent of Genesis 3. Perhaps more fundamentally, *gnosis* points to an awakening to the secret that our true selves are already divine. In that context, *gnosis* can also be understood as the first step in the process of self-apotheosis. For in *gnosis*, we learn, negatively, that the gross materiality of the world is more illusory than real and, positively, that the reality to which we can return is our share in the divine that is ours by right of origin and not simply as a divine gift.[10]

A. D. Nuttall has argued that what he generalizes as "the Gnostic heresy" resides at the visionary heart of *Paradise Lost*.[11] More specifically, Nuttall sees that heresy especially embodied in the concept of the "alternative Trinity" (or, perhaps more accurately, an alternative to the Trinity) in which "the crucial factor" is the "hostility of the Son to the Father" (20), at least the Father equated with the Demiurge if not with the true God who has sent the Son in the form of Jesus to lead us back to our origin. This privileging of the redemptive Son over the tyrannical Father is particularly odd given the way Milton actually represents this relationship. For, if anything, it is Milton's Arianism that more regularly comes through in his portrait of the Son, a figure at once subordinate and dutiful to the will of the Father.

Even more surprisingly and almost inexplicably, in building this case for Milton's Arianism against the very Gnosticism he claims to uncover, Nuttall remarks that "we do not find in Milton's poem a Promethean Son, heroically antagonistic to the Father" (136). But if the "crucial factor" for Gnosticism is, as Nuttall suggests, the "hostility of the Son to the Father," and if such hostility might be expressed in a heroically conceived "Promethean Son," how can Nuttall have missed Satan's role as Gnostic adversary to the poem's Yahwistic Demiurge? In suggesting that "Milton's reason resisted the Gnostic promotion of Satan while his imagination intermittently allowed it" (143), Nuttall seems resistant himself to what the poem obviously portrays: Milton's consciousness might have resisted the Gnostic Satan at least in terms of promoting him as a model of Christian spiritual conduct and right reason, but, as Bloom is right to recognize, the Miltonic imagination more than intermittently portrays Satan in the heroic light of the Gnostic rebel. Indeed, if, even as Nuttall occasionally recognizes, the fundamental Gnostic tenet is that our true selves are already divine, Satan's filial antagonism to and his open rebellion against the creator-father are premised precisely on his imagining, fantastical as this might be, of his own existence as ontologically equal to that of the creator.

Satan's Gnosticism as both heroic stance and delusional fantasy will be the subject of the next section. Before we move on, though, I would like briefly to align Milton's Gnostic depiction of Satan more explicitly with the Freudian issues that are at the center of this study. Nuttall is no doubt correct to suggest that Gnostics "loved to travel backwards to pre-history," for "they noticed that the only way to add to a revealed text giving an account of creation was . . . to add preliminaries to the creation itself, a pre-genetic theology" (7). In their flights of fancy, Gnostic mystics thus worked "by extending their beginnings, further and further back," a "pre-Creationism" to which "Milton seems to be drawn" (169, 171). But especially as read through the lens of the son's hostility to the father who precedes him, that interest in "pre-Creationism"—a time before time, the origin of origins—might suggest how a Gnostic understanding of Milton's imaginative commitments might then also view those commitments through the perspective of the issues we have encountered in previous chapters, and in particular the son's belated recognition that, in the person of his father, the origin always already lies elsewhere.[12] Indeed, we might call the uncanny the *gnosis* of Freudian psychoanalysis itself. As we shall see in the next section, in this portrait of the tardy son, Milton draws together the past in the Judeo-Christian tradition and his own future in Freud's vexed efforts to articulate the tension between fathers and sons as one of temporal precedence: the father comes first and the son can only exist ever afterwards in the paternal shadow.

IV

Satan's argument with Abdiel in Book 5 turns precisely on his desire to assert a temporal-ontological equality with God. He will effectively manufacture this equality by refusing to acknowledge that he is even created by God:

> That we were formd then saist thou? and the work
> Of secondarie hands, by task transferd
> From Father to his Son? strange point and new!
> Doctrin which we would know whence learnt: who saw
> When this creation was? rememberst thou
> Thy making, while the Maker gave thee being?
> We know no time when we were not as now;
> Know none before us, self-begot, self-rais'd
> By our own quick'ning power. (5.853–61)[13]

Clearly, to be "self-begot, self-rais'd" would be a negation of God's monopoly on "quick'ning power," a power he will subsequently assign in Book 7 to the Son for the creation of the world (7.162–67). More to the point, as Abdiel tells the rebel angels, God has *previously* assigned this power to the Son for the purposes of creating the entire angelic host:

> Thy self thou great and glorious dost thou count,
> Or all Angelic Nature joind in one,
> Equal to him begotten Son, by whom
> As by his Word the mighty Father made
> All things, *ev'n thee, and all the Spirits of Heav'n*[.]
>   (5.833–37; my emphasis)

Despite Satan's mockery—he refers to the result of God's transfer of creative power to the Son as "the work / Of secondarie hands"—we assume that Abdiel is telling the truth here: the angels are created beings and the Son created them.[14] But is it possible that the angels had never before learned this "Doctrin"? If so, it may also be that Abdiel is here offering a kind of prophetic utterance (paradoxically, revelation aimed toward what has come before): he is inspired to reveal a truth that, moments before, even he did not know. After all, chronologically speaking, the Son's role as creator of the angels has not previously been stated in the poem, and in that sense Satan is right to observe that Abdiel's "point" is both "strange" and "new."[15]

In that context, of course, Satan's incredulity might be understandable. But his retort to Abdiel's revelation suggests a certain desperation, as though he needed to come up with a reason, no matter how far-fetched, for rejecting it:

> who saw
> When this creation was? rememberst thou
> Thy making, while the Maker gave thee being?
> We know no time when we were not as now;
> Know none before us, self-begot, self-rais'd
> By our own quick'ning power.

Obviously, it is the very condition of being created to "know no time before": by definition, one who requires a "Maker" to give "being" cannot know the before-time. The angels cannot remember their making precisely because they were not there to see it. And Satan's subsequent leap from not remembering his creation to the assertion that he was "self-begot" not only fails to show a logical connection (why should *not remembering* one's creation mean that one is self-created?) but actually contradicts itself: he does not actually remember being "self-begot" (and how could he?) any more than he can remember being created. Satan cannot be "self-begot" because that would have required a state of existence prior to his existence, the possession of "quick'ning power" before he actually possessed the life that could employ it. Abdiel's point might be "strange and new," but Satan's own experience bears it out. The point is strange because it is new, and it is new because Satan wasn't in a position to have learned it, let alone observed it, while it was happening.

Leaning on without endorsing Bloom's celebration of the Gnostic Milton, William Kerrigan has noted that, as "the poem of genesis par excellence," *Paradise Lost* is particularly obsessed with "the prolonged observation of generative acts" (158, 161). But it is important to distinguish in this context what various characters in the poem are able to observe about such acts and what they are unable to observe, a distinction that, as we shall see in a moment, applies even to the narrator's perspective. Adam, for example, calls special attention to the fact that he did not observe his own creation; thus he describes his awakening into consciousness to the angel, Raphael:

> For Man to tell how human Life began
> Is hard; for who himself beginning knew?
> . . .
> As new wak't from soundest sleep
> Soft on the flourie herb I found me laid
> In Balmie Sweat, . . .
> . . .

> Strait toward Heav'n my wondring Eyes I turnd,
> And gaz'd a while . . .
> . . .
> My self I then perus'd, and Limb by Limb
> Survey'd, . . .
> . . .
> But who I was, or where, or from what cause,
> Knew not; . . .
> . . .
> Not of my self; by some great Maker then. (8.250–78)

We might contrast that account with Adam's very different cognitive experience during the creation of Eve:

> Mine eyes he [God] clos'd, but op'n left the Cell
> Of Fancie my internal sight, by which
> Abstract as in a transe methought I saw,
> Though sleeping, where I lay, and saw the shape
> Still glorious before whom awake I stood;
> Who stooping op'nd my left side, and took
> From thence a Rib, with cordial spirits warme,
> And Life-blood streaming fresh; wide was the wound,
> But suddenly with flesh fill'd up and heal'd:
> The Rib he formd and fashond with his hands;
> Under his forming hands a Creature grew. . . . (8.460–70)

In other words, Adam can be present for, even consciously aware of, the creation of another, but he can have no recollection of how he himself came to be. He can only infer that he was made by "some great Maker" at some point in the past. And he has no memory of this event—his own beginning—because he was necessarily, if paradoxically, absent from it.[16]

A similar situation faces the unfallen Uriel, the angel stationed on the sun. In their Book 3 encounter, he tells the disguised Satan that he actually witnessed the Son's creation of the world: "I saw when at his Word the formless Mass, / This worlds material mould, came to a heap" (3.708–09). Like Adam at Eve's creation, that is, Uriel can be present for and can thus bear witness to the creation of someone or at least something else. But the immediately preceding passage anticipates the very crisis at the heart of the Satan-Abdiel debate in Book 5: a created being cannot have any direct experience of its own creation. Still speaking to the disguised Satan, Uriel comments on what remains unknowable in "the works of God":

> Fair Angel, thy desire which tends to know
> The works of God, thereby to glorifie
> The great Work-Maister, leads to no excess
> That reaches blame, but rather merits praise
> The more it seems excess, that led thee hither
> From thy Empyreal Mansion thus alone,
> To witness with thine eyes what some perhaps
> Contented with report hear onely in heav'n:
> For wonderful indeed are all his works,
> Pleasant to know, and worthiest to be all
> Had in remembrance always with delight;
> But what created mind can comprehend
> Thir number, or the wisdom infinite
> That brought them forth, but hid thir causes deep. (3.694–707)

Even on a surface level, the passage as a whole and, more particularly, its final three lines attest to some discrepancy between Uriel's witnessing of the creation of the world and his inability truly to understand it. But while Uriel doesn't seem to be consciously aware of it (or else he is simply not troubled by it), the divine creation that is incomprehensible would necessarily include his own. In other words, although Uriel can take "delight" in the memory of what he witnessed but could not fully understand in the Son's creation of the world, the passage almost insists that we imagine another of the "works of God"—that is, another of the Son's acts of creating—that Uriel does not and cannot remember because he was not present to witness: his own origin and that of his fellow angels. And that origin is less incomprehensible than it is inaccessible, for its "cause"—*his / their* cause—is "hid . . . deep." What Uriel's praise of the incomprehensibility of God's creative power at once reveals and conceals is a missing—an inability to witness—that even the reader will only be able to register later when, in Book 5, the poem returns us to the point at which the angels become aware of their belated status relative to the Son. Of course, because Uriel's praise comes a full two books before Raphael's recounting of the actual incident that triggers Satan's rebellion, we can't at this stage fully register just how much Uriel is unwittingly anticipating what will set Satan off. But the linking of creation to what will "glorifie" the "Work-Maister" rather than his creatures, the distinction between what one might "witness" in person and what one might have to be "contented . . . [to] hear onely" ("with report"), and even the difference between what one might have "in remembrance" (because one was present at an actual event from which a memory might be formed) and coming upon an situation only later (as the disguised Satan does here) and in relation to which one can, at most, only see belatedly, all call attention to how Uriel's description of something that has already happened (the creation of the world) at once foreshadows and reenacts the heart of Satan's problem. For created beings, the origin itself is not only lost forever, but its revelation after-the-fact functions to demonstrate the power and priority of the Creator.

As tardy sons, then, neither Satan nor Uriel can remember a time when they were not as now. In relation to their own origins, they must therefore be "contented with report" precisely because, in the only sense that matters, they were effectively absent from their own creations. Even if Uriel himself doesn't fully register the implications, Satan will later reveal what is hidden in Uriel's praise of God: in his debate with Abdiel, Satan encounters the afterwards in which he exists and from which none of the angels can ever escape. Like any created being who bothers to notice, Satan can only discover his condition of afterwardsness belatedly because he was brought into existence by a Maker in relation to which he necessarily comes after.[17]

For the angels, then, we move from asking how it is possible for them not to know that they were created (and created by the Son) to wondering how they could have known what they were never told to begin with, at least until the belated present of Abdiel's revelation (Book 5's version of Uriel's "with report"). The angels, in short, experience their very existence as uncanny, what is at once familiar and hidden away, the secret of their own origins. Satan's denial before Abdiel points to Milton's reply to Augustine's assertion that the cause of evil is unknowable: the cause itself *is* knowable; it is the moment of origin that is not. And not just this specific denial of an origin elsewhere but the entire rebellion marks a collective disavowal among the rebel angels for whom the begetting of the Son and all that surrounds it has unleashed a burden of knowledge they cannot admit. Here, the burden entails the knowledge that they are "secondarie" beings, a term that Satan mockingly applies to the Son as a way of deflecting its more obvious application to himself and indeed to all angels even as *sons* of God. As much of a fantasy as Satan's position might be—that he is "self-begot, self-rais'd"—he and the other rebel angels need to assert their own "quick'ning power" in order to cope with the traumatic recognition that their origins belong elsewhere.[18]

And so, as Bloom notes, "Milton overtly assigns Satan a Gnostic stance": he rebels, in a sense, to insist that he is not merely "secondarie." Satan's own fantastical position is staked out in his debate with Abdiel, but it is God's earlier proclamation of the begetting of the Son, a passage that we've previously considered, that, as Bloom also observes, "shocks Satan into rebellion" (112). Here is the full proclamation:

> Hear all ye Angels, Progeny of Light,
> Thrones, Dominations, Princedoms, Vertues, Powers,
> Hear my decree, which unrevok't shall stand.
> This day I have begot whom I declare
> My onely Son, and on this holy Hill
> Him have anointed, whom ye now behold
> At my right hand; your Head I him appoint;
> And my Self have sworn to him shall bow
> All knees in Heav'n, and shall confess him Lord:
> Under his great Vice-gerent Reign abide
> United as one individual Soule
> For ever happie: him who disobeyes
> Mee disobeyes, breaks union, and that day
> Cast out from God and blessed vision, falls
> Into utter darkness, deep ingulft, his place
> Ordaind without redemption, without end. (5.600–15)

"Shock" is the right word and not only because of the terrible severity of what is threatened, a severity apparently not previously encountered in God. It is also shocking because the elevation of the Son over the angels is so radically unexpected and, from Satan's point of view at least, entirely unnecessary; so he declares in his first effort to rally his troops:

> Who can in reason then or right assume
> Monarchie over such as live by right
> His equals, if in power and splendor less,
> In freedom equal? or can introduce
> Law and Edict on us, who without law
> Erre not? (5.794–99)

Morally and spiritually, God's imposition of "Law and Edict" upon the angels is precisely what creates the freedom Satan so vigorously champions here. In the Miltonic cosmos, obedience is a willed act, and until there is a law to obey (whether the command to bow down before the Son or the prohibition against eating the fruit of a particular tree) there is, by definition, no choice that could form the basis of free obedience.

But even if Satan cannot conceptually accommodate this new reality, what is most shocking in this scene is that, until this very moment, the angels appear to have been completely ignorant of the Son's existence. Even some of Milton's earliest readers seem to have been disturbed by the strangeness of this representation. So one Charles Leslie could write in 1698: "To make the Angels ignorant of the blessed Trinity; and to take it ill to acknowledge him for their King whom they had always ador'd as their God; or as if the Son had not been their King or had not been begotten until that day. The scheme of the Angels revolt cannot answer . . . to the eternal Generation of the Son."[19] Setting aside the question of Milton's commitment to the orthodox notion of the "blessed Trinity," we might observe that, while the first part of Leslie's statement is accurate—Milton's angels are "ignorant" of some basic God-principle at the center of their own existence—the second part of the statement seriously misrepresents what the poem gives us. Milton's angels (whether they end up rebelling or not) clearly had *not* "always ador'd" the Son "as their God," the Son had *not* functioned as the king of the angels before this day, and, most important, to the extent that, in Book 5, the Son's begetting appears to mean his elevation to some new royal status (a point Satan and Abdiel actually agree on), in Milton's telling the Son had *not*, in fact, "been begotten until that day." Leslie may be correct in suggesting that, in terms of traditional Christian theology, the "Angels revolt cannot answer," but in terms of representing the uncanny origins of fallenness Milton's depiction answers quite a lot.

Indeed, the shock that there is such a being as God's "onely Son" is effectively linked to something even more disturbing, something similarly on display in the passages from Genesis and Exodus we encountered in the introduction to part III: the emergence of a boundary between the angels and God (a boundary precisely set in the person of the Son) and a changed relationship to God based on a previously unrecognized ontological hierarchy. Satan's "Gnostic stance" is actually new in the poem—it appears for the first time in Book 5—because prior to the Son's begetting he did not have to take such a stance. But with God's proclamation the angels are now—and only now—compelled to see that they are not the same as God, that they are not equal to God, that they are not themselves gods.[20] And they are not gods because a begetting and a creation (two acts of origin that the angels knew nothing about) mark what Leon Wieseltier, in a passage we considered in the introduction to part III, refers to as the "'was' before the beginning."[21] Until now, the angels did not know that this "was" existed.

That Milton is going out of his way to make this "was" as problematic as possible is borne out by a number of features of the story, both what he represents and what he chooses not to represent (or perhaps cannot represent). Bloom is certainly correct to observe that God's proclamation concerning the Son is what prompts the angelic rebellion. But we notice immediately that there is some confusion over precisely what the term begetting means here. Bloom himself incorrectly (or at least reductively) identifies it with God's announcement that the Son is his "onely Son" (5.604), a phrase that appears aimed at deliberately confusing both angels and readers about what the preceding line means: "This day *I have begot* whom I declare . . ." (5.603; my emphasis). Indeed, to the extent the begetting is being linked to what is described in 604–06 ("and on this holy Hill / Him have *anointed*, whom ye now behold / At *my right hand*; your Head I him *appoint*"), God's proclamation of the Son's special status as his "*onely* Son" is given either merely as the corollary of or perhaps as the main justification for the begetting-as-exaltation (anointing/appointing): the begetting itself must refer to that (the Son's elevation to the king of the angels) rather than to the Son's own coming into existence.[22] Milton's main source-text here, Psalm 2, suggests as much.[23] Of course, the proclamation itself—the "Law and Edict" concerning angelic subjection to the Son's authority—calls attention to that very discrepancy: the begetting that actually matters, what in *De Doctrina Christiana* Milton refers to as "literal, with reference to [the Son's] production," is not even narrated. In other words, the event (the past begetting) that is the very basis of the Son's Book 5 begetting (why the elevation happens at all) is so lost to the past that not only do the angels seem to know nothing about it but neither of the poem's two narrators (Raphael and Milton) can even describe it. Even aided by divine inspiration, poetic-prophetic vision cannot reach back that far.

We might also observe here that, to the extent the entire narrative of the begetting (elevation) of the Son is part of Raphael's account to Adam of the war in heaven, this account is marked, on multiple levels, as an *after*thought: it is not the primary focus of Raphael's charge—to warn Adam about Satan—and, within the design of epic as a whole, it is the original event that can only be narrated much later than it actually happens and then only in the highly mediated form of Raphael's telling. That said, it cannot be stressed enough that what Milton calls the "literal" begetting of the Son (Psalm 2:7's act of fathering) is not shown in the poem at all. Again, what is shown (at least as narrated by Raphael) is the announcement of the enthronement in which the phrase "This day I have begot" (5.603) refers to God's *anointing* of the Son as "Head" of the angels (5.605–06). The wording immediately following "begot"—"whom I declare / My onely Son"—might suggest that the other and earlier begetting (the Son's coming into existence *as* the "onely Son") is being included as part of the announcement (which, if true, would also effectively prove that the angels had not previously known about the Son's special status; indeed, they may not have known that he even existed until this moment). But to the extent the first or "literal" begetting can only be announced after-the-fact (and as something effectively lost sight of), we might reasonably ask whether, in Milton's poetic-theological consciousness, this first event cannot be or must not be represented. In short, for some reason its depiction exceeds the limits of his vision.[24]

In this context, the begetting that *is* narrated (God's proclamation of the Son's elevation, the anointing, the appointing) effectively problematizes the "literal" begetting of the Son as the origin of origins. What the poem has earlier called the Son's "Birthright" (3.309)—he alone is begotten not made—is precisely what makes the Son different from and prior to everything else in God's creation. And it is his special status that also makes the Son the creator of all else, including the angels, the very subject of Satan's debate with Abdiel. It is worth noting again that, if the original begetting itself cannot be represented, neither can the Son's creation of the angels: Abdiel proclaims it, but, as we have previously noted, it is never available in the poem except as revelation after-the-fact (revelation-as-*report*). Taken together then, those two events, the begetting of the Son and his subsequent creation of the angels, are what the poem itself can never quite catch up with.[25] Bloom remarks almost in passing that the poem "begins true time" "with God's proclamation" in Book 5. But this statement misses the fact that "true time" in the Miltonic cosmos always already begins elsewhere, in the "'was' before the beginning." The two events are constituted by their absence—they are what cannot be narrated—and they thus speak precisely to the question of origins at the heart of Satan's rebellion against the Judeo-Christian creator-god.

V

A final glimpse at the experience of one of the unfallen angels might help us understand just how radically committed Milton is to depicting Satan's Emersonian Fall, a discovery of existence that comes too late. The belated shock and shock of belatedness that prompt Satan's rebellion as psychic defense are powerfully reinforced by what Gabriel's comment about Satan in Book 4 tells us about Gabriel himself. How did *he*, a still unfallen angel, experience heaven before the fall of the rebel host or even before God's exaltation of the Son? Gabriel's disgust with Satan's prelapsarian conduct is as surprising a feature of the Book 4 exchange as the very conduct he describes:

> And thou sly hypocrite, who now wouldst seem
> Patron of liberty, who more then thou
> Once fawn'd, and cring'd, and servilly ador'd
> Heav'ns awful Monarch?

Minimally, Gabriel's comments suggest that, even earlier than we might have expected, all was not well among the heavenly host. After all, Gabriel seems to have been disgusted by Satan's obsequiousness before God—that is, he is remembering his earlier disgust with the situation of worship in heaven—even though obsequiousness before God is all there can be for a created being. The main element of Gabriel's charge (Satan's servile adoration of God) seems also to contain a note of jealousy or rivalry, as if he recalls Satan outhustling him on the worship scene. At the very least, he is rebuking Satan for violating some assumed decorum of devotion. More implicitly, though, and perhaps even unconsciously, Gabriel's disgust might also be directed toward God: his snapshot of the prelapsarian, pre-begetting Satan suggests in God a vain, all-too-willing recipient of his creatures' fawning and cringing. Gabriel seems to be remembering, in a pained way, that God is the creator of the situation in which even the greatest angels must servilely compete for his attentions.

Gabriel's disgust therefore masks a self-disgust, a kind of humiliation that is by definition the subject-position of the creature-worshipper before the creator-god. It is worth noting that the very behavior in Satan that so grates on Gabriel is simply assumed as right and natural by the newly created Adam who, in his later account to Raphael, describes the question that enters into his mind upon realizing that the animals he has just named could not have created him:

> O by what Name, for thou above all these
> Above mankinde, or aught then mankinde higher,
> Surpassest farr my naming, how may I
> Adore thee, Author of the Universe[?] (8.357–60)

It is difficult to imagine that the innocent Adam's desire to "Adore" his "Author" would be any different from the *servile adoration* previously performed by the unfallen Satan. Gabriel's need to imagine Satan's performance as the act of a hypocrite (and we observe that he doesn't here say that Satan was merely pretending to worship God) is thus more obviously an effort to reject the very state of affairs that governed (still governs) the relation of *all* faithful creatures to the "Author of the Universe." By calling Satan a hypocrite rather than, say, a liar or an actor, Gabriel suggests on one level that there's nothing wrong with adoring God if it is done in the right frame of mind (Adam's, for example). Rather, it is Satan's hypocrisy in adoring God in one instant and then wanting to dispossess him the next that is the problem: the implication is that Satan was already false somehow without actually having misrepresented his original feelings toward God. But the fact that Gabriel describes Satan's worship as fawning, cringing, and servile more strongly suggests that his effort to smear the unfallen Satan as a hypocrite is also a way for Gabriel to deny that his own behavior before God could not have been very different from Satan's or from Adam's: adoration is adoration. To hint that only a (future) hypocrite could have worshipped in such a publicly humiliating way is Gabriel's means of disavowing his own humiliating worship, a state of affairs that, for an unfallen angel, must be ongoing.

But why, we might ask, doesn't Satan himself recognize this humiliation earlier, when Gabriel does? Why, that is, does Satan only recognize his humiliation *after* the Son's exaltation if Gabriel so easily recognized it before? It may be that we have this situation backwards and that Gabriel is closer to Satan than we might have expected. For Gabriel's assessment of Satan's earlier behavior, behavior that appears to have occurred prior to the Son's exaltation, might actually be a judgment formed only in Gabriel's own post-exaltation consciousness. In other words, the poem's chronological displacements (it begins *in medias res* and only in Book 5 does it return to its chronological beginning) effectively cover over the fact that Gabriel's Book 4 *recognition* of Satan's earlier fawning and cringing (conduct that must in some way have mirrored Gabriel's own) itself comes late, after the Son's exaltation, an event that alters the angels' relationship to their own identities. Gabriel isn't among the Satanic legions, of course, but there is no necessary reason to think that the angels who remain loyal to God all accept the new reality as unquestioningly as Abdiel does. Gabriel's disgust at Satan's previous behavior would appear to mark, then, a disguised and belated self-disgust he cannot acknowledge. But until the begetting of the Son forced the issue (it forced all the angels to understand their relationship to God precisely as one organized around divine priority), did either Satan or Gabriel understand his behavior toward God as worship? Is what Gabriel calls Satan's fawning and cringing only a *later* interpretation of behavior neither could have initially viewed in those terms? Did Gabriel and Satan or any of the angels even understand themselves as God's creatures, different from and subservient to their creator because created by him (or, more to the point, created in the afterwards and as afterthought, in the belatedness of the "secondarie" Son)? Or is this precisely what the begetting of the Son opens their eyes to, a discovery that then compels them to understand their relationship to God as servile and humiliating, directed toward what previously had not even been perceived as fundamentally different from themselves?

Something changes at the moment of the Son's exaltation in Book 5: there is a change both in how Satan sees God and, more to the point, in his relationship to God (and thus also to himself). But it is Gabriel's portrait of a Satan (Lucifer) we cannot recognize that leads us to this understanding, which is why the exchange between Gabriel and Satan at the end of Book 4 is so critical. Again, and just as important, the exchange powerfully suggests that something similar happened to Gabriel even though he remains unfallen. It is interesting in this context that John Guillory accepts Gabriel's interpretation of Satan's pre-exaltation behavior toward God: that it was a ruse of some kind, performed "in hope / To dispossess [God], and thy self to reigne" (4.960–61). But the sheer illogic of that claim—how precisely was Satan going to dispossess God by pretending to adore him?—more obviously portrays Gabriel's statement as a *mis*interpretation and a misinterpretation that functions for Gabriel as the rebellion itself does for Satan: precisely to disguise or deny what he cannot face more directly. To impose upon the fawning and cringing Satan a motive he can evade in himself permits Gabriel to avoid confronting his own past behavior, behavior that clearly disgusts him.[26]

Of course, Gabriel's function at this point in the poem is to reveal something of Satan we could not have understood otherwise: what his experience was like prior to the begetting (exaltation) of the Son. And what the later (but chronologically earlier) parts of the poem reveal is that Satan's prelapsarian experience must somehow have been grounded in ignorance of what divine creation *entailed*, in both senses of that word: what it involved and what it imposed as a burden. From what Gabriel tells us we must assume that, prior to the Son's begetting, Satan was perfectly happy with his relationship with God. If not, we have no way of understanding how his servile adoration could become the burden of the "debt immense of endless gratitude." That is, given the profound contradiction between Satan's soliloquy at the beginning of Book 4 and Gabriel's observations at the end, we should imagine that God's command to the angels to bend their knees before the Son and "confess him Lord" forces into Satan's consciousness a deeply disturbing recognition of what was and so is always already true. With the Son's begetting, Satan (and perhaps also Gabriel) comes to see his pre-begetting behavior toward God as Gabriel *now* sees it: *as* servile adoration. In short, if we take seriously Gabriel's prelapsarian perspective, even if he can only recount this time from an altered later perspective, we must be willing to admit that the primary motivation for Satan's fall—its first and deepest cause (a cause Augustine could not imagine)—is shame, a shame that, in its displaced form, even

Gabriel now feels. Angelic embarrassment about the very nature of existence not only produces self-loathing but also leads to actions best understood as psychological defenses against the burden they do not want to acknowledge. In this context, Satanic pride (Augustine's sole motive for the fall) is best understood as a defense against that burden (Freud might have called this wounded narcissism). For Satan's discovery of his existential humiliation is coincident with the fall itself, and pride is his chief means of coping with it, a way of disavowing what he once was: a servile adorer, a fawner and cringer before "Heav'ns awful Monarch." The begetting of the Son is the condition of possibility for that discovery, the moment at which Satan discovers that he exists, that he exists within God's cosmos, and so has been created by another.

Bloom declares that, "as he starts downward" in the wake of the Son's begetting, the Gnostic Satan—and in this he is much like Hamlet and Freud—"declares that he has fathered himself" (112). It is in championing this "dark idolatry of self" that Bloom dismisses the remorse Satan expresses in his Book 4 soliloquy as unworthy because fundamentally un-Satanic (109–10):

> Forgetful what from him I still receivd,
> And understood not that a grateful mind
> By owing owes not, but still pays, at once
> Indebted and dischargd; what burden then?

We might counterpoise what Bloom calls Satan's "dark idolatry" to what Jentsch in his discussion of the discovery at the heart of the uncanny terms "dark knowledge," a knowledge that "dawns" only belatedly. Bloom too easily dismisses the possibility that Satan's Gnostic stance is a fantasy he cannot finally overcome. But the concluding question of Satan's soliloquy, "what burden then?," brings us back to Cavell's sense of tragedy as a burden of knowledge. In *Thus Spoke Zarathustra*, Nietzsche will claim that such a burden might reside in the impossible weight of what comes before, a weight that seems to describe the experience of the character we know as Milton's Satan:

> [W]hat is it that called, which claps even the liberator himself in chains? "It was": thus is called the will's gnashing of teeth and loneliest melancholy. Impotent against that which has been—it is an angry spectator of everything past. The will cannot will backward; that it cannot break time and time's greed—that is the will's loneliest misery. . . . Thus the will, the liberator, became a

doer of harm; and on everything that is capable of suffering it avenges itself for not being able to go back. This, yes this alone, is *revenge* itself: the will's unwillingness toward time's "it was."²⁷

Satan's drive for revenge against God is best understood as just such an expression of "ill will against [divine] time." Satanic vengeance is thus intelligible as at once a symptom of and a defense against his crisis of origins precisely as that crisis marks the recognition of his own inescapable belatedness in relationship to his creator-god.

As we saw at the close of chapter 2, Freud defines the "it was" in terms of an impossible debt against which consciousness rebels, and he locates that rebellion in the ambivalence bound up with the son's hostile relationship to this father: "When a child hears that he *owes his life* to his parents, or that his mother *gave him life*, his feelings of tenderness unite with impulses which strive at power and independence, and they generate the wish to return this gift to the parents and to repay them with one of equal value. It is as though the boy's defiance were to make him say: 'I want nothing from my father; I will give him back all I have cost him.'" Freud concludes the passage by observing that "all [the son's] instincts . . . find satisfaction in the single wish *to be his own father*" ("Contributions to the Psychology of Love" [1910], XI, 172–73; emphases in original). As if anticipating Freud, even as he falls, the Gnostic Satan, Bloom observes, "declares that he has fathered himself." But this in only a declaration, a posture: Freud himself knows that this is a wish and not reality. For the life any son "owes," at least as he owes it to the father, can only be repaid with the defiance that says he owes his father nothing. But the Satan of the Book 4 soliloquy sees more clearly: what he owes his father is a "debt immense" that can never be discharged. Unless one has the strength of Hamlet, the Gnostic stance can only ever be a Gnostic fantasy, a fantasy that one can be self-begot, that one can be one's own father. The remorse Bloom finds unpersuasive in Satan is the reality principle overriding the pleasure principle. And rebellion itself, even when the "dark idolatry of self" thrills the reader, can only be understood as a defense against the very impossibility of possessing oneself, of being present at one's own origin.

VI

If my reading of *Paradise Lost* has aimed at what Nuttall's only points toward—a full engagement in the poem's Gnostic vision—it does so precisely to the extent it interprets that vision in relation to Freud's thought: the way in which the son's estrangement from authority—from his very claim to be self-authored—is drawn up into the biblical notion of the primacy and priority of the father. More precisely, I have argued here that the Gnostic elements on display in Milton's story of Satan's rebellion are best understood not as a belated effort either to resuscitate or combat an ancient heresy but as a mythic representation of one of the deepest struggles in the human psyche, the struggle to cope with the fact that we have a beginning. In Satan, we see the experience of a son of God who only when it is "too late to be helped" runs up against the recognition of his absence from the scene of his own origin. In other words, Milton portrays in Satan the traumatic encounter with the very fact that we exist. Reading Satan as a Gnostic heretic, in short, we see Milton's portrait of a son truly antagonistic to his progenitor-father as at once an anticipation and a proleptic correction of Freud's grappling with the source of filial ambivalence, a problem that had vexed him since 1896: the son's resistance to paternal authority and priority initiated by and at the primal scene.

To the extent Milton would not have understood, let alone accepted, the premises of the very psychoanalysis he helped to invent, we can at least register, first, how Gnosticism functions in *Paradise Lost* to explain Satan's adversarial position (that is, the motive for the rebellion against God) and, second, how that motive, is lodged in a particular state of mind and one that makes most sense when understood as a psychological portrait (Milton invents a Satanic psychology). Although it is possible to understand Satan as a jealous brother (older or younger is not clear) displaced as God's favorite by the Son—and, indeed, that motive does seem to be suggested in Books 4 and 5—such antagonism towards his brother is itself a response to an even more primal loss. Translated from the theological to the psychological, the first cause of Satan's revolt is not jealousy against the Son but the shock Satan experiences at the discovery that he is (as all creature's must be) merely a son of God (not of the same essence, not of the same age). Satan's Gnosticism is a fantasy both in the general sense that the Miltonic universe is not as Gnostics imagine it and in the specific sense that Satan fantastically longs to reclaim something he never had to begin with. Both the act of Satan's discovery and the ongoing condition are belated: the "loneliest melancholy," as Nietzsche puts it, stems from time's curse, the paternal "it was" that is never our own.

Milton's representation of Satan's Gnostic crisis—his longing to be "self-begot" and the vexed question of whether beings created by God can be, as the poem suggests, "Authors to themselves" (3:122)—is a reminder both that Shakespeare was not the only early-modern writer capable of anticipating Freud and that what we might call the proto-psychoanalytic perspective of early-modern thought was densely interwoven into the period's religious discourse.[28] We might remind ourselves that, as we saw in chapter 3, in his "providence in the fall of the sparrow" speech Hamlet's loss of the father is marked by his allusion to Matthew 10. And what we saw is that, for Shakespeare, the struggle for the son to say "I am, I exist" in the face of paternal authority is inseparable from a movement away from the religion of God-the-father: both fathers are strangely forgotten. I would argue more broadly that, for a writer in a Judeo-Christian culture, an anxiety of origins cannot be disentangled from a religion of origins, especially where that religion's sense of origin, duty, command, and identity are so bound up in the father-son relationship.

The Gnostic Satan of *Paradise Lost* rebels in a fantasy that he can father himself. For his part, Freud will give voice to Hamlet's twofold rebellion (against the human father and against God-the-father) in a note in the *Interpretation of Dreams*, a passage that is particularly relevant as a way of understanding the formative, albeit repressed, presence of Judeo-Christianity at the origins of psychoanalysis:

> Here is some further interpretive material. Handing [my father] the glass [urinal] reminded me of the story of the peasant at the optician's, trying glass after glass and still not being able to read. . . . The way in which the father in Zola's *La terre* was treated among the peasants after he had grown feeble-minded.— The tragic requital that lay in my father soiling his bed like a child during the last days of his life; hence my appearance in the dream as a *sick-nurse*. . . . This recalled a strongly revolutionary literary play. . . in which God the father is ignominiously treated as a paralytic old man. In his case will and deed were represented as one and the same thing, and he had to be restrained from cursing and swearing by one of the archangels . . . My making *plans* was a reproach against my father dating from a later period. And indeed the whole rebellious content of the dream, with its . . . derision of the higher authorities, went back to rebellion against my father. (IV, 217n1)

What Freud refers to here as "derision of the higher authorities" marks a critique of Judeo-Christianity that is symbolically related to the "rebellion against his father": God-the-father is a paralytic old man; Jacob Freud soils his bed like a child. The phrase translated here as "with its derision" (German: *verhöhnende* [tauntingly, jeeringly]) also strangely echoes two moments in *Paradise Lost* in which Milton uses the word "derision" in relation to Satan's rebellion: the first to refer to Satan's mockery of the angels who remain loyal to God (6.607–08) and the second, more famously, to refer to the Son's mockery of the futility of the rebellion (5.735–37). Milton's paired uses of the word suggest the mutual contempt of the warring sides, rebellious sons against an all-powerful father with his still dutiful sons at his side. It is precisely in that sense that Freud speaks of the derision he experienced in the form of a dream: disdain for the authority of the father where that father is inseparable from a higher, cosmic power (the father-god or the father-as-god).

Perhaps more tellingly, the "reproach" against his father appears to represent more honestly the nature of the vexed feelings Freud experienced at the time of his father's death. As we observed in chapter 3, in his 1896 letter to Fliess Freud had referred to his feelings as "self-reproach" in the wake of his father's passing as a kind of survivor guilt. But the note in the *Interpretation of Dreams* suggests his revised recognition that if "self-reproach" was an apt description of his feelings in 1896 it was only because of the ambivalence he felt over his own sense of rebellion against his now deceased father, a personal feeling that by 1914 is more generally theorized as a "mental constellation of revolt." That rebellion, we might now surmise, was precisely against the forced recognition that the beloved father stood at the point of origin, the origin marked, in the Judeo-Christian tradition, in terms of the father-God and one that the son—any son (dutiful or not)—could never have chosen for himself. The complexity of this interrelationship, Freud's personal investment in it, and, in particular, his effort to refute his origin by choosing his own father—all recorded in his final major work, *Moses and Monotheism*—will be the subject of our final chapter.

6

Choosing the Father in *Moses and Monotheism*

> A hospital for sick and needy Jews,
> For those poor mortals who are triply wretched;
> With three great maladies afflicted:
> With poverty and pain and Jewishness
> . . .
> Will Time, eternal goddess, some day end it,
> Root out this dark misfortune that the father
> Hands down to the son?
>
> —Heinrich Heine, "The New Jewish
> Hospital in Hamburg"

> He who is willing to work gives birth to his own father.
>
> —Kierkegaard, *Fear and Trembling*

I

Early in *Moses and Monotheism*, his last major work, Freud reflects almost casually that "everything new must have its roots in what was before" (22). He makes the statement as part of his summary of the origins of the proto-monotheism of the Egyptian Eighteenth Dynasty, but it could just as easily apply to *Moses and Monotheism* itself. For in many ways *Moses and Monotheism* marks a return to his own earlier work, even to the very roots of that work. What is new in this strange text is an attempt to theorize "the origin of monotheism among the Jews" (81), but Freud quite openly acknowledges that he is building on work he had done a quarter-century earlier in *Totem and Taboo* where he had explored more broadly the psychoanalytic foundations of primitive religion.[1] In both texts Freud views religion as a social-psychological neurosis deriving primarily from and in turn fueling the filial ambivalence—the tension between identification and hostility—at the heart of the son's (or sons') vexed relationship to his (their) father.[2] Moving back even further in Freud's intellectual itinerary, we might remind ourselves that ambivalence toward his own recently deceased father, Jacob Freud, was what Freud had grappled with in 1896 at the very beginning of psychoanalysis. Some forty years later in *Moses and Monotheism*, he returns to this starting point to (re)discover that "ambivalency belongs to the essence of the father-son relationship" (172).[3] Now raised to a cultural force through "mass psychology" (163), such "ambivalency" provides a psychoanalytical explanation for the peculiar neurosis Freud equates with Jewish identity itself and particularly with the mysteriously compulsory force of Jewish faith.

Precisely because of the way it privileges the father-son relationship, many have interpreted *Moses and Monotheism* through lens of Freud's Oedipal theory and applied it to his relationship to his own father, Jacob Freud.[4] Given the growing threat to European Jews during the time he was writing the book (1934–39), it is difficult to read it purely as disguised autobiographical confession. But it is not out of the question that Freud himself might have accepted that verdict, as though his work on Jewish identity were the final chapter of his life-long self-analysis. Of course, an Oedipalized understanding of virtually all human experience was the very centerpiece of psychoanalysis as he understood it, an understanding Freud extended to religious experience as well.

That said, in focusing on how the father-son relationship becomes the main focus of *Moses and Monotheism*, I stand by my study's core claim that the theory of the Oedipus complex is itself a distortion. From the very beginning, that is, the theory marked Freud's attempt to provide an explanation for filial ambivalence and thus functioned as a disavowal of what that ambivalence signified if not consciously to Freud then within what we might call the interstices of Freudian rhetoric. As we have seen in many of his writings—*The Interpretation of Dreams*, "Theme of the Three Caskets," "Remembering, Repeating, and Working-Through," "Mourning and Melancholia," "From the History of an Infantile Neurosis," "The Uncanny," *Beyond the Pleasure Principle*, *Inhibitions, Symptoms and Anxiety*—Freud consistently interpreted filial ambivalence through the interlocked aspects of the Oedipal condition: infantile sexuality, the son's desire for the mother and the corresponding sexual rivalry with the father, repression of forbidden sexual wishes and the fear of castration at the hands of the father, a son's drive to be in the place of the father leading to both identification with and hostility toward the father. But I have argued throughout that filial ambivalence derives not from a forgetting that comes from repression but precisely from a primal absence, a missing at the point of origin, and thus from a crisis of belatedness in relation to the father who necessarily comes before the son. The persuasiveness of that claim is the burden of the study as a whole and the special and concluding burden of this chapter.

II

Before taking up the details of *Moses and Monotheism*, it is worth reflecting on how Freud arrived there. Many works written after the *Interpretation of Dreams* have a share in the evolution in Freud's thought, but by way of transition to a final consideration of *Moses and Monotheism* we shall look at just two, his 1914 essay "The Moses of Michelangelo" and his 1930 preface to the Hebrew translation of *Totem and Taboo*.

Published anonymously in *Imago* in 1914, the essay is a highly speculative analysis of Michelangelo's famed statue for the tomb of Pope Julius II. Although we shall touch on a few details from the analysis itself, it is the short introduction to the essay that is of most interest for our purposes. To begin, the introduction reads as a kind of meditation on the very work of psychoanalysis, for Freud treats the interpretation of art as an analogy to his own disciplinary practice. Noting the "paradoxical fact that precisely some of the grandest and most overwhelming creations of art are still unsolved riddles of our understanding," Freud argues that it is the proper task of critical analysis "to show that behind them . . . lie concealed," just as in the human psyche, "all that is most essential" (XIII, 211, 214). Just as important, as though he were interpreting one of his own dreams, Freud is intrigued by how the "state of intellectual bewilderment" that so often derives from the encounter with works of genius is typically accompanied by a "powerful [emotional] effect" that is just as hard to explain. In regard to this latter mystery, he brings the same determination he would to the analysis of psychical phenomena. He thus tells us that he often must "spend a long time trying to apprehend . . . i.e. to explain to [him]self what their effect is due to," a labor he pursues doggedly because his own peculiar "turn of mind . . . rebels against being moved by a thing without knowing why [he is] thus affected and what it is that affects [him]" (211–12).

Before he gets to the specifics of the "powerful effect" produced in him by Michelangelo's statue, Freud offers two examples from literature to demonstrate the value of "the application of psychoanalysis" to artistic analysis. Not surprisingly, these examples come straight out of his own earlier work: "Let us consider Shakespeare's masterpiece, *Hamlet* . . . I have followed the literature of psychoanalysis closely, and I accept its claim that it was not until the material of the tragedy had been traced back by psychoanalysis to the Oedipus theme that the mystery of its effect was at last explained" (XIII, 212). The statement is charmingly disingenuous since that "tracing back" had been Freud's own work, but he must engage in the charade to preserve a perhaps pointless anonymity as the essay's author. Still, this recollection of the Freudian Hamlet is significant in that it opens up the possibility that what he will be most attentive to in his analysis of the statue's own inscrutability might return us to a foundational moment from his own past, something related to his peculiar investment in Shakespeare's play.

While on the surface nothing either in the introduction or in essay as a whole immediately suggests "the Oedipus theme," Freud's description of his personal viewing of the statue hints that what he associated with *Hamlet* (or Hamlet) might still be haunting him in 1914. This haunting is most pointedly marked in what we might call, following his phrasing in the "non vixit" dream (discussed in detail in chapter 3 above), the paired *revenants* or ghosts of the essay's introduction:

> Another of these inscrutable and wonderful works of art is the marble statue of Moses, by Michelangelo, in the Church of S. Pietro in Vincoli . . . [N]o piece of statuary has ever made a stronger impression on me than this. . . . How often have I mounted the steep steps from the unlovely Corso Cavour to the lonely piazza where the deserted church stands, and have essayed to support the angry scorn of the hero's glance! Sometimes I have crept cautiously out of the half-gloom of the interior as though I myself belonged to the mob upon whom his eye is turned—the mob which can hold fast no conviction, which has neither face nor patience, and which rejoices when it has regained its illusory idols. (XIII, 213)

The dreary setting—the "lonely piazza," the "deserted church—comes back again and again to Freud but only because, to satisfy some unexplained need, he keeps returning to it. And then there is the unsettling feeling produced by the statue itself, for Freud experiences this Moses as strangely alive, its eyes turned upon him—and the invisible mob of which he feels himself a part—in "angry scorn."[5]

That said, the main link here between what he had previously encountered in *Hamlet* and his current fascination with Michelangelo's statue is mediated through the essay's echoing of the "non vixit" dream. For what he keeps coming back to in his repeated viewing of the statue—what we might call Moses's look of reproach—strangely recalls the figure of his mentor, Ernst Brücke and, more particularly, the old man's "terrible blue eyes with which he looked" at Freud in an expression of controlled anger, disappointment, censure. Even during that dream, as we noted in chapter 3, he knew that he was "dealing . . . with people who were dead" (V, 422). Now the reencountering of Brücke's withering gaze within the stone figure suggests that something from the past that is not truly alive in the present except in Freud's own mind is what has returned to judge him.[6] That figure who will not properly stay dead—a *revenant* or a lost one that keeps coming back (V, 486)—points to the real import of Freud's reference to *Hamlet*. Michelangelo's lifeless statue, that is, expresses something from the past that continues to impose a burden on the living Freud, a *revenant* that draws together the figures of Moses and Brücke in Freud's mind: the dead father, the deceased Jacob Freud.

It is Freud himself who draws *Hamlet* into this ghostly return, but precisely in the figure of King Hamlet rather than in Prince Hamlet. For behind the association of Brücke's "terrible eyes" and the "angry scorn" from the eyes of Michelangelo's Moses lies the moment from 3.4 of *Hamlet* when, confronted a second time by the ghost of his father, the Prince feels the judgment from beyond the grave now directed at him rather than at either Claudius or Gertrude:

QUEEN: Whereon do you look?

HAMLET: On him, on him! look you *how pale he glares*!
His form and cause conjoin'd, preaching to stones,
Would make them capable.—*Do not look upon me*,
Lest with this piteous action you convert
My stern effects, then what I have to do
Will want true color. (3.4.124–30; my emphases)

On the one hand, the Ghost's *pale* glare (in 1.2 Horatio had referred to its *pale* countenance [1.2.31–34]) anticipates how in the "non-vixit" dream Freud fixes Joseph Paneth with "a piercing look" so that "*under my gaze he turned pale*; his form grew indistinct and his eyes a sickly blue—and finally he melted away." It is at this stage that Freud first introduces his notion of the *revenants* or ghosts who might be wished out of existence; and so he adds: "I annihilated P. with a look" (V, 421–22). But in Shakespeare it is the Ghost's fixing of his eyes on Hamlet that causes this son to feel such discomfort that it is he who turns pale ("Do not look upon me / Lest . . . what I have to do / Will want true color"), an image that seems closer to the description of how the father-figure Brücke "levelled [his] reproach" at Freud (V, 481). For Freud's account of the scene at Brücke's laboratory puts Freud very much in Hamlet's position in respect to the Ghost's return in 3.4: "What overwhelmed me were the terrible blue eyes with which he looked at me and by which I was reduced to nothing." And in Freud's addition that "no one who can remember the great man's eyes, which retained their striking beauty even in his old age, and who has ever seen him in anger, will find it difficult to picture the young sinner's emotions" (V, 422), we find another similarity: Hamlet and Freud are both "young sinners" being reproached by their respective ghosts, dead fathers both, and thereby reduced to nothing.

As the essay's introduction has it, this experience is akin to what Freud also felt under the force of the glare of Michelangelo's Moses, the perspective of the one being reproached (the young sinner) rather than of the one doing the reproaching.[7] But the analysis in the essay proper takes the opposite perspective. There, Freud focuses exclusively on Moses's own complex feelings in the face of the Israelites' worshipping of the Golden Calf (Exodus 32). The very detailed reconstruction argues that what Michelangelo is quite radically depicting is Moses in the process of containing his wrath and so choosing, against the explicit narrative of the biblical account, not to smash the two tablets of the Law.[8] In this sense, Freud's analysis of Michelangelo's intentions exists in opposition to the "powerful effect" the statue has produced in him, the interpretation of which he must trace to its source because, as we have noted, his natural "turn of mind . . . rebels against being moved by a thing without knowing why [he is] thus affected and what it is that affects [him]." For, again, what Freud says he responds to (and he feels compelled to repeat the experience by going to see the statue again and again) is precisely what is not depicted in the statue, "the angry scorn of [Moses's] glance" as it is *directed at and felt by* the Israelite "mob upon whom his eye has turned." It is his own feeling of being among the accused that moves Freud, even haunts him; he discovers himself as a member of a group that "can hold fast no conviction, which has neither faith nor patience" (XIII, 213). In other words, the source of the statue's effect on Freud and thus also the meaning that can be gained by an act of interpretation that is akin to psychoanalysis itself is the experience of being reproached as just another one of those sinners who, briefly liberated from Moses's authority, immediately disregard the very foundation of that authority, the voice of the Law itself.

We might be even more precise in saying that what the Israelites violate in their making of the Golden Calf (what makes them the model of Freud's own faithlessness) is the very boundary between Hebrew monotheism and paganism. With the Golden Calf they break both the first and second commandments, but more broadly they reject the very notion of the Mosaic religion and so return to something even more fundamental to paganism than the simple worship of idols and false gods. For by making the very god they will worship—"[T]he people gathered against Aaron and said to him, "'Come, *make us a god* . . .' . . . Early next day, the people offered up burnt offerings and brought sacrifices" (Exodus 32:1, 6; my emphasis)—they threaten to traverse the gap discursively produced by the emergence of monotheism, the very separation of human and divine. Effectively reversing what the bible variously recounts in Genesis 1–3 (the Creation and Fall), Genesis 11 (the Tower of Babel), and Exodus 19 (the Theophany of Sinai)—God's repeated attempts to establish the boundary that will enshrine his fundamental difference from his creatures—the Golden Calf story shows the Israelites putting themselves in the place of the creator so as to make themselves, as was feared in Genesis 3:22, like gods. In that sense, as human beings they refuse to come *after* the act that created them; or, as the people of Israel, they refuse their own chosenness. Lurking behind Moses's wrath is thus the (re)assertion of an act of ontological and temporal distinction and the divine authority that inheres in it. The slaughter of the 3,000 at the hands of Moses's tribe, the Levites, at the conclusion of the Golden Calf story (Exodus 32:25–29) symbolically renders forceful reminder as violent subjugation: the rebellious children of Israel will be overawed and so compelled to submit in the face of Moses's and God's precedence (in both senses of that word). The founding principle of Hebrew monotheism, man is not God, is thereby renewed.

Yet in Freud's interpretation of Michelangelo's version of the scene, defiance of such precedence rears its head once more. Most obviously, Michelangelo's Moses (or at least Freud's version of it) does not act: he controls his wrath and thereby becomes passive in a way that he is not in Exodus 32:19. But this change also means, as Freud himself observes, that Michelangelo quite deliberately defies the authority of biblical tradition itself: "[T]he artist, in depicting the reaction of his hero . . . deviated from the text" (XIII, 232).⁹ Michelangelo's infidelity would thus necessarily be Freud's as well, and both here in the essay's abbreviated form and in the much longer account in *Moses and Monotheism* Freud will, like Michelangelo, not only break with the basic narrative but, more fundamentally, make an "alteration" in the very "character of Moses" (233). If Freud thereby claims the right to tell a new story, there is something even more radical at play. For while the Moses of the essay is not explicitly rendered as a father-figure as he will be in *Moses and Monotheism*, in siding with the gentile Michelangelo's revision against the very words of the Exodus account Freud now offers a story different from what he would have inherited through Jewish tradition and so would have been bequeathed to him by his own father.

As we shall see, in *Moses and Monotheism* Freud will call this tradition—Judaism itself—the "Father religion" in contrast to Christianity as the "Son religion" (111). But perhaps more significantly, in his preface to what was to have been the 1930 Hebrew translation of *Totem and Taboo* Freud will refer to Judaism as the "religion of his fathers" (German: *väterlich[en] Religion*), a group that, we would surmise, includes Jacob Freud and from which, Freud tells us, he is personally "estranged" (XIII, xv). Here is the full English text of that preface as provided in the *Standard Edition*:

> No reader [of the Hebrew version of] this book will find it easy to put himself in the emotional position of an author who is ignorant of the language of holy writ, who is completely estranged from the religion of his fathers—as well as from every other religion—and who cannot take a share in nationalist ideals, but who has never yet repudiated his people, who feels that he is in essential nature a Jew and who has no desire to alter that nature. If the question were put to him: "Since you have abandoned all these common characteristics of your countrymen, what is there left to you that is Jewish?" he would reply: "A very great deal, and probably its very essence." He could not now express that essence clearly in words; but some day, no doubt, it will become accessible to the scientific mind.
>
> Thus it is an experience of a quite special kind for such an author when a book of his is translated into the Hebrew language and put into the hands of readers for whom that historic idiom is a living tongue: a book, moreover, which deals with the origin of religion and morality, though it adopts no Jewish standpoint and makes no exception in favor of Jewry. The author hopes, however, that he will be at one with his readers in the

conviction that unprejudiced science cannot remain a stranger to the spirit of the new Jewry. (XIII, xv)[10]

This preface is especially important as a precursor text to *Moses and Monotheism* for a variety of reasons. First, while *Totem and Taboo* had been published in 1913, the new preface shows Freud recalling the subject matter of what will become central once again in *Moses and Monotheism*, what here he calls "the origin of religion" (*Ursprung von Religion*). And while he adds that *Totem and Taboo* itself "adopts no Jewish standpoint," *Totem and Taboo* does in fact make several nods in the direction of the Judeo-Christian tradition. Just as important, the occasion of the Hebrew translation and Freud's own references in the new preface both to the appearance of his work in "the language of holy writ" (*heilige Sprache*) and, despite his own claimed estrangement from it, to "the religion of his fathers" suggest that he was once again thinking about religious origins, but this time precisely from a Jewish standpoint.

More conceptually, the preface marks how, at the beginning of the last decade of his life, a series of phrases, ideas, even self-revelations are swirling together in Freud's thoughts (or perhaps, more accurately, swirling together *once again*). The phrase, "religion of his fathers" (or father[ly] religion) is a metonymy for Judaism, of course, but it also serves as a reminder of why Judaism is a part of Freud's life at all: it was the religion of his own father. But if, as he hints, the *väterlich[en] Religion* is still part of his own life because it was his father's before him, it is not simply something that belonged to and then ended with his father. In the first place, despite his overt estrangement from it, Jewish tradition is still a foundational element of his own personal-familial heritage from which he derives an essential if indefinable aspect of his own identity, a point to which we shall return in a moment. Beyond that more limited familial context, the openness of the German *väterlich[en]* (the plural of the English "religion of his *fathers*" perhaps captures this idea more effectively) takes us even further back in time to an inheritance that emanates from an ancient past and that has come down to Freud over countless generations. And while he takes a very obvious pride in this cultural-religious legacy (a theme that will be central to *Moses and Monotheism*), his estranged condition might also suggest that he feels the weight of those generations as a kind of burden he might otherwise choose to shake off.[11]

Minimally, this mingling of pride in his Jewish identity and his pushing away of it points to yet another manifestation of ambivalence regarding an aspect of experience Freud here otherwise inexplicably associates with his relationship to the father(s). Further exploration of this ambivalence will come in *Moses and Monotheism*, but the 1930 preface clarifies something of the process by which thoughts of his own father (and his father's religion) might have become entangled in newly imagining the founder of that religion, Moses, in a way Freud had not viewed him in the essay on Michelangelo's statue: as a father, indeed as the great father of the Jews. The preface also hints at what, as we have seen throughout this study, is the real source of filial ambivalence. Freud observes, as we have noted, that *Totem and Taboo* "deals with the origin of religion," but that phrase is in complex dialogue with his identification of Judaism as the "religion of his fathers," an identification that points at once to a time-of-the-before (the time of one's forefathers) and thus to something from the deep past that yet imposes itself in the present. A reformulated conflated phrase, "the origin of the religion of his fathers," would remind us that Freud understands religion and the ambivalence that attends it (especially in Judaism, the "Father religion") as constantly traversing the vexed terrain of the origin more abstractly conceived. In other words, to investigate the origin of the religion of his fathers would necessarily entail investigating the problem of the origin itself to the extent that religious experience is, for Freud, always caught up in the son's vexed relation to his father. Thus how religion begins, historically speaking, raises the more philosophical questions of what an origin is at all, what it means to have—to possess or to be possessed by—an origin, and what it means to have an origin that comes to us from another.[12]

In short, Jewish identity is for Freud something that comes down from the father(s), something familiar yet strange, something whose "essence" he recognizes though he "cannot express clearly in words."[13] What Freud is unwittingly registering here, I would venture, is that the essential in his Jewish identity is what in it cannot be expressed precisely because its familiar inaccessibility *is* its essence: what it means to be Jewish (or at least what it means, psychoanalytically, to be a Jewish son) is to experience the inaccessible origin that belongs of necessity to the father(s). In other words, what defines this son of a Jewish father is an inherited identity as a situation of estrangement in which identity is experienced not just through *what* his father bequeathed him (the *väterlich Religion*) but through the very fact that it was bequeathed by the father.[14] In the early 1930s, such is the burden, one emanating from the past and experienced in the present as ambivalence, that (re)imposes itself on Freud. It is a burden drawing together the figures of Moses and his own dead father, Jacob Freud, and their shared Jewish identity as this had been bequeathed to a son who had never chosen it for himself. Now in the last decade of his life, first, in the new preface of 1930 and then more fully in *Moses and Monotheism*, Jewish identity as the very place of his father(s) is the final form of Freud's most tenacious *revenant*, what had haunted him since 1896.

III

In part no doubt because Freud recognized the purely speculative nature of his account, *Moses and Monotheism* starts with a bombshell: Moses, the greatest of the ancient Israelites, was most likely an Egyptian. The claim is actually less outrageous than it first appears.[15] Freud cites the Egyptian origins of the name "Moses" (*Moses and Monotheism*, 4–6)—a fact recognized by both ancients and moderns—and he also calls attention to the clumsy handling of the myth of the birth of the hero (what Freud terms the "exposure myth" [11]) in Exodus 2. In the typical folktale version, a child from a royal family is lost or abandoned and subsequently raised by another family, usually peasants, only later to discover and return to his true parents, often, as in the Oedipus-story, with violent consequences (6–13). As Freud notes, however, Exodus 2:1–10 tells the story in precisely the opposite way: the child of slaves (a "man of the house of Levi" and "a Levite woman" [2:1]), Moses is raised as the son of Pharaoh's daughter only to return to his people as an adult. Rhetorically, as Freud is right to argue, the biblical account shows all the signs of a folktale motif or type-scene being rewritten with the express purpose to claim for Moses a hidden Israelite origin. Such evidence would only be necessary to counter the obvious but embarrassing truth: that Moses was an Egyptian, perhaps one of high standing (if not the adopted son of Pharaoh's daughter then maybe a priest or regional governor as Freud suggests or an army commander as is suggested, by Josephus and others, in the various legends of Moses's conquest of Ethiopia).[16]

But if some rhetorical sleight-of-hand is necessary to make the greatest of the Israelites an Israelite by birth, Moses's actual ethnic origins quickly cease to matter. When the adult Moses arrives in Median, for example, the daughters of Reuel immediately identify him as an Egyptian (Exodus 2:19), a statement neither he nor the J-narrator bothers to refute. And when he returns to Egypt, there is no mention of, let alone a teary-eyed reunion with, his biological parents, Amram and Jochebed. In short, by the time he returns to Egypt, his origin is simply not an issue. Whether an Israelite or an Egyptian or even a Medianite, when he returns to Egypt he is simply the vehicle through which Yahweh will act to (re)claim his people. He is the liberator, leader, and lawgiver of the Israelites. And the rest, so the Bible tells us, is history.[17]

That said, Freud wants or needs Moses to be an Egyptian or, perhaps more accurately, *not* to be an Israelite.[18] Much of the rest of this chapter will be taken up with Freud's complex way of responding to the question he seems to have conceptually borrowed from the opening line of Ernst Sellin's 1922 *Mose und seine Bedeutung für die israelitisch-jüdische Religionsgeschichte*: "Wer war Mose?" (Who was Moses?). More to the point, we shall consider what Freud understood Moses's identity as representing at the center not just of the origins of Jewish monotheism but of Jewish tradition as a whole.

Yet the basic question lingers: if it really doesn't matter to Judaism and Jewish history more broadly what Moses's ethnic origins were, why does Freud care about Moses's origins at all? Although he elsewhere acknowledged that "Moses being an Egyptian" was the "starting point" of his researches on the origins of Jewish monotheism, it was "not the essential point."[19] Thus, while part I of *Moses and Monotheism* focuses quite explicitly on Moses's ethnic origins, the text as a whole takes up Sellin's "Who was Moses?" by considering other perspectives on the question's complex relation to the paired issues of identity and origins. For Freud, Moses is even more fundamentally in the paradoxical position of being at once a son and a father, and in that dual form he effectively embodies the "ambivalency" Freud describes as "the essence of the father-son relationship." Moses's origins matter, in short, because he is peculiarly expressive of the agon that had always been the central dynamic of Freudian psychoanalysis itself.

At first Moses is a son; so *Moses and Monotheism* begins with this sentence: "To deny a people the man whom it praises as *the greatest of its sons* is not a deed to be undertaken lightheartedly" (3; my emphasis). Throughout part I (first published with part II in 1937) Freud understands Moses precisely as someone's offspring: his very name essentially means "child" (5), and in the analysis of the exposure myth Freud consistently imagines Moses as the archetypal hero-son in relation to his parents.[20] By part III, however, Freud has reconceptualized Moses's role. There he becomes a parent or more precisely a father: he is now "an eminent father-substitute" (113; *Standard Edition*: "an outstanding father-figure" [XXIII, 89]); and as the "father imago" he takes on the "poor Jewish laborers . . . [as] his dear children" (140). Near the very close of the text Freud will definitively assert that Mosaic Judaism marks a restoration and final submission to "the Great Father," the God of Judaism who incarnates even as he substitutes for the people of Israel's earlier relation to Moses himself (172).

That said, if in the person of Moses, father and son are somehow identified if not precisely identical—at one point Freud observes that "the father was also once a child" (141)—Freud's very application of the exposure myth to Moses's birth-story more directly calls attention to the tension that inheres in the father-son relationship. The initial positioning of Moses as the son within the hero's birth-legend, we thus note, permits Freud to (re)introduce the core theme not just of *Moses and Monotheism* but of the entire psychoanalytic project: the father-son rivalry, that perpetual battle in which, despite the Oedipal implications he constantly rediscovers, Freud can find almost no place for the mother.[21] As he goes further into the conventions of the exposure myth he notes that the oracle or dream "warns the father of the *child's birth as containing grave danger* . . . in consequence *the father . . . gives orders for the new-born babe to be killed* or exposed to extreme danger." But then "saved . . . by animals or poor people . . . when full grown [the son] rediscovers his noble parents . . . [and] *wreaks vengeance on his father*" (8; my emphases).[22] Freud's extended analysis of the mythic conventions suggests that his real aim in introducing these folktale elements is less to provide evidence for Moses's actual Egyptian heritage and more to situate the larger argument of *Moses and Monotheism* within some familiar psychoanalytic territory:

> A hero [the chief character represented in the exposure myth] is a man who stands up manfully against his father and in the end victoriously overcomes him. The myth in question traces this struggle back to the very dawn of the hero's life, by having him born against his father's will and saved in spite of his father's evil intentions. . . . The inner source of the myth is the so-called "family romance" of the child, in which the son reacts to the change of his inner relationship to his parents, especially that to his father. The child's first years are governed by grandiose over-estimation of his father . . . Later on, under the influence of rivalry and real disappointments, the release from the parents and a critical attitude towards the father set in. (9–10)

Whether he was an Egyptian or an Israelite by birth, Moses's first role in *Moses and Monotheism* is as a son, particularly a son of a father toward whom he must have felt, as do all sons in the Freudian universe, an almost murderous hostility.

But precisely because Moses sits on both sides of the father-son divide, when he returns to this filial hostility in part III Freud complicates matters again, this time by positioning Moses on the receiving side of the son's aggression. Whereas in part I Freud had addressed the father-son dynamic in relation to Moses's birth (with Moses presented as the vengeance-seeking son of a hated father), part III portrays Moses as a tyrannical father-figure who, as leader of an unruly populace, faces violent rebellion at the hands of his figurative sons. The collective opposition to Moses's demands—his disciplinary rigor and strictness in theological, ritual, and ethical matters, and his many other impositions (3, 4, 25, 30, 57, 74, 86, 92)—prompts his followers to slay him just as the sons in the pre-totemic society had slain the clan father. Revisiting the prehistorical situation he had theorized in *Totem and Taboo*, Freud muses that "after these considerations I have no qualms in saying that men have always known . . . that once upon a time they had a primeval father and killed him" (129). By the end of the *Moses and Monotheism*, Moses is no longer (or no longer simply) a son-hero "who stands up manfully against his father and . . . overcomes him" but is rather (or is also) the father-founder who is overcome, his oppressive domination resisted by the united sons who finally rise up and slay him.[23]

That said, if in Freud's reconstruction one binary of Mosaic identity (Egyptian or Jew) subtly morphs into a second (father or son), it is because the second calls attention to an even more vexing issue hidden away in the first: what does it mean to come before or after? For the paradox Freud discovers in Sellin's question—"Who was Moses?" becomes in Freud's reformulation how can the great *father* of the Jews also be the greatest of their *sons*?—returns us to the existential crisis of temporal priority and belatedness that had been at the heart of Freud's grappling with the father-son agon since the death of Jacob Freud. Whether he fully realized it or not, in *Moses and Monotheism* Freud stumbled again into that crisis by (re)locating it at the origin of Jewish identity itself. That is, in the question of Moses's ethnic origins Freud does not simply ask whether the great father of the Jews was actually an Egyptian by birth and upbringing but whether this father-founder preexisted the very people who would later claim him as their son and who, as a son, would necessarily have come *after* rather than *before* them. In other words, the real question is who precisely were the Jews before Moses came to them. In that context, what Freud calls "the fateful content of the religious history of the Jews" (57) turns back to the key question Freudian psychoanalysis had articulated without ever truly confronting: what does it mean to have an origin that always already belongs to another?

Even in relation to the origin of the monotheism Moses would bequeath to the people of Israel, Freud shows that there is something baffling in the very attempt to locate a beginning. While Moses brings Egyptian monotheism (the Aton religion) to the Jews, the origin of that monotheism is itself obscure, seemingly lost to time. Freud highlights the role of one pharaoh, Amenhotep IV (thereafter Ikhnaton), but Ikhnaton's own father, Amenhotep III, seems rather inexplicably to have initiated this shift in Egyptian religion. And even his first stirrings in this direction may have been influenced by the importation of concepts from Syria or the surrounding area. To put this another way, despite emphasizing Moses's founding role in the origin of Jewish monotheism, Freud shows that Moses himself is not even the origin of monotheism, for he too is belated in relation to an earlier act of founding. Freud thus works back from Moses to Amenhotep IV and then to Amenhotep III and then even further back: what he imagines as the Egyptian origins of monotheism might actually have come, paradoxically, from areas closer to biblical Canaan, especially under the influence of "Asiatic princesses" taken as wives of various pharaohs (23). The key here is that, in trying to locate the origin of monotheism, Freud stumbles into the possibility not just that Judaism's Egyptian origins had been covered up but that the very origin of the monotheism at the core of Judaism is fundamentally unknowable. The origin, that is, has been lost somehow even as it continues to exert its force (and more powerful for being lost) in the present. What I am suggesting is that, as Freud conceives without fully acknowledging, Jewish identity is itself in some necessary or foundational way inaccessible because its origin is what can never be possessed. It belongs elsewhere and so defines Jewish cultural identity as always already belated.

How then did the Jews begin? Not surprisingly, Freud hedges on his answer. On the one hand, he takes for granted that the Jews lived in Egypt prior to the Exodus and had a collective ethnic identity defined, in part at least, through the practice of a Canaanite religion traceable to a time before their captivity. We've already noted how Freud imagines Moses coming to these "poor Jewish laborers" (140), but much earlier he imagines the "Jewish people" as "immigrants" ("the Jews settled in Egypt") collectively practicing "some kind of religion" prior to Moses's imposition of "a new religion" (18). And in saying time and again that Moses "chose the Jews" (33, 38–39, 43, 53–55, 75 and *passim*) and subsequently "delivered them from Egypt" (136 and *passim*), he simply accepts the basic tenets of the Exodus-story: the descendants of the Hebrew patriarchs settled in Egypt, were eventually enslaved there, but then, having been liberated by Moses, returned to their ancestral homeland.[24]

On the other hand, Freud counters that traditional view in suggesting that the Jews in Egypt were not quite the Jews as the bible and Jewish history would lead us to imagine. While at one point he casually remarks that "the immigrants had probably been in [Egypt] long enough to develop into a numerous people" (43), he later wonders how Moses could have forged "out of indifferent individuals and families *one* people" (136), a description more suggestive both of a smaller group and one not yet constituted by a definitive collective identity. And even if "a people" did live in Egypt, in referring to "those who *later* [that is, post-Exodus] became the Jewish people" (43; my emphasis), Freud also leads us to consider more seriously the precise ethnic identity of the original pre-Mosaic group: Freud variously depicts them as "Semitic tribes" (32, 74), "Semitic Neo-Egyptians" (38, 46), "former Egyptians" (45), people (perhaps even in some form *a* people) Moses will only later make into a "nation" (34, 135, and *passim*).[25]

That said, whatever wavering we might find in his position, for the most part Freud views Moses as interacting with a defined group of some kind even if the biblical associations between those living in Egypt and earlier generations that lived in Canaan under the leadership of the patriarchs were only added later. And so we get this summary speculation as to what happened initially:

> Moses was a noble and distinguished man, perhaps indeed a member of the royal house, as the myth has it. He must have been conscious of his great abilities, ambitious, and energetic; perhaps he saw himself in a dim future as the leader of his people, the governor of the Empire . . . The dreamer Ikhnaton had estranged himself from his people, had let his world empire crumble. Moses' active nature conceived the plan for founding a new empire, of finding a new people, to whom he could give the religion that Egypt disdained. . . . Perhaps he was at the time governor of that border province (Gosen) in which . . . certain Semitic tribes had settled. These he chose to be his new people. . . . He established relations with them, placed himself at their head, and directed the Exodus. (31–32)

Moses's paired acts of "finding a new people" and then choosing them "to be his new people" appear mainly to have entailed his imposing upon a previously existing group traits, ideas, and practices they did not possess before: laws, circumcision, the concept of a single god as this might have been part of the new Aton religion Moses had acquired from Amenhotep IV.[26] Thus, at the opening of part I Freud remarks that "the man Moses, the liberator of his people . . . gave them their religion and their laws" (3); and at the close of part I he refers to "the legislation and religion [Moses] gave the Jewish people" (15). Moses, in short, "stamped" the people with what was new to them (135), "forced" it all upon them (142), "burdened" (35) them with what was foreign, something new and difficult that came to them unbidden "from outside, from a great stranger" (63).[27]

Later, however, Freud will locate something even more fundamental in Moses's imposition: "[S]ince we know that behind the God who chose the Jews and delivered them from Egypt stood the man Moses, who achieved the deed, . . . I venture to say this: *it was one man, the man Moses, who created the Jews*" (136; my emphasis). Freud clearly understood that this was a foundational claim of *Moses and Monotheism*, with implications more far-reaching and potentially more disturbing than the seemingly more provocative one that Moses was himself an Egyptian. We previously noted Freud's observation in a letter to Arnold Zweig that his hypothesis of Moses's Egyptian origins was the "starting point" of the book's argument. But in an earlier letter to Zweig (September 30, 1934) he presented his first impulse in a slightly different fashion: "The starting point of my work is familiar to you . . . Faced with the new persecutions, one asks oneself again how the Jews have come to be what they are and why they have attracted this undying hatred. I soon discovered the formula: Moses created the Jews."[28] This other starting point, we note, is not concerned with Moses's particular identity but rather takes up the question of the origins of Jewish people themselves ("how the Jews have come to be"). Understood in this context, Freud's exploration of Moses's origin doesn't simply unearth his Egyptian roots but also unveils the intriguing contention that the Jews only came into being through Moses. But just what is at stake in this second claim?

In Freud's account, we recall, Moses forced, stamped, and burdened this new people with his Egyptian religion in all its moral and spiritual rigor. But following Freud's more provocative insight—"Moses created the Jews"—I would argue that the chief burden imposed by Moses inhered in the very radicality of that act. Moses created the Jewish people, Freud tells us, by choosing them "to be his new people." But I would amend this claim: *pace* Freud, that is, Moses did not simply choose an already existing people to be his people; rather, he made a new people by choosing them.

Reminding ourselves of the question posed by Milton's Satan, we might then ask, "what burden then?" In the recollection of Satan's anguish we return to Freud's "starting point . . . the formula: Moses created the Jews" and ask: who are the Jews? Freud insists on giving them a descriptive title almost as though it were an alternative name: the chosen people.[29] But in line with his earlier assertion that Moses "chose them [certain Semitic

Neo-Egyptian tribes] to be his new people," Freud concludes that the Jews are not, in fact, *God's* chosen people:

> Still more astonishing is the conception of a god suddenly "choosing" a people, making it "his" people and himself its own god. I believe it is the only case in the history of human religions. . . . Sometimes, it is true, we hear of a people adopting another god, but never of a god choosing a new people. Perhaps we approach an understanding of this unique happening when we reflect on the connection between Moses and the Jewish people. Moses . . . had made them his people; they were his "chosen people." (54–55)[30]

Whatever he found in the poor laborers of Egypt, "the great stranger" Moses did not simply impose upon an already existing people a collection of laws, ideas, and practices that would thereafter be part of their shared identity. Rather, he created their very identity as a people: "*he declared them to be holy*," and they thereby became "the chosen people of God" (135; my emphasis). What burden indeed? Through his act of choosing that was at the same time an act of creation, Moses burdened a people with their very origin by bringing into existence what did not exist before. And the identity with which he burdened a people meant that *his* people could only exist in the ever-afterwards defined by the choice of the great stranger, the great father. In this context the Jews' very status as the chosen people more properly means—could only ever have meant—the *having been chosen people*, a status forever reminding them that they are perpetually and ineluctably belated in relation to a choosing from which they were always already absent. More needs to be said on this topic, but we must first make a brief detour through Freud's own explicitly formulated understanding of the key issues involved.

IV

If, as Yosef Hayim Yerushalmi has argued, the "true axis" of *Moses and Monotheism* is the "problem of [Jewish] tradition, not merely its origins, but above all its dynamics," this is because Freud is intrigued by how the experience of passing on of tradition from one generation to the next is strangely bound up with "compulsive conviction" (*Moses and Monotheism*, 108).[31] Freud had first broached this subject in *Totem and Taboo* where he had asked "what are the ways and means employed by one generation in order to hand on its mental states to the next one?" (XIII, 158). He would return to and clarify the problem in *Moses and Monotheism*: "A tradition based only on oral communication [of ideas] could not produce the *obsessive character which appertains to religious phenomena*" (130; my emphasis). It is precisely with an aim toward a psychological understanding of "in what exactly consists the . . . nature of a tradition, and in what resides its peculiar power, . . . [and] from what sources certain ideas, especially religious ones, derive the power to subjugate individuals and peoples" that Freud takes up the "particular case of Jewish history" (65).[32] For this case—what he says "may be properly termed a traumatic experience" (65)—exemplifies for him how a religious tradition becomes a burden on a people, how it "take[s] . . . hold" of them with an "irresistible claim to be believed, against which all logical objections become powerless" (107–08). But even if one might understand an original traumatic experience at the origin of Judaism, by what psychosocial mechanism could that trauma subsequently have been passed down with the same compulsory force? How, in short, might the trauma have been transmitted transgenerationally as what Freud had once called an "inherited psychical endowment" (*Totem and Taboo*, XIII, 31)?

To understand how Freud theorizes this process we need to return once more to what he referred to in a 1937 letter as "the earliest beginnings" (*Letters*, 439). As Freud understands it, as a body of doctrines, precepts, practices, and, more broadly, a new spiritual orientation, Jewish monotheism began as the Egyptian Aton-religion, initially developed by the priests at the Sun Temple of On and later formally established as the official Egyptian state-religion at the very end of the Eighteenth Dynasty by Amenhotep IV, who renamed himself Ikhn*aton* in honor of the one universal god.[33] But Ikhnaton's reign was all too brief (c. 1375–1358 BCE), and its end saw the vengeful resurgence of traditional Egyptian pagan-polytheism. As a devoted adherent to Ikhnaton's failed reforms, Freud's Moses ("a distinguished Egyptian—perhaps a prince, priest, or high official" [17–18]) gathered around him a people on whom he could impose and so perpetuate the new religious vision:

> [Moses] must have been conscious of his great abilities, ambitious, and energetic, perhaps he saw himself in a dim future as the leader of his people, the governor of the Empire. . . . With the king's death and subsequent reaction he saw all his hopes and prospects destroyed. If he was not to recant the convictions so dear to him, then Egypt had no more to give him . . . In

this hour of need he found an unusual solution . . . the plan of founding a new empire, of finding a new people, to whom he could give the religion that Egypt disdained.

As Freud concludes, Moses "established relations" with these people "placed himself at their head, and directed the Exodus"; those "with whom he left his native country were to be a better substitute for the Egyptians he left behind . . . a holy nation." (31–34).

Stiff-necked as they were, however, these "culturally inferior immigrants" (18) (to be distinguished from Moses's own original Egyptian followers, the Levites) did not easily accept the yoke of the Aton-religion and especially its demands to renounce magic, anthropomorphic depictions of the gods, their cherished fertility and death cults, and perhaps most of all the hope of an afterlife.[34] In opposition to the rigor of the new religion as well as to Moses's particularly uncompromising personality (37–38, 57–58), the newly constituted people constantly rebelled against Moses's leadership (e.g., the story of the Golden Calf and the various uprisings against Moses and Aaron as recounted throughout the books of Exodus and Numbers) until they finally overthrew him and killed him.[35]

It is this event that for Freud particularly explains the "compulsive character" (65) of Jewish monotheism, especially as distinct from the earlier Egyptian rejection of Ikhnaton's reforms. Drawing again on the earlier account he had offered in *Totem and Taboo* on the prehistoric origins of human religion, he argues that the slaying of Moses reawakened in the people of the Exodus archaic memories of the hordic sons' murder of the primeval father and with these memories the same remorse the sons had experienced in its aftermath. Within those primitive tribal groups remorse would turn eventually to guilt, longing and, finally, denial only to give rise in turn to the creation of the totemic system to commemorate the slaying: at once an act of appeasement of the slain father and a ritualized expression of continuing hostility to his authority—in short, another manifestation of the original filial ambivalence though now in highly distorted form of religious practice (103–07, 164–70). And just so the guilt-ridden Jews would deny their deed—"There came a time when the people regretted the murder of Moses and tried to forget it. . . . [T]he painful fact of his violent removal was . . . successfully denied" (58–59)—only to return to the scene of the crime after a centuries-long process of transformation. Their slain founder (leader, lawgiver, educator) would thus be reborn as the Father-God by a fusing of the barely remembered Mosaic doctrines, laws, and rituals (e.g., circumcision) with the volcano-god, Yahweh, which the wandering Jews had appropriated from kindred Semitic tribes in Median.[36]

In Freud's understanding then, the compulsory force that he finds so particular to Jewish monotheism (a monotheism "treasured by them as their most precious possession" [108]) thus derived from a double experience of the return of the repressed. First, the overthrow of Moses awakens repressed memories regarding the slaying of the primeval father: murderous hostility toward followed by the guilt for actually killing him.[37] Second, the new repression of the guilt following the slaying of Moses repeats and in that way intensifies the original primeval forgetting. This repetition at once transfers the deeply repressed filial ambivalence of archaic man to the father-founder Moses and over time, through the process of distortion that at once reveals and obscures the continuing repression, opens the door to a new return of the repressed in the beliefs and practices associated with the father-god, Yahweh.[38] Or, as Freud succinctly puts it, in the person of the father-founder Moses "the figure of the great man has grown into a divine one" (141).[39] The "Father religion" (111) Freud calls Judaism would thereafter become an expression, though a necessarily distorted one, of the longing for the slain father. And submission to the deified father (now in the form of the god Yahweh) through obedience to the Law and adherence to tradition more generally would ever-after fuel even as they would be fueled by collective repression and its attendant neurosis.[40]

By early in part III of *Moses and Monotheism*, Freud feels confident enough in the relation he has asserted between the psychopathology of the neurotic individual and the mass psychological qualities of religious experience to say that the "analogy . . . approximating to identity is rather in the nature of an axiom" (90–91). But in order to theorize and then apply the notion of collective neurosis Freud must make a leap of psychoanalytic faith to the scientifically untenable assumption that "existence of memory traces of the past in the unconscious" can be transmitted across generations. And so, he is forced to conclude, "the masses, too, retain an impression of the past in unconscious memory traces" (119–20), for only as memories return from repression in their distorted form can the Mosaic religion become a tradition.

That said, although he reasons that "if we accept the continued existence of such memory traces in our archaic inheritance, then we have bridged the gap between individual and mass psychology and can treat peoples as we do the individual neurotic," Freud also recognized that such a theory was scientifically ungrounded and had already been widely discredited "by the present attitude of biological science" (128). On one level what he calls a "bold step" is "inevitable" to Freud's way of thinking (the translation in the *Standard Edition* perhaps gets the idea more clearly: "the audacity cannot be avoided" [XXIII, 100]) simply because his theory of Jewish tradition-as-neurotic compulsion requires it. That is, he simply cannot theorize that tradition could have "force[d] the masses under its spell" (130) without the concept of the return of the repressed functioning on a cultural level.[41] But on a different level his sense that Jewish tradition can yet hold the people's collective imagination centuries upon centuries after the religion's founding and in a form still "inaccessible to consciousness" (121) suggests that Freud accedes to the unscientific theory on other grounds.

Although he never mentions him by name, Freud is here rather notoriously applying to human psychology the pre-Darwinian theory of evolution most associated with the French biologist Jean-Baptiste Lamarck (1744–1829), who had argued that an organism can pass on acquired characteristics to its offspring (a theory sometimes referred to as "soft inheritance"). Darwin rejected this theory, and early twentieth-century genetic science eventually disproved it, facts that Freud no doubt knew by the time he wrote *Moses and Monotheism*.[42] Freud's earlier interest in Lamarckism had largely been confined to inheritance among prehistoric humans of the kind he had theorized in *Totem and Taboo*.[43] In *Moses and Monotheism*, by contrast, he attempts to apply psychological-Lamarckism in the context of historically specific events from the relatively recent past and developed over a short historical span (roughly eight centuries), a shift in context that made an already discredited theory even more untenable. But even if we understand that Freud needed this notion of the quasi-genetic passing down of experiential imprints ("memory traces") to make sense of the "spell" of tradition, why was he so attached to the idea in his exploration of the origins of *Jewish* tradition?

Yerushalmi offers purely as speculation that "Freud's Jewishness . . . played a role in his Lamarckian predilections"; "I am not implying that Lamarckism is 'Jewish,'" he writes, but "rather have in mind its subjective dimension, the feeling harbored and expressed by committed and alienated modern Jews alike of the *enormous weight . . . of the Jewish past*, whether it be *felt as an anchor or a burden*. Deconstructed into Jewish terms, what is Lamarckism if not the powerful feeling that, for better or worse, one cannot really cease being Jewish . . . because *one's fate in being Jewish was determined long ago by the Fathers*."[44] The final italicized phrase might be productively aligned first, with Freud's own metonymy of Judaism as the "väterlich[en] Religion" ("the religion of his fathers") and second, with Yerushalmi's earlier observation that those he calls "psychological Jews" (among whose number he would certainly count Freud) grapple with the realization that "vital parts of their lives are still *determined by ancestral choices* they may no longer understand."⁴⁵ We might then bring together those interanimating phrases and with them take up once again the key questions of the preceding section: what does it mean, psychoanalytically, to think of Jewishness as a burden and how did Freud attempt to theorize that notion in *Moses and Monotheism*?

In the previous section I linked that burden to the Jewish sense of chosenness or, more precisely, the *having been chosen* as the experience of belatedness. I would now like to revisit that idea by drawing on the related perspective offered by Cathy Caruth in her effort to retheorize Freud's notion of trauma and apply it the psychohistory offered in *Moses and Monotheism*. Building on Freud's own position that the Jewish "people passed through what may properly be termed a traumatic experience," Caruth reconsiders the idea of "latency" or delayed effect that Freud himself had associated with the time-gap between the murder of Moses and the subsequent (re)emergence of Mosaic tradition some eight centuries later (*Moses and Monotheism*, 82–117). Although Caruth will come to explain the psychological process at work in such a situation differently than Freud himself does (more through dissociation than through repression), in her first attempt to treat the issue of latency in Jewish tradition she simply follows Freud in locating the originary traumatic moment in the murder of Moses: "it is this latency of the event that . . . explains the peculiar, temporal structure, the belatedness of the Jews' historical experience: *since the murder is not experienced as it occurs*, it is fully evident only in connection with another place, and in another time."⁴⁶ But when she returns to this issue later in her study, the starting point of Jewish trauma has rather inexplicably morphed into an experience that *predates* the murder: "Thus, we might say, on the basis of [Freud's] understanding of traumatic repetition . . . , that the murder of Moses, . . . ultimately leads to a belated attempt to return to *the moment before the murder, to Moses' doctrine of chosenness*" (69; my emphasis). In short, Caruth now locates the originary trauma in the experience of chosenness itself, rather than, as Freud would have it, in the guilt and ambivalence derived from the act of violence perpetrated against Moses.⁴⁷

Caruth is not especially clear as to why the experience of chosenness would be traumatic. But this is not an isolated assertion on her part as the following passages amply demonstrate:

> The history of the Jews in *Moses and Monotheism* . . . resonates
> in significant ways with the theory of trauma in its attempt to

understand the actual experience of the Jews—their historical development—in terms of *an experience they cannot claim fully as their own*, the passing on of the monotheistic religion. This passing on of monotheism is the experience of a determining force in their history that makes it not fully *a history they have chosen, but precisely the sense of being chosen by God.*

***

Arguing that monotheism is truly operative in Jewish history only as a "tradition," Freud suggests that the *sense of being chosen is precisely what cannot be grasped in the Jewish past*, the way in which the past itself has imposed itself upon it as a history that it survives but does not fully understand. . . . Monotheism, in shaping Jewish history . . . thus becomes, in the history of the Jews, *the crucial and enigmatic query, What does it mean to be chosen?*

***

If monotheism for Freud is an "awakening," it is not simply a return of the past, but of the fact of having survived it, a survival that, in the figure of the new Jewish god, appears *not as an act chosen by the Jews, but as the incomprehensible fact of being chosen* . . . *Chosenness is thus not simply a fact of the past but the experience of being shot into a future that is not entirely one's own.* (67, 68, 71; my emphases; original italics deleted)

Several intriguing concepts swirl together in this formulation; these especially include the paired notions, first, that tradition is a passing on (or return) of a traumatic state into the present of what began in the past and, second, that the chosenness associated with God's action in history is an experience of having a condition imposed from outside and defined precisely in relation to a temporal existence that one can never truly claim as one's own. Just as important for Caruth, the origin of Jewish monotheism does not become an ongoing trauma for the reason Freud had cited: a violent act, forgotten and so denied, that only after many centuries returns from repression in distorted form. Rather, basing her understanding of latency and return on an analogy for Jewish experience that Freud himself explicitly rejects (the "train accident" [*Moses and Monotheism*, 84]), Caruth locates the force of trauma in a constitutive missing at the point of origin:

> The experience of trauma, the fact of latency, would thus seem to consist, not in the forgetting of a reality that can hence never be fully known, but in an inherent latency within the experience itself. The historical power of the trauma is not just that the experience is repeated after its forgetting, but that it is only in and through its inherent forgetting that it is first experienced at all. And it is this inherent latency of the event that paradoxically explains the peculiar, temporal structure, the belatedness of the Jews' historical experience. (17)

Although Caruth is not as clear as she could be, in her terms chosenness as the experience of *having been chosen* (by God) is traumatic because the "inherent latency" of the original event constitutes a foundational absence within Jewish history, religious tradition, and even consciousness. This absence—linked to the very "belatedness of the Jews' historical experience"—means, as Caruth later writes, that Jewish historical experience (tradition itself) is a trauma without end because it can *never* be claimed as one's own.[48]

Following Caruth's lead, we might return to Freud's commitment to psychological Lamarckism and especially to Yerushalmi's notion that, for Freud and indeed for many modern Jews, Jewish tradition and Jewish identity are experienced as "the enormous weight" of history itself: "the Jewish past" as what "was determined long ago by the Fathers." Whether as what Yerushalmi calls "an anchor or a burden" (perhaps both at once), Jewishness is something one can never escape because the "vital parts" of one's own life "are still determined by ancestral choices." Going beyond what Caruth herself states, I would suggest that Yerushalmi's rather vaguely formulated "ancestral choices" becomes absolutely central to the Freudian problem of Jewishness precisely to the extent those choices emanate from a past inaccessible to the present, determined elsewhere and by others in a time and a place from which the son was necessarily absent. To align Caruth's views with my own, we might say that the ancestral choices determined in the time of the Fathers (and particularly in the time of the great-father, Moses) transform Moses's act of choosing into an experience of chosenness that becomes the trauma of "being chosen." Indeed if, as Caruth claims, "the nature of chosenness . . . resonates with the sense of being possessed by one's past," it is because the "inherent latency" of a traumatic experience as it is first encountered or lived through (what she calls the "inherent forgetting" by which that initial traumatic moment "is first experienced at all") becomes the "peculiar, temporal structure" of that historical experience locked into its own "belatedness" (135n17, 17).[49] To the extent Judaism and Jewish experience generally are viewed as inextricably linked to the very notion of a tradition that both begins and is sustained in trauma, the trauma that is chosenness becomes more foundational to Jewishness than is monotheism itself. Viewed from this perspective, chosenness is thus also the answer to Freud's effort to come to understand the nature of Judaism's "compulsive character." Chosenness is, in short, the Ur-trauma in a way that the murder of Moses is not, a point that, as we saw in section III, *Moses and Monotheism* actually demonstrates even against Freud's explicit argument.

That said, while Caruth helps us understand the insight that Freud himself had registered without recognizing, she does so without herself understanding precisely how or where or even why *Moses and Monotheism* equates chosenness with trauma. Revising Freud's notion of monotheism's historical latency through the concept of a foundational missing or "inherent latency" coincident with the originary traumatic encounter, Caruth imagines that such missing yet points to an actual "being there" that, for no apparent reason, the Jewish people found so painful that their collective experience underwent dissociation, a psychical breach in time that subsequently prevented the development of normal memory (trauma stood in its place). Freud himself saw a kind of dispossession at the heart of Jewish history whereby Jewish identity itself became weighed down by a past the people could never quite claim as their own.[50] But *pace* Caruth, without perhaps being aware of the significance of the assertion and thus of the full meaning of his own argument, Freud locates this dispossession in the fact that, paradoxically, the Jewish people were not present for their own beginning; they were absent because they did not yet exist (they did not, as Caruth would put it, merely dissociate their beginning). Yerushalmi aptly refers to this lost origin as what was "determined by ancestral choices" (though we might correct that to call it the choice of a single [non-]ancestor, the great stranger, Moses). This determination becomes the burden or trauma of Jewish identity because, as Freud insists, it was the Ur-ancestor Moses's act of choosing them that created the Jews in the first place. Moses, that is, created the Jews by imposing on what did not yet exist through an act that belonged to him alone. That choice came to define what Freud calls "the fateful content of the religious history of the Jews" because it would inhabit the people, haunt them ever afterwards, with the burden of an origin that could never be theirs.

Caruth aims to make a similar argument, but she can do so only by vaguely and unconvincingly equating the "inherent latency" of the Ur-trauma with a dissociative state (her revision of the forgetting that Freud himself aligns with neurotic repression). But the true absence of the Jewish people—the inherent latency of their actual traumatic origin—lay not in a dissociative missing of a *divine act* of religious calling but rather in a literal "not having been there" at the time of very human one, Moses's act of choosing. The Jewish people's being created by having been chosen (by Moses) marks Jewish history as traumatic to the extent it created a burden of consciousness that would thereafter invade and sustain a particular historical identity as always already defined by an essential afterwardsness in relation to its own beginning.[51]

To disavow that burden, Jewish tradition tells a new story, one that begins by inverting the conventions of the myth of the birth of the hero. Moses thereby becomes a Jew rather than an Egyptian, but he also thereby becomes a son and precisely the son of a Jewish father. He thus also becomes a member of a group, a scion of the tribe of Levi and so, more generally, of the people of Israel as a whole who existed from ages past. And no matter his greatness, Moses as the founder of the Jewish people can then be reduced to just another person within the collective line of descent referred to in the opening line of Exodus: "These are the names of the *sons of Israel* who came to Egypt with Jacob" (1:1; my emphasis). In that context, Moses himself, who doesn't even make an appearance until chapter 2, must necessarily come after.

Yet the very role thereafter attributed to him—he is the *greatest* of the sons of Israel—also turns Moses into hero. As the heroic son, Moses will once again expose what Jewish tradition sought to disavow in him: the deep ambivalence that emerges in the son whose very existence can but testify to his own afterwardsness. Any son in Freud's formulation necessarily feels ambivalence. On the one hand, he identifies with and even longs for the father (at least he longs to be in the place of the father); on the other hand, he is profoundly, murderously hostile. Knowing that the son threatens him, the father opposes his very existence (warned in a dream, the father knows that "the child's birth" holds "grave danger . . . In consequence, the father . . . gives orders for the new-born babe to be killed" [8]). If he is to exist, then, the son will "be born against his father's will" (9). What could be more heroic than to come into existence in opposition to the person who brings one into existence? In choosing to be born in spite of his father, the heroic son calls himself into existence; he thus makes possible the fantasy of Milton's Satan, to be self-begot, self-made. In so doing, the son becomes, in effect, his own father.

"Who was Moses?" Ernst Sellin had asked in 1922, and from 1934 to 1939 Freud tried to answer that question in a way that only a psychoanalytic approach could. For what *Moses and Monotheism* is, finally, is a vexed meditation upon the identity of Moses that becomes a meditation on the origins of an entire people. As Freud's meditation crosses a terrain of ambiguity—*how is a father also a son?*—it comes at once to express and to expose on a cultural level the central Freudian dynamic, the perpetual agon between those two figures that, from the son's perspective at least, always marked the crisis of what it means to come after. In composing *Moses and Monotheism*, Freud would rediscover that same ambivalence in the very identity of the Jewish people as a whole. Throughout the text, Freud clearly registers that there is something inaccessible in Jewish identity, something present yet absent, something impossible to grasp yet strangely familiar. What I am arguing, then, is that in *Moses and Monotheism* Freud comes to recognize, despite his own explicit argument, that what we might call the existential urgency residing at the heart of Jewish identity was nothing other than a collective experience of the uncanny: the people's very origin was never possessed because always belonging elsewhere, imposed by another whose very act of choosing them into existence necessarily defined them as coming too late.

V

What then of Freud himself as another son of Israel, whose other name, so Genesis 35:10 tells us, was Jacob? How did this son of Israel-Jacob experience the burden of the Jewish uncanny?

In his 1930 preface to *Totem and Taboo*, Freud recognized his Jewishness both as an indelible part of his identity, something bequeathed to him from earlier generations, and as an essence (he was "essentially a Jew") he could not put into words. In short, his Jewishness was at once deeply familiar, comforting even, and inexplicably elusive.[52] It gave him a sense of who he was but bound him to a past to which he belonged without knowing how or why: what was his own and not his own simultaneously. In 1938 letter to his grandson Ernst Freud he would write only half-jokingly that "it is typically Jewish not to renounce anything and to replace what has been lost" (*Letters*, 440). If was still "essentially a Jew," eight years later was he also *typically* so? As he neared completion of his last major work could *he* renounce and replace what his fellow Jews could not? And if in 1930 he already felt estranged from the religion of his fathers, was this because he was already in the process of moving beyond its traditions and tradition itself as what needed to be renounced so that it could be replaced? And is his invention of a new genealogy what renunciation and replacement might look like?

Yerushalmi asks rhetorically of such a view of the Freud of *Moses and Monotheism* whether "an Egyptian Moses [would] make Freud any less a Jew?" and then again, "is the denial that Moses was a Hebrew a projection of Freud's own yearning for a different lineage?"[53] The answer to both questions is yes, though for reasons other than what Yerushalmi might imagine. Marthe Robert gets to the crux of the issue in arguing that what she had termed in relation to the *Interpretation of Dreams* Freud's "imaginary filiation" is still central to his thinking over three decades later: *Moses and Monotheism*, she thus writes, "was rooted in [Freud's] most remote past [both the cultural past of Jewish history and his own personal-familial history], in his need to reconsider the facts of his birth, to change them at least in his imagination and so become master of his fate." And she makes the astute observation that Freud there makes a final push to "break the chain of generations and so free himself forever from all the fathers . . . and ancestors who conspired to remind him of man's intolerable limitations."[54] The problem with this argument is that, as we noted earlier, Robert views the process of self-liberation through the lens of a lifelong Oedipal conflict with Jacob Freud. Thus, she simply has no particular meaning in mind for what those "intolerable limitations" are except to accept rather tamely Freud's own general verdict: that for him as for any son the causal chain from incestuous desire for the mother to murderous hostility for the father functions as the determining factor of his entire life.[55]

Nevertheless, Robert is on to something when she refers to Freud's anguished engagement in the "old wound of Jewish existence and the fundamental question of his origins" and then later to the fact that in *Moses and Monotheism* he is "still obsessed by the problem of origins."[56] But it is the work of my own project to offer a different understanding of Freud's obsession with that problem, of the "intolerable limitations" the "old wound of Jewish existence" imposed on him, and thus why he was led to invent a new genealogy in the figure of the Egyptian Moses. Most succinctly, he needed to discover (or invent) the Egyptian Moses precisely to disavow the psychic inheritance of Jewishness itself as what came down from the father(s).

Against Freud's own explicit argument, what *Moses and Monotheism* shows is that the problem of Jewish existence *is* the problem of the origin itself because the origin is for Freud, in the most primal sense, what is passed down from the father(s) to the son(s). In the form of their "ancestral choices," Jewish fathers impose the burden of pastness upon their sons who thereafter belong to that past without being able to claim it as their own except by submitting to it as tradition. In so submitting, any such Jewish son dooms himself to an agentless afterwardsness in which, as we saw in section III, his own place among the chosen people can only be understood in the passive voice: as a having been chosen. In opposition to the sons of Israel, Freud depicts Moses, the (non-)Jewish Ur-father, as possessing a peculiarly "active nature" (32) because this Egyptian prince or "great stranger" who came "from outside" (63) created the Jews by choosing them. In contrast to the active Moses (father/founder), Freud portrays the Jewish people themselves as akin to the "helpless, intimated son[s] of the father of the [primeval] horde" (172) and as such, as he had earlier put it, "dispossessed" by the "burden . . . that had been forced on them" (58)—dispossessed, that is, because first possessed by what was chosen for them and thus by a choice that would always come "from outside."

Moses's act would thus create not just the Jewish people but also the Jewish uncanny—Jewishness *as* uncanny—because he foisted upon the newly chosen sons the burden of their absence from the scene of their own origin. It is no wonder that Jewish tradition would try to forget this experience or, rather, forget their recognition of something they had never actually experienced. In this sense, Moses's choice of them could not have been repressed because the very people so created did not yet exist to have formed a memory. They could only recognize their own belatedness, what Emerson had called the discovery of an existence that always comes too late. Jewish tradition's writings about Moses would thus need to begin by (re)telling his birth story so as to reimagine him as just one son of Israel among countless others. If, despite his greatness, he is but one son among their already existing number, but one son of an ordinary Jewish father and mother, he could not have come before them. And if he did not come before them, the Jewish people would not now and forever after be confronted with an existence that did not belong to them, an act of origination forever lost because what was absent at the scene of origin was their own choice to exist.

But *Moses and Monotheism* would tell a new story, just as Michelangelo's narrative in his statue of Moses, as Freud recognized (or at least claimed to recognize), "deviated from the [biblical] text." "This Moses," Freud's writes in 1913 as though he were foreseeing his own vision of the late 1930s, "must be quite a different man, a new Moses of the artist's conception; so that Michelangelo [is he but a Freudian-imago?] must have had the presumption to emend the sacred text and to falsify the character of this holy man. Can we think him capable of a boldness which might almost be said to approach an act of blasphemy?" Yes, of course, is Freud's answer. And so if Michelangelo's Moses will "not [be] the Moses of the Bible" (XIII, 230) then neither will Freud's.[57]

In the opening section of his last major work Freud will thus invert the very inversion of the story of the hero's birth that, following Otto Rank, he had located in the ancient Jews' account of Moses. That is, he reverses the process by which the birth-legend had turned an Egyptian prince into a son of Israel. He thereby restores the hero to his true origin. On the one hand, then, Moses is no longer a Jew because no longer the son of Jewish parents. On the other hand, to the extent the Jewish people had claimed him as their greatest son, the Egyptian, which is to say non-Jewish, Moses becomes a hero in the way Freud had defined that term: "A hero is a man who stands up . . . against his father, . . . [one who is] *born again against his father's will.*" We might take the italicized phrase in a more symbolic fashion very much in keeping with the spirit of the book to mean the one who refuses to be created by his father's choice or perhaps the son who refuses the father's choice in him.[58] If the heroic Moses creates by choosing, Freud himself, we might say, seeks to repeat this heroic act. He invents a genealogy not just so that Moses will become an Egyptian but so that he himself might be (re)born against the will of his own father. For by choosing a non-Jewish (great-)father he also locates a new origin in something other than the "religion of his fathers," which is at the same time his father's religion and so the father himself.[59] In his very act of choosing the non-Jewish Moses as the great father of his people, Freud cannot truly have been fathered at all: even as one who necessarily comes late, if he is present to make this choice he must have been there from the beginning.

By retelling the (hi)story of the Jewish people in the origin of monotheism, Freud's discovery or invention of the Egyptian Moses thereby becomes the story of a new hero, Freud himself. But what of his fellow Jews, those "helpless, intimidated son[s]" dispossessed of their own origin by an act in which they played no part? Are they to be forever after excluded from the possibility of heroism? Jewish tradition's revision of the hero's birth-legend not only creates a Jewish Moses but also marks the people's acceptance of their own belatedness: the absolute cleavage between God and man established at the heart of monotheism thus now also becomes the temporal division of the origin and the afterwards. The sons of Israel will then always exist in the latter—the afterward subsequently (re)enacted through adherence to tradition—because created by a great father-stranger (God is now a distorted image of Moses himself) who alone can create and choose and exist at and even before the beginning. But even in lamenting that "we Jews have been reproached for growing cowardly," Freud can yet look back to a past when they were members of "a valiant nation" (*Letters*, 453).⁶⁰ If such a nation only existed "once upon a time," as he puts it, what the Jews actually did to distinguish themselves in that ancient past was not insignificant. If they were chosen by Moses to carry the bright torch of monotheism into a pagan darkness, they yet had to reciprocate that choice with a choosing of their own, accepting from Moses and so making their own precisely "the religion that Egypt disdained" (*Moses and Monotheism*, 32). "Monotheism has not taken root in Egypt," he will observe later in the account, "a failure [that] might have happened in Israel" as well (141). But prompted by their noble prophets who had been "seized by the great and powerful tradition," the Jewish people would establish, albeit in distorted form, what they had been given by Moses as "the permanent content of the Jewish religion." "It is honor enough for the Jewish people," Freud adds with real sincerity, "that it has kept alive such a tradition and produced men who lent it their voice, even if the stimulus had first come from outside" (63).⁶¹

But their unique role as caretakers of what Moses offered is something more, for it is also, and more fundamentally, "the proof of a special psychical fitness in the mass which had become the Jewish people that it could bring forth so many persons who were ready to take upon themselves the burden of the Mosaic religion" (142). Paradoxically, the burden of having been chosen becomes "the reward of believing that their people was a chosen one" precisely by the *taking on*—the very choosing—of the burden itself.⁶² For Freud, in other words, it was only through the people's response to Moses's choice of them, something approaching a heroic choice of its own, that the Jews could make real what the great father, the great stranger, had imposed on them. If as belated sons they could not all be a Freud, let alone a Moses, Freud yet finds in the Jewish people a more modest form of heroism, one worthy of its own acknowledgment and toward which he can still feel an ancestral pride.

Epilogue

> I'll . . . stand
> As if a man were author of himself
> And knew no other kin.
>
> —Shakespeare, *Coriolanus*

I

At the beginning of the end, I take up a text from Freud's beginning that, on the surface at least, deals with his end (death). It is one of the longest dreams Freud recounts in the *Interpretation of Dreams*:

> Old Brücke must have set me some task; STRANGELY ENOUGH, it related to the dissection of the lower part of my own body, my pelvis and legs, which I saw before me as though in the dissecting room, but without noticing their absence in myself and also without a trace of any gruesome feeling. Louise N. was standing beside me and doing the work with me. The pelvis had been eviscerated, and it was visible now in its superior, now in its inferior aspect, the two being mixed together. Thick flesh-colored protuberances (which, in the dream itself, made me think of hemorrhoids) could be seen. Something which lay over it and was like crumpled silver-paper had also to be carefully fished out. I was then once more in possession of my legs and was making my way through town. But (being tired) I took a cab. To my astonishment the cab drove in through a door in a house, which opened and allowed it to pass along a passage which turned a corner at its end and finally led into the open

air again. Finally, I was making a journey through a changing landscape with an Alpine guide who was carrying my belongings. Part of the way he carried me too, out of consideration of my tired legs. The ground was boggy; we went round the edge; people were sitting on the ground like Red Indians or gypsies—among them a girl. Before this I had been making my own way forward over the slippery ground with a constant feeling of surprise that I was able to do it so well after the dissection. At last we reached a small wooden house at the end of which was an open window. There the guide set me down and laid two wooden boards, which were standing ready, upon the window-sill, so as to bridge the chasm which had to be crossed over from the window. At that point I really became frightened about my legs, but instead of the expected crossing, I saw two grown-up men lying on wooden benches that were along the walls of the hut, and what seemed to be two children sleeping beside them. It was as though what was going to make the crossing possible was not the boards but the children. I awoke in a mental fright. (V, 452–53; original italics deleted)

The dream concerns a journey and a difficult one at that: hence, the consistent concern with body-problems (dissected pelvis and legs, "tired legs"), the need to be carried (in a "cab" or by an "Alpine guide"), the quality of the ground ("boggy," "slippery"), and finally, the dilemma of how to "bridge the "chasm" to the "small wooden house" (the boards laid out for the purpose are already a problem because of his tired legs, but the boards then turn into two sleeping children). In the subsequent analysis, Freud makes it clear that the journey carries him toward death: the " 'wooden house' was . . . , no doubt, a coffin, that is to say, the grave"; the house reminds Freud of a "an excavated Etruscan grave" he had once been in ("a narrow chamber with two stone benches along its walls, on which the skeletons of two grown-up men were lying"); and these details come immediately after a reference to Rider Haggard's novel, *She*, from which Freud recalls a "perilous journey . . . leading into an undiscovered region" (perhaps also recalling the "undiscovered country" of Hamlet's "To be or not to be speech") that results, not as one might have hoped, in "finding immortality" but rather in "perish[ing] in the mysterious subterranean fire" (454). In this context we might infer that the opening image of dissection in which Freud peers into his own body is connected to the dream's "two grown-up men lying on wooden benches" that itself recalls the skeletal figures from the Etruscan grave.[1] In one sense, then, the dream appears to represent Freud's anticipation of his own death, an image that repels him ("I awoke in a mental fight").

That said, even in following Schopenhauer that "the problem of death stands at the outset of every philosophy" (*Totem and Taboo*, XIII, 87), Freud himself had taught us to be wary about making facile assumptions. Thus, for example, in pondering the nature and origin of the fear of death in his *Inhibitions, Symptoms and Anxiety*, Freud observes that "the unconscious seems to contain nothing that could give any content to our concept of the annihilation of life. . . . [N]othing resembling death can ever have been experienced; or if it has, as in fainting, it has left no observable traces behind" (XX, 129–30). In regard to the "dissection/wooden house" dream, we might note that Freud is not dead but only tired (feeble perhaps). Our sense that the dream-thoughts might be more concerned with getting old is confirmed in his later observation that, while in the dream itself he "missed the gruesome feeling ['*Grauen*'] appropriate to" the experience of being dissected, "the other sense of the word" is "grey," as in grey hair; Freud thus associates with the dream his wish "to miss growing grey" though he knows he is "already growing quite grey" (V, 477–78).

But even the simple anxiety over aging expressed through the dream (and the journey suggests Freud working through some kind of temporal process or life-narrative) appears as shorthand for another, more complex concern. Thus he writes that "the grey of my hair was another reminder that I must not delay any longer. And . . . the thought that I should have to leave it to my children to reach the goal of my difficult journey forced its way to representation at the end of the dream" (V, 478). In other words, the "mental fright" experienced as he awoke did not point to a fear of getting old *per se* or even of dying but of getting toward "the end" (the end of the dream as the end of life) without having reached his goal and thus "hav[ing] to leave it to [his] children." And when shortly thereafter in summing up another dream Freud will write "after all, I reflected, was not having children our only path to immortality" (487), we might surmise that the goal of his difficult journey, a goal he may not be able to reach on his own, is immortality itself; that is, in his life-journey he will have failed to have achieved the immortality he sought on his own and will instead have to rely on "having children" as the "only true path to immorality."[2] We might note in this context that the previously mentioned reference to the novel *She* also suggests that what Freud fears is precisely not "finding immortality," as he had thought he would, through his own exertions: thus the "tired feeling in my legs" (and the question: "How much longer will my legs carry me?"), the "tired mood," and the "doubting thought" are all suggestive of an anticipatory fear *not* of coming to his end in death but of failing to have lived the life he had imagined for himself and thereby achieving the immorality he had expected. If the dream is about a journey *toward* death (so life itself), the question at the heart of the dream is what sort of life will Freud have led before he dies, what will he have accomplished? Will what he has left behind as his legacy just be his children (otherwise "our only path to immorality") or some other monument, like that Etruscan grave about which his dream-thoughts say, " 'If you must rest in a grave, let it be the Etruscan one' " (454–55), a monument subsequently excavated and admired by others?

Even if Freud might eventually rest in an Etruscan grave, what form would that monument take? Why must he "not delay any longer"? What do the boards stand for by which he might make his crossing on his own (albeit all the time "frightened about [his] legs" as though they may not be sufficient), boards that might otherwise be replaced by children? The reference to his former mentor, Ernst Brücke, at the very beginning of the dream puts the drive for immorality, initially at least, into a professional context. If the task imposed by Brücke in the dream, "a dissection *of my own body*," is his own "*self-analysis*" (V, 454), what Freud seems most concerned with is how that analysis will translate into professional accomplishment through publication: "I reflected on the amount of self-discipline it was costing me to offer the public . . . my book on dreams" (453); "the dissection meant the self-analysis which I was carrying out . . . in the publication of this present book about dreams—a process which had been so distressing to me . . . that I had postponed the printing of the finished manuscript" (477). Whether Freud explicitly means that the "wooden boards" in the dream (the means by which he should have properly reached his grave-as-monument and so a self-achieved immortality) should have been his published writings, in the dream he analyzes immediately after (the "train to Marburg" dream) he clearly understands writing as a path to social status (he mentions Adam Smith's *Wealth of Nations* by title and makes a general reference to the great Schiller), even a kind a vengeance on "first-class" types who might otherwise look down upon him.[3] We might thus assume that the "dissection/wooden house" dream expresses Freud's anxiety either that he won't finish his planned writing or that it won't be publically accepted in such a way that he might gain by it a proper monument to professional success. The image that he otherwise inexplicably associates with his greying hair, "a reminder that I must not delay any longer," makes particular sense in relation to the figure of "Louise N." who assists Freud in the "dissection/wooden house" dream. In the analysis, Freud explains that, in response to her request for "something to read," he had "offered . . . Rider Haggard's *She* . . . '[a] *strange* book, but full of hidden meanings'" (perhaps like the *Interpretation of Dreams* itself). But Louise had asked instead "'Have you nothing of your own?'" To which Freud tellingly responds, "'No, my own immortal works have not yet been written'" (453). The acknowledgment that he hasn't truly yet started down his path to immortality combined with his obvious concern that, even if he does publish, he will not find a receptive audience—Louise then replies, "with a touch of sarcasm," that she and others "'expect these so-called ultimate explanations . . . which you've promised that even *we* shall find readable'"—together suggest that at the heart of the "dissection/wooden house" dream is his anxiety that, in the end, he will not be able to "cross over" to his grave with a noteworthy, publically recognized achievement to his credit. All he will leave behind to ensure his immortality will be his children.

Still, if the dream suggests something of Freud's feelings governing his parental relation with his children (however abstractly conceived), we might turn the dream around and consider Freud in the role of a son rather than that of a father. There are several reasons to contemplate such a reversal. First, in previous dreams (e.g., the "non vixit" dream), "old Brücke" is typically a father-figure and, more precisely, a substitute for Jacob Freud. We might especially recall the look of reproach Freud had to face in the "non vixit" dream in Brücke's "terrible blue eyes"; he had received this reproach because he had arrived late at the laboratory, an experience, I argued earlier, that pulled together the feeling of (self-)reproach Freud felt in the 1896 dream because he had arrived late at his father's funeral and the image of *Hamlet* 3.4.124–30 where the Ghost of King Hamlet reproachfully gazes upon his prince-son for failing to do his filial duty. The recollection of that moment in *Hamlet* might partly explain the reference to the "undiscovered region" from Haggard's *She* in the "dissection/wooden house" dream. Although Hamlet says that "no traveller" has ever returned from the "undiscover'd country" (3.1.78–79), his strange forgetting of the Ghost's visitation in 1.4–5 suggests that through the intermediary of Haggard's novel Freud's allusion to *Hamlet* points to his Hamlet-like effort to avoid recognizing the continuing presence of his father in his life.

We might, moreover, give some attention to the way Freud's ends his initial analysis of the "dissection/wooden house" dream: "I woke up in a 'mental fright,' even after the successful emergence of the idea that children may perhaps achieve what their father had failed to—a fresh allusion to the strange novel [*She*] in which a person's identity is retained through a series of generations for over two thousand years" (V, 455; original italics deleted).

Freud appears to feel that the "emergence" in the dream of the idea that a child's success in achieving what the father could not should have worked against his waking up in "mental fright"; that is, he would have expected that idea to have been a source of pleasurable affect.[4] But since the dream appears to view in negative terms the possibility that Freud's (the father's) only immortality will be in his children and not, as he had hoped, in his own professional success, he should only have expected to have felt pleasure in the idea of a child's surpassing its father if he had been identifying with the child against the father. That is precisely an idea (though one he experienced with great ambivalence) Freud would take up in his 1936 essay, "Disturbance of Memory on the Acropolis":

> It must be that some sense of guilt was attached to the satisfaction in having gone such a long way. There was something about it that was wrong, that from earliest times is forbidden. It was something to do with a child's criticism of his father, with the underevaluation which took the place of the overevaluation of earlier childhood. It seems as though *the essence of success was to have got further than one's father*, as though to excel one's father was still something forbidden. . . . The very theme of Athens and the Acropolis in itself contained evidence of the son's superiority. . . . [But] what interfered with our enjoyment of the journey to Athens was a feeling of filial piety. (XXII, 247; my emphasis)

In short, in the context of Freud's full life at least, the idea that emerges in the "dissection/wooden house" dream of a child's achieving more than its father puts Freud as much in the former position as in the latter. Behind the anxiety in the dream we might then also wonder if Freud is worried less that he won't be professionally successful than that, in his fantasy at least, he will be so successful that he will cross into "something forbidden" by claiming a "superiority" to his father ("the essence of success"—and perhaps of immortality—"was to have got further than one's father"). To the extent the dream ends with the image of a grave as a kind of monument to the dead (which is how Freud appears to understand the Etruscan grave he had once visited), in it we see Freud still grappling with where he had been four years previously when first prompted to self-analysis by his father's death. In the dream of 1896 he felt the self-reproach of a son who had not done his filial duty in mourning his dead father properly. And in the "dissection/

wooden house" dream recorded in 1900 the grave-as-monument might be disturbing because in his own planned success he transgresses against a proper filial piety in the expectation of a body of professional work that will at once render him immortal and leave his father behind.

The question here is whether the final image of the dream—"It was as though what was going to make the crossing [the immortality of the father] possible was not the [two wooden] boards but the children"—can be taken to present Jacob Freud as the father in search of crossing into death and Freud himself as the child(ren) through whom the father will achieve immortality (in this case not just through the mere act of siring his son, Sigmund, but also vicariously through his son's fame).[5] The fact that in the dream it is the father-figure, Brücke, who imposes on Freud the task of the dissection that Freud then recognizes as the self-analysis (precisely what was prompted by Jacob Freud's death) suggests, minimally, that behind his own longing for professional achievement with its attendant "immortality" is filial ambivalence. What his own father had imposed on him, including the desire for greatness that will start with the writing of his own strange book full of hidden meanings, conflicts with the feeling that by achieving his own greatness he will necessarily diminish his father.

Might we then restore to the "dissection/wooden house" dream the figure of the father or, more precisely, the son's filial ambivalence toward the father, his need at once to honor and to surpass him? If we can, we might then also revise the final meaning Freud assigns the dream. As we noted, Freud ends his initial attempt at analysis as follows: "I woke up in a 'mental fright,' even after the successful emergence of the idea that children may perhaps achieve what their father had failed to—*a fresh allusion to the strange novel [She] in which a person's identity is retained through a series of generations for over two thousand years.*" Freud seems to mean by the phrase I have italicized that it is its own kind of immortality to have a share in "a series of generations"; that is, in what is no doubt a particularly Jewish conception of life-after-death, even in death one might retain identity not only through having one's own children (their very existence keeps the parents alive regardless of what they might accomplish) but through a much longer line of descent: "over two thousand years." Freud himself is not particularly pleased by the prospect—it doesn't prevent his awakening in fright—and we might observe in this context that, especially through the "fresh allusion" to *She*, the measure of time ("two thousand years") appears to look to the past as much as much to the future. (In Haggard's novel, Ayesha or "She-who-must-be-obeyed" *has lived* for over two thousand years, which means that her identity as retained "through a series of generations" points toward her past rather than toward her future; and, in fact, she dies at the end of the story, which suggests that she does not find immortality in the sense Freud intends.) Viewed from this perspective, Freud's *not* taking pleasure at the possibility of retaining identity across countless generations might have less to do with his needing to surrender his hope of professional success (to exchange that immortality for the simple fact of having children) than with the weight of time he feels pressing upon him, a weight imposed "through a series of generations for over two thousand years": in short, the burden coming down through time from the mere existence of his ancestors or forefathers.[6] To feel oneself belonging to such a series would be its own kind of immortality, but it is not, the dream reminds him, what Freud seeks for himself. For instead of achieving through his own efforts what might be worthy of admiration, he fears that he will live on only because he is part of something larger than himself, something that defines and limits him even as he lives his life. Without accomplishment, the very accomplishment by which he would diminish his own father as what came before, what immortality he could experience would derive from his share in a collective rather than from his own personal identity. And to the extent a long past ("over two thousand years") burdens him with the most lasting portion of his identity, even at the moment of death he would not be able to truly claim his existence as his own.

If some strange notion of immortality is being expressed through the dream (a grave that is more like a quaint little house, an identity that lasts millennia, etc.), we might go further to say that such immortality, even where it might also mark an outlasting of the father and an outstripping of his achievements, feels uncannily akin to being buried alive in one's own life. Even if the "children may . . . achieve what their father has failed," the successful child is yet locked into a "series of generations" that points backwards in time rather than forwards. The small wooden house of the dream (a coffin, a grave) is thus not death so much as the past itself and the identity it imposes, bound as it is and so binding the child to what comes before, to generations of ancestors stretching back to time immemorial. The most horrifying part of the dream is the suggestion that the child, Freud himself, the son of his father, has lived, unknowingly, for two thousand years inside that grave. Even when he is alive he has only the life imposed by the presence of the (fore)father(s) he cannot escape.[7] Even while living he is, like Hamlet at the funeral of Ophelia in 5.1 of Shakespeare's play, already in the grave.

II

In the person of his father and particularly in his ambivalent response to his father's death in 1896, Freud confronted a personal psychical crisis that is best understood as an experience of existential unease. A year later he would write to his colleague, Wilhelm Fliess, that he had uncovered the secret of that ambivalence in what would come to be known as the Oedipus complex (letter of October 15, 1897, *Origins*, 223–24). It has been one of the central arguments of this study that Freud's eureka-moment was misleading (to himself and to his followers), for what he felt in the wake of his father's death was not the result of the Oedipus complex as traditionally conceived. The most obvious reason to take this position is that, despite his later specification that the son's desire to kill his father arose "*because* of his passion of his mother" (*Origins*, 224; my emphasis), in work after work Freud comes back to the son's vexed and varied feelings for the father (hostility, submission, duty, obedience, identification, love, guilt, remorse, etc.) without even trying to show except by the loosest of analogies—and these largely determined by his need to reassert the near universal applicability of his core theory—that incestuous desire was a factor in these feelings, let alone their chief cause.

In short, what Freud understood as the Oedipal economy as both theorized and applied had always been a diversion, a way of deflecting his thought away from the real source of filial ambivalence. Over his long career, Freud consistently pointed to this other source, but he could only ever address it indirectly either because he was professionally over-committed to the notion of the Oedipus complex or because he never truly recognized his own best insight. I have argued, moreover, that this insight had been anticipated in many of the texts in which Freud claimed to find support for his theory, texts that he interpreted through a psychoanalytic and usually an Oedipal lens: the Moses story, *Hamlet*, Hoffmann's "The Sandman," etc. We might say, then, that these texts not only anticipated Freud's work (a position Freud himself no doubt would have openly acknowledged) but also proleptically corrected it. Still, the fact that in the interstices of Freudian rhetoric we find their intuitions and his appearing over and over again demonstrates that Freud had not completely failed to learn the lessons these texts were teaching him. In a sense, without fully recognizing it, Freud arrived at his own best insight through the act of *mis*interpreting them. At the very least, his (mis)interpretive work points us to a different way of understanding filial ambivalence even in the context of a Freudian mode of analysis.

If then his Oedipal theory obscures as much as it reveals, what Freud's writings constantly circle back to without ever being able to directly acknowledge is that the unease he felt in the wake of his father's death marked his recognition of what it meant for the son to have come after his father and thus to *have been* fathered. The pairing of passiveness and belatedness lurking in that "have been" also meant that, in relation to what came before, the son was necessarily absent from the scene of his own origin.

To the extent Freud is explicitly interested in the origin, his Oedipal theory imagines an experience from infancy that "happens" and is then "forgotten" in the unconscious through repression only to be retroactively configured at a later stage so as to form the basis of a neurosis. (In its most specific form this is the primal scene: a witnessing of parental copulation coded as a sexual-aggressive act.) From that point of retrospection (or retroactive interpretation), what can never quite be properly remembered is dealt with psychically either through repetition (a "positive" attempt to revive the initial traumatic experience) or through "defensive reactions" (a "negative" attempt to inhibit them [*Moses and Monotheism*, 93–95]).[8] But the crisis of belatedness or afterwardsness that I have attempted to document as the deeper meaning of Freud's interest in the origin cannot be understood through the sequence of event—forgetting/repression—return (in distorted form) because the absence or missing that initiates the trauma of coming after can only have "happened" when the subject (always the son for Freud) was not present to have experienced it at all. For the father's act of choosing brought into being what did not yet exist. And from the perspective of the son thus compelled to live with the burden of the ever-afterwards, what was precisely absent or missing from the scene of the origin was his own capacity to choose, to call himself into existence, to father himself.

The primal scene as the moment of recognizing that one must always come after means that self-fathering is excluded from the start even if that fact is not recognized until some later triggering event, what Emerson had called the "discovery we have made that we exist." Hence, the primal scene also marks the advent of the uncanny into consciousness. For the primal scene brings to light from the past and *as* one's own past what is both familiar—even too familiar—and inaccessible. The origin that is one's own and not one's own is always just out of one's grasp but in a way that constantly beckons. What Freud felt in 1896 only to explain away in 1897 and for the rest of his career was precisely how his father's death awakened in him the fact that his own origin was forever lost to him, not something he had experienced and then forgotten but rather something he would never be able to remember because it was not something he ever had to begin with.

As he would say in *Beyond the Pleasure Principle*, what is truly traumatic is our confrontation with a force that brings us out of our inanimate state into conscious life, "a force of whose nature we can form no conception." And what makes this moment truly uncanny is that it also carries the recognition that, if *we* can form no conception of its nature, someone else can. The choice of our existence always already belongs to another.

Nevertheless, as we saw in chapter 6, in his final major work, published in the last year of his life, Freud is still searching without knowing how or why to claim that choice as his own. He would, as we observed, resist the imposition from the Jewish father (his own father and the Moses of biblical tradition and so also tradition itself) to claim that the Jewish Moses was in fact a "great stranger," an Egyptian, one who "came from outside" and who created the Jews (who never existed before) precisely by choosing them. In many ways, the new (hi)story Freud told still bore the marks of the ambivalence he had never fully faced let alone completely overcome. Moses was both the great father of the Jews and, as the opening of *Moses and Monotheism* reminds us, the greatest of their sons. Freud powerfully identified with this figure—who himself, in Freud's account, had identified with Ikhnaton, the Pharaoh who had not only started a new religion but had also refused the name (Amenhotep IV) bequeathed to him by his father. And Freud made this identification in part by discovering (or inventing) and thereby choosing the non-Jewish Moses. If Moses was not to be among the sons of Israel then neither would Freud. Like Moses, then, he would be a true hero, a son born against his father's will and so in defiance of the father's choice. If the tortured son, Nathanael, in Hoffmann's "The Sandman" had been traumatized by the recognition that his origin belonged to the "old man" (*Der Alte*) whose presence was forever hidden away in a past to which Nathanael and indeed the story itself had no access, in *Moses and Monotheism* Freud would be more like another tortured and equally belated son, Hamlet, who refused to live in the shadow of his paternal namesake by resisting what the dead father imposed.

As we saw in chapter 5, Milton's portrait of Satan suggests that, in the Judeo-Christian tradition at least, such self-authorizing could only ever be a Gnostic fantasy. And for Freud to be able to choose his own father (not the Jewish father, Jacob Freud, but the Egyptian Moses as the great father) would be tantamount to bringing himself into existence in the sense that the very act of choosing would be, as *Moses and Monotheism* is at pains to suggest, an act of creation (to be "self-begot," as Milton's Satan puts it). More to the point, to have existed at the place where he could choose the father could only mean that he had been there, like the divine Son of John's quasi-Gnostic gospel, at or, paradoxically, even before his own beginning. Even if this self-fathering or the refusal of any father is itself a fantasy, it is yet a choice. More to the point, even as an expression of filial ambivalence, it certainly does not manifest the Oedipal son's desire to slay the father, let alone to sleep with the mother. It marks, rather, the son's desire to be free of paternal authority-as-priority. It marks, in short, the refusal to come after.

In 1896, Freud had the uncanny intuition that his dead father was not truly dead and indeed continued to exert a pressure that in some inexplicable way was related to his very absence. Some four decades later in *Moses and Monotheism* he translated that burden into Jewish ethnic-cultural terms in the experience of having been chosen by a great stranger who himself seemed to confuse what it meant to be a father or a son, what it meant to come before or after. *Moses and Monotheism* is thus, finally, a meditation on the problem of filial ambivalence that had vexed Freud since 1896 because the new (hi)story of the Jewish people (and especially the origin of Jewish monotheism) was caught up in the question of how Jewishness itself—as history, as faith, as culture, as tradition—expressed the experience of missing at the point of origin, an absence that came home in full force only through the father's death (whether for the Jews, for Hamlet, or for Freud). Jewish identity, in short, as least as recounted in *Moses and Monotheism,* is the very experience of filial belatedness carried over into a cultural mythology and played out in the terrain of mass psychology. It was the Egyptian Moses who imposed this identity, and for the Jews he created the experience of having been chosen became an inherited psychosocial property in which tradition would thereafter mark a dispossession at the origin and offer a simultaneous compensation for and disavowal of that very dispossession.

If as Yosef Hayim Yerushalmi suggests, *Moses and Monotheism* cannot be read "merely as psychological autobiography" (let alone as "psychoanalytic confession"), it can be, perhaps should be, understood as the "final chapter in a Freud's lifelong case history."[9] For the story of Jewish origins provides both an example of and evidence for the ongoing impact of an insight, perhaps just a vague intuition, that had been displaced into Freud's writings for his entire career as a psychoanalyst. *Moses and Monotheism* is an expression of the quest to lay to rest the ghost of the dead father, if not for all Jews then at least for Freud himself. It was a quest Freud had set in motion in the *Interpretation of Dreams*, his first foray into the mode of interpretation that would become the centerpiece of Freudian psychoanalytic practice. The ambivalence that he discovered in his response to his father's death was not about Judaism itself (which Freud clearly admired) or even directly about the human person we know as Jacob Freud. But the ambivalence did concern what in 1930 Freud would refer to as the *väterlich[en] Religion* ("the religion of his fathers" [XIII, xv]), a phrase that metonymically yokes together Judaism as Freud's own religious heritage (if not his actual religion), the religion of his own father and thus the figure of Jacob Freud as a Jewish father, and the very notion of Jewishness as something passed down over time and bequeathed to the son(s) as both imposition and loving gift, a bequest that carried with it the burden of eternal belatedness at both the personal and the cultural level (in a word: tradition).

What Freud's personal-familial life shared with the larger Jewish legacy he both celebrated and rejected was the sense of a burden emanating from the past and, in a sense, coincident with that past. It was a past that had a beginning the present could neither claim nor simply ignore precisely because it was determined by that beginning. For Freud, the father resided at that beginning and, from that position, chose the son's origin, indeed chose the son into existence. But through force of will a son who was not helpless and intimidated could become a hero by claiming the origin for himself. Like Hamlet, Freud could only make this choice at the very end of his life, and he did so in *Moses and Monotheism* by choosing and then identifying with a non-Jewish father.

What *Moses and Monotheism* reveals, finally, is the remarkable staying power of the struggle with filial ambivalence that, in a very real sense, had been the origin of psychoanalysis itself. The existential crisis at the heart of Freud's project would in 1939 produce a study of Jewish ethnic-cultural origins as the crisis of what it meant for an entire people to come too late. At the personal level, in the Egyptian Moses he created for himself a new genealogy, one in which, succeeding where Milton's Satan could not, he could be self-begot, unfathered, never belated.

Notes

Introduction

1. The painting is part of the permanent collect of the Museum Boijmans Van Beuningen, Rotterdam, The Netherlands: http://collectie.boijmans.nl/nl/object/4232.

2. I borrow this term from Jean Laplanche's translation of the Freudian term "*Nachträglichkeit*," more typically translated into English as "deferred action": see, for example, "Notes on Afterwardsness," in *Essays on Otherness*, ed. John Fletcher (New York, 1999), 260–65.

3. We might compare Lacan's musing that the "'I think' to which it is intended that presence be reduced, continues to imply, no matter how indeterminate one may make it, all the powers of reflection by which subject and consciousness are confounded" ("Maurice Merleau-Ponty," *Le Temps Modernes* [1961]; qtd. in Jacques Lacan, *The Language of the Self: The Function of Language in Psychoanalysis*, trans. Anthony Wilden [New York, 1968], 106n49). In a related context, Paul Ricoeur makes the more general observation that psychoanalysis opens up a new chapter in the "philosophy of the subject" because "it imposes the dispossession of the subject as it appears primarily to itself in the form of consciousness. It makes consciousness not a given but a problem." Ricoeur adds that, after Freud, "one can no longer establish the philosophy of the subject as a philosophy of consciousness" precisely because "reflection and consciousness no longer coincide" ("A Philosophical Interpretation of Freud," trans. Willis Domingo, in Paul Ricoeur, *The Conflict of Interpretations: Essays in Hermeneutics*, ed. Don Ihde [Evanston, IL, 1974], 161, 172).

4. "Experience," in *Selections from Ralph Waldo Emerson*, ed. Stephen E. Whicher (Boston, 1957), 269. Subsequent page references will be cited in the text.

5. For a variety of responses to the essay's way of representing loss, see B. L. Packer, *Emerson's Fall* (New York, 1982), 148–79; Richard Poirier, *The Renewal of Literature: Emersonian Reflections* (New Haven, CT, 1988), 134–81; and Stanley Cavell, "Finding as Found: Taking Steps in Emerson's 'Experience,'" in *This New Yet Unapproachable America: Lectures after Emerson after Wittgenstein* (Albuquerque, NM, 1989), 77–118.

6. For discussion of how Emerson's essay treats the "problem of time" as an experience of self-alienation—a "quality of being lost, of losing one's place"—see T. S. McMillin, *Our Preposterous Use of Literature: Emerson and the Nature of Reading* (Urbana, IL, 2000), 140–41.

7. For a nuanced account of how mourning for his son informs the entire essay, see Sharon Cameron, "Representing Grief: Emerson's 'Experience,' " *Representations* 15 (1986): 15–41.

8. "The Animal That Therefore I Am (More to Follow)," trans. David Wills, *Critical Inquiry* 28 (2002): 380–81.

9. Emerson makes only a single passing reference to his dead son, Waldo: "The only thing grief has taught me is to know how shallow it is. . . . In the death of my son, now more than two years ago, I seem to have lost a beautiful estate,—no more. . . . I grieve that grief can teach me nothing" (256).

10. In his first use of the term *Urszenen* in a letter of May 2, 1897, Freud was referring to a variety of traumatic infantile experiences without explicitly connecting these to parental coitus. Three years later in the *Interpretation of Dreams* he stressed the role of the observation of parental coitus in the generation of anxiety but without explicitly using the term (V, 584–85). In a letter to an Open Forum in 1912, again without using the term Freud asked his colleagues to send to him any accounts of "patients' dreams whose interpretation justifies the conclusion that the *dreamers had been witness to sexual intercourse in their early years*" (qtd. XVII, 4; italics in original). That request was clearly connected to his current analysis of the patient subsequently known as the Wolf Man. It is in this context that the more familiar understanding of the term "primal scene" ("From the History of an Infantile Neurosis," XVII, 39 and *passim*) was first developed and given its most extended treatment. For related discussions of the term, see Henry Edelheit, "Mythopoesis and the Primal Scene," *Psychoanalytic Study of Society* 5 (1972): 212–33; and Harold Blum, "On the Concept and Consequences of the Primal Scene," *Psychoanalytic Quarterly* 48 (1979): 27–47.

11. Freud hypothesizes that the one-and-a-half-year-old Wolf Man was stimulated in the anal zone and was so sexually excited by his parents' intercourse that he passed a stool (XVII, 80–81).

12. Freud at times imagines the latent operation of this psychical residue as a form of instinct—a "phylogenetic heritage" (XVII, 97)—akin to that found in animals.

13. *The Sacred Complex: On the Psychogenesis of Paradise Lost* (Cambridge, MA, 1983), 163.

14. Late in the case history, as a kind of summation, Freud writes: "about the time of the boy's fourth birthday, . . . the dream brought into *deferred operation* his observation of intercourse at the age of one and a half . . . The activation of the picture, which, thanks to the advance in his intellectual development, he was now able to understand, operated not only like a fresh event, but like a new trauma" (XVII, 109; my emphasis). Reflecting on this scenario earlier, he had commented: "it may seem comic and incredible that a child of four should be capable of such

technical judgments and learned notions. This is simply another case of *deferred action*. At the age of one and a half the child receives an impression to which he is unable to react adequately; he is only able to understand it and to be moved by it [more literally "grasped by it": *von ihm ergriffen*] when the impression is revived in him at the age of four" (45n1; my emphasis).

15. At the very end of the case history, Freud makes that very general statement that the "Oedipus complex . . . comprises a child's relation to his parents" (XVII, 119). But despite a slightly earlier suggestion that the Wolf Man's womb-fantasy was "in all probability . . . a softened substitute . . . for the phantasy of incestuous intercourse with the mother" (XVII, 101–02), overall he has almost nothing to say about his patient's infantile erotic attachment to his mother. To the extent Freud sees heterosexual/maternal inclinations in the Wolf Man, these are almost always directed toward maternal substitutes of one kind or another: his sister, his nurse (Nanya), the nursery-maid (Grusha), and other servants and peasants from the estate (90–94 and *passim*). But for the most part Freud's analysis centers on "another person as a sexual object . . . his father," an "object-choice, which . . . had taken place along the path of identification" (27; also 35, 64). At one point Freud even refers to this attachment as "an inverted Oedipus complex" (119).

16. *Sacred Complex*, 163; for Freud's own summary, see XVII, 46–47.

17. Freud writes that, subject to the revisionary process, the primal scene rematerializes in an "inexhaustible variety of new shapes" (XVII, 51). In the case of the Wolf Man, his retrospective/reenacting "dreams gave an impression of always working over the same material in different ways" (19).

18. On the question of the status of the primal scene, in his account of the Wolf Man Freud acknowledged his uncertainty as to whether the primal scene was an actual event or a fantasized one, a psychical idea that existed only in backward-looking imposition of meaning especially as mediated by the son's newly Oedipalized vantage: see especially XVII, 48–60, 97–103. Partly no doubt because he grew frustrated by the pressure placed on him to state once-and-for-all whether the scene had actually occurred, in the end, Freud was content to fall back on the two notions: first, that primal fantasies were real to the mind (and thus, within the analytical situation, needed to be treated as though real whatever their actual status as events) and second, that the reality of the event in some sense created that identity grounded in sexuality as necessarily "splintered" (43–44).

19. *The Language of Psycho-analysis*, trans. Donald Nicholson-Smith (New York, 1974), 335; subsequent page references will be cited in the text. In the case of the Wolf Man, Freud observes that "these scenes from infancy are not reproduced during the treatment as recollections, they are the products of construction" (XVII, 51). At the very end of the study he reflects on how the child's psyche continually works over "the re-activated primal scene," which at first at least exists in the mind as "some sort of a hardly definable knowledge, something, as it were, preparatory to an understanding" (120).

20. Rainer Nägele remarks that, in the context of the primal scene, Freud consistently "designates a first position as the effect of something," which is "the

point of a *Nachträglichkeit*." But he also observes how, paradoxically, the position that initiates the "representing [of the] primal scene . . . constitutes itself as a primal scene of belatedness" (*Reading after Freud* [New York, 1987], 183–84).

21. Freud, of course, already knows—the wound is always the mark of castration: "Here, then, he [the Wolf Man] was playing the part of his father, and was connecting his mother's familiar haemorrhages with the castration of women, which he now recognized,—with the 'wound' " (XVII, 86).

22. *Sacred Complex*, 166–67.

23. Kerrigan: "The primal scene is the site at which the issues of ego differentiation become translated into the issues of the Oedipus complex. The entire complex unfolds within its structure . . . the primal scene includes the complex" (164). Reflecting on the "predominant part that is played in the formation of neuroses by . . . libidinal motive forces" (XVII, 9), Freud will locate those forces precisely within the Oedipal economy whose role in shaping identity-as-sexual is granted full explanatory force.

24. In short, what Freud narrates to the Wolf Man may be nothing more than what Nägele calls a "symptom of a fantasy" (184), a belated interpretation that imposes meaning on a scene that remains hidden, elusive, never quite directly available.

25. Freud is inconsistent in how he understands the psychical retention of the primal scene. At one point he states quite emphatically that "these scenes from infancy" are not held as "recollections" in the normal sense (XVII, 50–51). But earlier he had observed quite broadly that one of the functions of (later) fantasies is not just to reveal the reality of previous (real) events but also "to efface *the memory*" of such events (20; my emphasis).

26. Although he does frequently return to the notion that what he calls the primal scene may be a fantasy (see XVII, 49–51, 97–103), it is clear that, in the case of the Wolf Man at least, Freud wants to maintain that the term refers to a real event in the child's past. It is in this sense that, though subsequently forgotten, primal scenes were originally embedded in the mind only to be returned through a complex array of screen mechanisms (33–34, 42, 55–57).

27. *Primal Scenes: Literature, Philosophy, Psychoanalysis* (Ithaca, NY, 1986), 36–37; subsequent page references will be cited in the text.

28. Freud's own description suggests that he cannot imagine going beyond the primal scene: "only in such cases do we succeed in descending into the *deepest and most primitive strata of mental development* and in gaining from there *solutions for the problems* of the later formations" (XVII, 10; my emphases). The primal scene is the "solution" for—because it is the first cause of—the "problems of the later formations" Freud finds in the Wolf Man's obsessional neurosis. Lukacher, wrongly I think, suggests that in "reveal[ing] a more primordial concealment than he has ever imagined" (26), Freud thought that there could be something *more* primordial, *more* concealed than the primal scene itself. That idea is certainly suggested by certain elements of Freud's thought, but this is not how Freud explicitly understands the issue.

29. Freud was notoriously slippery on the question of reclaiming what had been (allegedly) forgotten of the primal scene. In later interviews, the patient known as the Wolf Man (Sergei Pankejev) revealed that Freud had told him that the past events he found so hard to accept would eventually return to him as memories: "And that's really how he described it. But no recollection came in my case" (Karin Obholzer, *The Wolf-Man: Conversations with Freud's Patient—Sixty Years Later*, trans. Michael Shaw [New York, 1982], 38). In his own study, Freud claimed that, in the therapeutic process, dreams functioned as "absolutely equivalent to a recollection," for their "analysis . . . invariably leads back to the same scene." But in a somewhat different vein he also noted that primal scenes "are as a rule not reproduced as recollections but have to be divined—constructed—gradually and laboriously from an aggregate of indications." And, against what the Wolf Man himself reported of Freud's position, Freud concludes that rather than actual memories "the patients themselves gradually *acquire a profound conviction of the reality* of these primal scenes, a conviction which is in no respect inferior to one based on recollection" (XVII, 51; my emphasis). This very problem of how memory appears to fail in the face of the primal scene led Freud to create a special category of repression: "by means of a process that can only be equated with a repression [*Verdrängung*], a *repudiation* [*Verwerfung*] of the new element" (109; my emphasis). Freud appears to mean by repudiation, as distinct from repression, a refusal in the face of an impossible contradiction, a refusal that results in a splitting of the ego different from that occurring in a neurosis (where the split occurs between the ego and the id). Just as important, because repudiation, while operating consciously, marks psychotic detachment from reality, the repudiated experience exists in a form from which memories can never truly be retrieved; as a special form of repression, that is, repudiation either prevents access to memories of the primal scene or, if the primal scene is not precisely encoded in the mind as a memory (Freud's "unconscious memory traces" [36]), prevents the disorganized form of the memory trace from taking shape as an organized recollection. After 1923, repudiation will be reconceptualized in other terms: e.g., "disavowal" (*Verleugnung*: XXIII, 204) and "isolation" (*Isolierung*: XX, 119–21).

30. At one point in the case of the Wolf Man, Freud refers to this mental trace as an "impression" (*Eindruck* [45n1]).

31. When Lukacher refers to the "radical ontological undecidability of the primal scene" (41), he is primarily calling attention to how, from the retrospective position, it is impossible to locate a beginning *of interpretation*; what comes later "points toward the origin, but interpretation cannot reveal the origin" (26).

32. Even at his conclusion Lukacher can still write: "Freud feels compelled to explain the inexplicable *forgetfulness* that always conceals the origin. The wolf dream conceals the origin, but it also reveals that the origin presents itself as concealment and *forgetfulness*" (41; my emphases).

33. In the *Interpretation of Dreams* Freud cites the dream of a patient who saw himself watching his parents copulating while he was still in the womb (V, 399–400). But even this example just makes my point: the earliest of all possible

witnessings paradoxically suggests an inescapable lateness—he already existed prior to having been born.

34. Claiming that the "primal scene establishes the originary function of nonoriginary temporal difference," Lukacher argues that "at the origin one discovers not a single event that transpires in one temporal sequence but a constellation of events that transpire in several discrete temporal sequences" (36).

35. *The Seminar of Jacques Lacan, Book III: The Psychoses (1955–56)*, ed. Jacques-Alain Miller; trans. Russell Grigg (New York, 1993), 104.

36. Elizabeth Bellamy, "From Ficino to Freud: Egyptian/Greek/Jew in Cultural History," in *Repossessions: Psychoanalysis and the Phantasms of Early Modern Culture*, ed. Timothy Murray and Alan K. Smith (Minneapolis, MN, 1998), 24. We might distinguish an immanent critique from what Ricoeur once referred to as a "philosophical reflection" on Freud, a "relocating [of Freud's] work in a different discourse, . . . reflective philosophy" (162).

37. As Laplanche and Pontalis note, Freud "never offered a definition, much less a general theory, of the notion of deferred action." But "it was indisputably looked upon by Freud as part of his conceptual equipment" (111). It is really to Lacan, especially his 1953 *Discours de Rome*, that we owe the first theoretical elaboration of the term especially in relation to the fundamental temporality of human consciousness, a temporality grounded in the experience of loss: see *Language of the Self*, especially 9–27.

38. As Nägele observes in relation to the sense of temporal alienation informing psychoanalytic theory and practice, the work paradoxically reveals "the presence of something which *itself is not*, and which is yet the foundation of presence." He adds that the realness of the primal scene as a past event is, even for Freud, "a necessary supposition or presupposition," and, as such, "appears only in the form of a limit, a threshold, a resistance which forbids trespassing . . . It cannot be represented, because it is the foundation and limit of representation" (174, 178).

39. "To Open a Question," in *Literature and Psychoanalysis: The Question of Reading Otherwise*, ed. Shoshana Felman (Baltimore, MD, 1982), 8–9.

40. Felman: "[L]iterature, by virtue of its ironic force, fundamentally deconstructs the fantasy of authority [in psychoanalysis] in the same way, and for the same reasons, that psychoanalysis deconstructs the authority of the fantasy—its claim to belief and to power as the sole window through which reality can . . . reach our grasp, enter into our consciousness" ("To Open a Question," 8).

Part I Introduction

1. *Remnants of Auschwitz: The Witness and the Archive*, trans. Daniel Heller-Roazen (New York, 1999), 148, 150; my emphases.

2. *The Birth of Tragedy and the Genealogy of Morals*, trans. Francis Golffing (Garden City, NY, 1956), 29.

3. As part of the transitional ground here, Freud points out that even in the *Merchant of Venice*, this original scenario is revealed in Bassanio's choosing among the three caskets, which, according to Freud, stand in for women (245–46). That is, this later form of the myth still shows vestiges of the original precisely by inverting it. Freud variously refers to these transformations as "inversions" (245–46), "displacements" (250), "replacements by the exact opposite" (253), and "reversals" (254).

4. For an attempt to read Freud's deployment of reversal in the essay as a kind of evasion or displacement of his own personal stake in the Shakespearean material, see Marjorie Garber, *Shakespeare's Ghost Writers: Literature as Uncanny Causality* (New York, 1987), ch. 4. As Garber puts it, the "theme" Freud addresses is actually "his," or rather "a problem only for him" (85). Garber is not always clear on what this problem is for Freud. At times, she hints that the essay's focus on the "old man" (Lear) expresses even as it masks his complex feelings toward his own father, Jacob Freud, an issue we shall take up more directly in chapter 3. At other times, however, Garber seems to be suggesting that Lear is a cover for Freud himself, the "old man" in relation to a youngest daughter (Cordelia standing in for Anna Freud). Either way, Garber's biographical-allegorical reading of the essay depends theoretically on Freud's Oedipal-castration model, a model that my own study aims to present as Freud's chief displacement, his effort to explain away a more primal concern with belatedness.

5. Combined with his interest in the sisters, this realization leads Freud to another claim: that if we know that "the third of the sisters is the Goddess of Death, we know the sisters" as a group: "they are the Fates, the Moerae, . . . the third of whom is called Atropos, the inexorable" (250).

6. For reasons that become clear over the course of the essay, Freud relates the folk-tale motif of the favored third daughter or third sister (Cordelia, Cinderella, etc.) to the substitution of love (beauty, kindness) for death; so he concludes: "[T]he Goddess of Death was replaced by the Goddess of Love and by that which most resembles her in human shape. The third of the sisters is no longer Death, she is the fairest, best, most desirable and most lovable among women" (253).

7. Some of the more specific gender-implications of this formulation, in particular the dual role of the mother as both birth and death, will be taken up briefly in chapter 2.

Chapter 1

1. "The Intrusive Past: The Flexibility of Memory and the Engraving of Trauma," in *Trauma: Explorations in Memory*, ed. Cathy Caruth (Baltimore, MD, 1995), 158. Subsequent page references will be cited in the text.

2. Van der Kolk and van der Hart write: "Freud's ambivalent position vis-à-vis trauma and dissociation is reflected in his concept of repression. . . . [S]ometimes he used the term in the sense of actively repressed conflictual instinctual

wishes: a defense against primitive, forbidden, Id-impulses, especially of a sexual nature.... With regard to trauma, the use of the term 'repression' evokes the image of a subject actively pushing the unwanted traumatic memory away" (168). Van der Kolk and van der Hart do not reject the concept of repression entirely; rather, they prefer "to reserve the use of the concept . . . for the defense against primitive, forbidden, Id-impulses" (168).

3. For their discussion of dissociation as an inability to integrate experience into an evolving life-history and for broader discussion of the links between the temporal structure of trauma and the failure of narrative memory, see van der Kolk and van der Hart, 169–77. For discussion of the notion of narrative selfhood, see Richard Kearney, *On Stories* (London, 2002), 125–56; and for discussion of this idea in the context of cognitive neurobiology, see Kay Young and Jeffrey L. Saver, "The Neurology of Narrative," *SubStance* 30 (2001): 72–84. Young and Saver observe that memory is more like a narrative system than a storehouse of images; thus, neurologically speaking, narrative patterns preexist and, in effect, create memory precisely to the extent that new experiences can be assimilated into those patterns (flexible as these must be). Although Saver and Young are not addressing trauma *per se*, one might extrapolate to say that an event becomes traumatic because it is experienced outside of normal memory (what van der Kolk and van der Hart call "narrative memory"). The trauma or "traumatic memory" stays outside of narrative memory precisely because it cannot be organized within the preexisting narrative patterns by which identity is created and sustained.

4. Whatever the objective reality of an event, it continues to exist only as a mental event (as "memories *stored* in the mind"); these "*actual memories*," as van der Kolk and van der Hart, observe, "may form the nucleus of psychopathology and continue to exert their influence on current experience by means of the process of dissociation" (158–59; my emphases). While in their discussion of "Deferred Action" Jean Laplanche and Jean-Bertrand Pontalis assert the necessity of getting away from the notion of "some kind of storing procedure" as central to the delayed manifestation of trauma (*The Language of Psycho-analysis*, trans. Donald Nicholson-Smith [New York, 1974], 114), elsewhere Laplanche notes that, for Freud, traumatic experience's movement "from past to future . . . implies the deposit of something in the individual which will only be reactivated later"; the "traces" of an earlier experience have been "retained and preserved" in the mind (*Essays on Otherness*, ed. John Fletcher [New York, 1999], 261–62).

5. *Unclaimed Experience: Trauma, Narrative, and History* (Baltimore, MD, 1996), 3–4; subsequent page references will be cited in the text. Although, as we shall see, she has a much different understanding of what the repetition of traumatic experience means, Caruth accepts the basic Freudian terms of how it is experienced (via repetition compulsion): "Faced with the striking occurrence of what were called the war neuroses in the wake of World War I, Freud is startled by the emergence of a pathological condition—the repetitive intrusion of nightmares and relivings of battlefield events—that is experienced like a neurotic pathology but whose symptoms seem to reflect, in startling directness and simplicity, nothing

but the unmediated occurrence of violent events. . . . Unlike the symptoms of a normal neurosis, whose painful manifestations can be understood ultimately in terms of the attempted avoidance of unpleasurable conflict, the painful repetition of the flashback can only be understood as the absolute inability of the mind to avoid an unpleasurable event that has not been given psychic meaning in any way" (58–59).

6. Having previously quoted Pierre Janet's statement that "memory is an action: essentially it is the action of telling a story," van der Kolk and van der Hart go on to quote Lawrence Langer's statement that Holocaust survivors cannot order a normal chronological life-history "because they know that their most complicated recollections are unrelated to time" (175, 177; Langer, *Holocaust Testimonies: The Ruins of Memory* [New Haven, CT, 1991]). Caruth similarly observes that "the barrier of consciousness is a barrier of sensation and knowledge that protects the organism by placing stimulation *within an ordered experience of time*. What causes trauma, then, is . . . *a break in the mind's experience of time*" (61; my emphases).

7. Although they do not mention repetition compulsion, Laplanche and Pontalis anticipate Caruth and van der Kolk and van der Hart in observing that a "deferred" response to a past experience acts on "whatever has been impossible in the first instance to incorporate fully into a meaningful context. The traumatic event is the epitome of such unassimilated experience" (112).

8. The idea that the ego might discover something "too late" was first formulated in Freud's *Project for a Scientific Psychology* (I, 358–59).

9. For Freud's own formulation, see *Moses and Monotheism*, 84, a passage Caruth quotes (70).

10. I quote from Caruth's revealing endnote (and the fact that she isolates this assertion in an endnote may itself be significant): "One can . . . understand Freud's description of the death drive . . . in terms of the very specific death described in the dream of the burning child, the death, that is, of a child. For what Freud defines as the death drive . . . could be seen generally as a sense that death is late, that one in fact dies only too late. And what could it mean to die too late, except to die after one's child? *It is important to note, here, a crucial shift that is not articulated in Freud's text, but is implied by Lacan's reading, from the notion of trauma as primarily a relation to one's own death to the notion of trauma as primarily a relation to another's death*. Freud's own shift from *Beyond the Pleasure Principle* to *Moses and Monotheism* [a shift Caruth explores in chapter 4] *may suggest . . . that the death of the other was always inseparable from his notion of one's 'own' death*" (142–43n10; my emphases; original emphases deleted).

11. Caruth acknowledges that the locating of all trauma as a response to another's death is but "implied by Lacan." It might be more accurate to cite the work of Laplanche as her main authority for this assertion. Discussing "death's entry on the Freudian scene" in *Beyond the Pleasure Principle* (and inflecting all of Freud's thought thereafter), Laplanche at first views the Freudian "maxim"—"if you would endure life, be prepared for death"—as meaning preparation "for *your* death," that is, the solitary and necessary end of each individual. But because he follows Freud in believing that "our unconscious is . . . inaccessible to the idea of our own death,"

Laplanche reorients his argument: "In the unconscious, death would always be the death of the other, . . . and we would accede to some intuition of our own mortality only through an ambivalent identification with a loved person whose death we simultaneously fear and desire: essentially in mourning." Laplanche thus reframes the maxim: " 'If you want life, prepare for death' might be translated as 'If you want life, prepare for the death of the other' " (*Life and Death in Psychoanalysis*, trans. Jeffrey Mehlman [Baltimore, MD, 1976], 5–6).

12. This is Caruth's slightly modified translation (64–65) of what appears in the *Standard Edition*, XVIII, 38. Apart from the change I will discuss, the only other change is Caruth's use of the word "drive" where the *Standard Edition* uses "instinct."

13. As we noted, Caruth will make the same claim later: "Freud . . . moves . . . to an explanation of the origins of life *as an 'awakening' from death* that precisely establishes the foundation of the [death] drive and of consciousness alike" (104; my emphasis).

14. Freud makes this point several times in *Beyond the Pleasure Principle*: "all instincts tend towards the restoration of an earlier state of things" (XVIII, 37); "on our hypothesis the ego-instincts arise from the coming to life of inanimate matter and seek to restore the inanimate state" (44); "If we are to take it as a truth that knows no exception that everything living dies for *internal* reasons—becomes inorganic once again—then we shall be compelled to say that '*the aim of all life is death*' and, looking backwards, that '*inanimate things existed before living ones*' " (38).

15. The German *erwecken* has the literal meaning of "to awake or arouse" (from sleep or lethargy). In a religious sense, the verb can be used to mean to resurrect or revive. Freud, no doubt, would have been aware of the latter meaning, but he appears to avoid the Christian connotation as much as possible precisely by employing the qualifying phrase "by the action of a force of whose nature we can form no conception."

16. It is noteworthy that immediately after the longer passage I have just cited, Caruth refers to the primary causes of trauma, precisely as Freud himself imagined it, "in relation to the *origins* of consciousness" rather than in relation to the *survival* of consciousness. But this slippage from origins to survival is part of the same misreading of Freud that permits her to write that in *Beyond the Pleasure Principle* Freud finally explains trauma in terms of "*the origins of life itself as an 'awakening' from death* that precisely establishes the foundation of the [death] drive and of consciousness alike" (104). We might observe, moreover, that, from the very start of her study, Caruth appears intent on substituting survival for origin as central to her revision of the Freudian death drive. In her introduction, for example, she asks: "Is the trauma the encounter with death or the ongoing experience of *having survived it?*" (7; my emphasis). In other words, even though she will eventually consider *Beyond the Pleasure Principle*'s own locating of the origin of trauma in the "origins of consciousness," she sets the stage from the outset for rejecting this key Freudian insight and for replacing it with a theory of trauma as originating in the response to death, specifically the death of another and the enigma of survival one necessarily encounters in relation to this death.

17. *Essays on Otherness*, 265.

18. For a very different conceptualization of the ethical possibilities of what we might call a psychoanalytically conceived otherness (and in this case positioned precisely within the Freudian father-son agon and more particularly in relation to the "mutual recognition" of the death of the other), see Paul Ricoeur, "Fatherhood: From Phantasm to Symbol," trans. Robert Sweeney, in *The Conflict of Interpretations: Essays on Hermeneutics*, ed. Don Ihde (Evanston, IL, 1974), especially 471–81, 491–95.

19. Caruth seems to be drawing on Laplanche's notion that there is "a certain *ethic* in relation to death" precisely to the extent that there is some "irreducible meshing of my death with that of another" (*Life and Death in Psychoanalysis*, 5–6).

20. Santner, *On the Psychotheology of Everyday Life: Reflections on Freud and Rosenzweig* (Chicago, 2001), 5–7.

21. Justin Martyr, *First Apology* in *Ante-Nicene Fathers*, ed. and trans. Alexander Roberts and James Donaldson, 10 vols. (Buffalo, NY, 1885–87), I, 183.

22. *On the Psychotheology of Everyday Life*, 9.

Chapter 2

1. Lupton and Reinhard associate this "three part fable of the feminine"—or, more precisely, "of the feminine object in male desire"—with Lacan's Imaginary, Symbolic, and Real: *After Oedipus: Shakespeare in Psychoanalysis* (Ithaca, NY, 1993), 146, 151, 153. Subsequent page references to this work will be cited in the text. In relation to Shakespeare's work, the post-Oedipal understanding of the mother-as-threat has been most thoroughly addressed in Janet Adelman's *Suffocating Mothers: Fantasies of Maternal Origin in Shakespeare's Plays* (New York, 1992).

2. Writing about Lear's experience specifically, Lupton and Reinhard observe that in his "regressive fantasy" Lear "return[s] to the idylls of infancy as the first casket lapses into the third" (152). This is the moment that, as Freud puts it, "the silent goddess of Death" takes her beloved son "into her arms" once again.

3. Lupton and Reinhard argue that the fantasy being worked out in the male life-narrative "only imagines the regressive pleasures of pre-Oedipal unity from within the frame of gendered desire; . . . infantilization is always disclosed as Oedipal fantasy" (149). Even in the final phase, what they understand as the eruption in male consciousness of maternal monstrousness is yet constituted "under the law of Oedipus" (154). We might observe here Paul Ricoeur's very broad comment that "Oedipal structures constitute a level of instinctual articulation for the entire life of man" ("Fatherhood: From Phantasm to Symbol," trans. Robert Sweeney, in *The Conflict of Interpretations: Essays on Hermeneutics*, ed. Don Ihde [Evanston, IL, 1974], 491).

4. In this regard my summary of Lupton and Reinhard's reconstruction of "man's life . . . in terms of the declension of the feminine object" (152) is somewhat reductive. In their interest in the male subject's final return to the pre-Oedipal, for example, their understanding of return in terms of "regressive fantasy"

turns as much on the notion of fantasy as on the notion of regressive. Although, in their interpretation, the male life-narrative does work its way back to the lost origin (the full maternal presence of Lacan's Imaginary), this return happens in a fantasmatic way: an attempt to reclaim from loss what the subject never truly had to begin with. Thus, much of their reading of the third casket's relation to the first is conceptualized as an instance of the Freudian fetish, that which "figures the *lack* of 'something' that was always already *lost*—it indicates not a lost thing, but *the Thing as loss*" (154). That said, while they are similarly engaged at a theoretical level with Freudian belatedness, their argument centers on originary absence less in terms of a crisis of being (the subject's existential helplessness in relation to the other's prior stake in the self) than in terms of a crisis of representation or signification. In short, committed as they are to the textuality of psychoanalysis, Lupton and Reinhard understand what is always already lost at the origin is the possibility of representation itself especially in terms of self-identity. Subjectivity then emerges as an ever-after governed by a fantasy-relation to what it never possessed.

5. In returning to the staples of his own thought, Freud was also reasserting the primacy of the father, and the threatening presence of the father in his relationship to the son, in the constitution of psychical life. As we shall see in greater detail in parts II and III, that vexed relationship, one governed by the son's ambivalent attitude towards the father, will be the key element in Freud's formulation of the crisis of belatedness even when he believes that he is merely reasserting the Oedipal model of experience.

6. Otto Rank, *The Trauma of Birth*, trans. James E. Lieberman (New York, 1952), 199. Subsequent page references will be cited in the text.

7. As Freud himself will later write, "what happens is that the child's biological situation as a foetus is replaced for it by a psychical object-relation to its mother" (*Inhibitions, Symptoms and Anxiety*, XX, 138). It is from within the experience of substitution that separation becomes trauma.

8. Rank thus claims that, after birth, the psyche is governed by a longing for the pleasures of reunion with the mother either in the form of womb-fantasies or in the form of various substitutions for the primal pleasure of the womb including symbolic representations in dreams, myth, ancient religious forms, and art as well as in neurotic manifestations of many types: "the rest . . . consists in replacing this lost paradise in the . . . highly complicated round-about ways of the libido, the primal state being . . . no longer attainable" (187).

9. For Rank, a wide variety of experiences of separation (personal as well as social) return us to and indeed reenact the original traumatic moment. We might especially note here Rank's view that the fear of castration is just the second such reenactment after weaning, a minimalizing of the central importance of castration that Freud will later reject.

10. *The Birth of Tragedy and the Genealogy of Morals*, trans. Francis Golffing (Garden City, NY, 1956), 29.

11. In the final chapter of his study, Rank writes: "According to our conception the newborn individual would immediately fall back into the abandoned state,

that is, practically expressed, would die, unless Nature undertook the first 'therapeutic' intervention and prevented the striving back by the anchoring of anxiety." He concludes: "The psychical anchoring in consciousness of the anxiety perception at parturition acts biologically as a therapeutic means against the backward striving tendency, and determines, as we have attempted to show, the actual process of becoming a human being. And consciousness is the human characteristic *par excellence*" (204, 216).

12. Rank will quote this passage in the *Trauma of Birth* (192).

13. Ernest Jones quotes from the minutes of the November 17, 1909, meeting of the Vienna Psycho-Analytical Society: "We expect it would turn out that the severe neuroses all have their prototypes in childhood life, so that we should find the kernels of the later neuroses in the disturbances of the development of childhood. . . . In the matter of anxiety one has to remember that children begin their experience of it in the act of birth itself" (*Life and Work of Sigmund Freud*, 3 vols. [New York, 1953–57], II, 443, 445). In the first of his "Contributions to the Psychology of Love" (1910), Freud will essentially repeat this statement: "Birth is both the first of all dangers to life and the prototype of all later ones that cause us to feel anxiety, and the experience of birth has probably left behind in us the expression of affect which we call anxiety" (XI, 173; cf. Rank, *Trauma of Birth*, 188, 204). He will deal with the issue at some length at the opening of Lecture 25 of *Introductory Lectures* (1916–17; XVI, 392–411). Even after the publication of the *Trauma of Birth*, Freud will make two generally approving statements regarding Rank's theory: "Rank's view of the effects of the trauma of birth seems to throw special light upon the predisposition to anxiety-hysteria which is so strong in childhood" (X, 116n3 [added in 1923]); "Rank has traced attachment to the mother back to the prehistoric intra-uterine period and has thus indicated *the biological foundation of the Oedipus complex*" (VII, 226n1 [added in 1924]; my emphasis).

14. This is precisely Freud's point when, towards the opening of chapter 8, he notes that, "in man, birth provides a prototypic experience of this kind, and we are therefore inclined to regard anxiety-states as a reproduction of the trauma of birth." Initially, we might assume that he is here endorsing Rank's view. But Freud is really just restating his earlier point that anxiety-states take the *form* of the first anxiety-state (birth), where peculiar sensations "connected with the respiratory organs and with the heart" are in evidence. Thus he observes that "an anxiety-state is the reproduction of some experience which contained the necessary conditions for such an increase of excitation and a discharge along particular paths," in short, the breathlessness and heart palpitations that are typical in anxiety attacks (61–62). As though to clarify the distinction he is drawing, Freud will add: "I am driven to the conclusion that the earliest phobias of infancy *cannot be directly traced back* to the impressions of the act of birth" precisely because "anxiety, instead of being at its maximum immediately after birth and then slowly decreasing, does not emerge until later, as mental development proceeds" (65; my emphasis).

15. Some of Freud's other objections seem almost frivolous, as though he were making up reasons to reject Rank's theory. For example, in chapter 10 (XX,

152) Freud will overstate Rank's position (Freud calls it a "formula") on the correlation between a particularly "difficult and protracted birth" (for the child at least) and the likelihood that this child will develop some form of neurosis. Rank does suggest such a correlation but he hardly insists on it. Moreover, his criticism that, were Rank's theory true, other mammals should evince the same "disposition to neurosis" because they too experience birth (even difficult ones) is founded on the completely untenable position that other mammals necessarily have the same mental-psychic structures as humans (complete with the same Conscious/Unconscious division and the same sexual-gender constructions), a position Freud himself will effectively reject in the last paragraphs of chapter 10 (XX, 154–56). Moreover, this objection regarding the similarities between humans and other animals at least partially contradicts Freud's earlier statement: in chapter 8 he notes that "anxiety is a reaction which, in all probability, is common to every organism, certainly every organism of a higher order." Freud clarifies his position only to muddy his perspective on Rank's theory when he concludes: "We do not know, besides, whether anxiety involves the same sensations and innervations in organisms far removed from man as it does in man himself. Thus there is no good argument here against the view that, in man, anxiety is modeled upon the process of birth" (XX, 134). See Jones, *Life and Work*, III, 56–74, for a full account of Freud's wavering attitude towards Rank's theory.

16. Freud will add that the "danger of birth"—even if, biologically speaking, it does mark a "real danger to life"—"has as yet no psychical content. We cannot possibly suppose that the foetus has any sort of knowledge that there is a possibility of its life being destroyed. It can only be aware of some vast disturbance in the economy of its narcissistic libido" (XX, 135).

17. At other times, however, Freud appears to be restoring Rank's notion that the newborn has real memories, if not of life in the womb than at least of the moment of birth itself. Speaking of situations in early infancy in which the child longs for its mother if only because "it already knows from experience that she satisfies all its needs without delay," a "situation of non-satisfaction in which the amounts of stimulation rise to an unpleasurable height without its being possible for them to be mastered psychically or discharged must for the infant be *analogous to the experience of being born*" (XX, 137; my emphasis). But Freud will go on to qualify what he means by "analogous to" by saying that it is not the separation from the mother that the infant (re)experiences so much as the simple feeling of nonsatisfaction; it is, in other words, the "situation of danger" in its purest form—"a *growing tension due to need*, against which it is helpless" (137; emphasis in original)—that leads both the newborn and the infant to "an accumulation of amounts of stimulation which require to be disposed of" and in response to which, "in both cases the reaction of anxiety sets in." Rather inexplicably, Freud then juxtaposes two statements that appear to offer different conclusions about the relationship between birth and (subsequent) anxiety: "It is unnecessary to suppose that the child carries anything more with it from the time of its birth than *this way of indicating the presence of danger*" (i.e., the feeling of anxiety as a response to danger); "When the

infant has found out by experience that an external, perceptible object [what at one point Freud calls the "apparatus" of the mother's body] can put an end to *the dangerous situation which is reminiscent of birth*, the content of the danger it fears is displaced from the economic situation onto the condition which determined that situation, viz., the loss of object. It is the absence of the mother that is now the danger" (XX, 137–38; my emphases; original emphasis deleted). To the extent that "analogous to . . . being born" becomes "reminiscent of birth," we might wonder if Freud cannot bring himself to reject completely what was, in fact, his own theory. We might note, finally, that, in one of his earliest efforts to theorize the birth trauma, Freud's use of the words reminiscence and reminiscences does in fact suggest something akin to memory: in hysterical attacks, for example, a reminiscence is the nonconscious recollection of a preceding event (an event still carried in the Unconscious); see the "Minutes of the Vienna Psycho-analytic Society," November 17, 1909, qtd. in Jones, *Life and Work*, II, 444–45.

18. Rank had made this point quite explicitly: "So the later childish Oedipus complex proves to be an immediate derivative, that is, the psychosexual elaboration of the intrauterine Oedipus situation—which proves to be the 'nuclear complex of the neuroses'" (194). Rank's revisionary position on the core issue of Freud's psychoanalysis was not lost on Freud and his other disciples. Summarizing the main contention of the *Trauma of Birth*, Jones writes of Rank's theory: "Clinically it followed that all mental conflicts concerned the relation of the child to its mother, and that what might appear to be conflicts with the father, including the Oedipus complex, were but a mask for the essential ones concerning birth." He adds the following personal observation: "These ideas of Rank had germinated slowly. It stayed in my mind that in March, 1919, when I met him with his pregnant wife in Switzerland, he had astonished me by remarking in a dismal tone that men were of no importance in life; the essence of life was the relation between mother and child" (*Life and Work*, III, 58).

19. Although, at the end of that chapter, Freud concludes that castration anxiety is "not the sole motive force of the defensive processes that lead to neurosis," it appears to be the sole motive force for men. He notes that a "castration complex" is still operational for "the female sex," though women are traumatized less by "losing the object itself" than by "losing the object's love" (XX, 143). Either way, it is castration rather than birth trauma that provides the motive force for defensive processes. Freud's earlier account had similarly left it unclear whether castration is the primal loss so that even birth might be said, in a kind of *hysteron proteron*, to be a repetition of genital severing: "The statement I have just made, to the effect that the ego has been prepared to expect castration by having undergone constantly repeated object-losses, places the question of anxiety in a new light. We have hitherto regarded it as an affective signal of danger; but now, *since the danger is so often one of castration*, it appears to us as a reaction to a loss, a separation" (XX, 130; my emphasis). In short, even as Freud here states again that "the first experience of anxiety which an individual goes through . . . is birth," castration rather than birth is the model on which all other separation-induced anxieties are founded.

20. It would be more accurate to say that Rank is echoing a point Freud had only recently made in the *Ego and the Id*: "death is an abstract concept with a negative content for which no unconscious correlative can be found" (XIX, 58).

21. Rank is following Freud on this point. As we have seen, in the *Interpretation of Dreams* Freud remarks that "the deepest unconscious basis for the belief in survival after death . . . merely represents a projection into the future of this uncanny life before birth."

22. Echoing Freud's own metaphorical description of death as "Mother Earth" ("Theme of the Three Caskets"), Rank refers to death both as "a second mother" and as "Dame World" (187, 197). Rank goes on to comment: "Here is not only the root of the popular idea of death as a deliverer, but also the essential factor in all religious ideas of deliverance. . . . How seriously the Unconscious conceives dying as a return to the womb may be concluded from the death-rites of all nations and times, which punish the disturbance of the eternal sleep . . . as the greatest iniquity and the most malicious crime" (197–98). Rank's position in 1924 might be viewed as an elaboration on a remark made by Freud just one year earlier. In the *Ego and the Id*, Freud had suggested that our encounter with death (he is rather vague on what this encounter entails) might in some way point us back to our original separation at birth: "[W]hen the ego finds itself in an excessive danger which it believes itself unable to overcome by its own strength, it . . . sees itself deserted by all protecting forces and *lets itself die*. Here, moreover, is once again the same situation as that which underlay the first great anxiety-state of birth and the infantile anxiety of longing—the anxiety due to *separation from the protecting mother*" (XIX, 58; my emphases). In 1923, in short, Freud, like Rank, saw the impulse to death as a fantasy of reunion with the lost mother.

23. This resistance, a willed reenactment of separation from the mother, might best be understood as an effort to abreact the birth trauma, what Freud himself would call "a sort of inoculation, submitting to a slight attack of the illness in order to escape its full strength" (*Inhibitions, Symptoms and Anxiety*, XX, 162). But Freud is inconsistent on this point. He explicitly rejects the "inoculation" model when it comes to Rank's idea of birth trauma: "We do not rightly know what is meant by abreacting a trauma. Taken literally, it implies that the more frequently and the more intensely a neurotic person reproduces the affect of anxiety the more closely will he approach to mental health—an untenable conclusion" (XX, 151).

24. As Rank puts it tersely, "Man depreciates her [the woman/the mother] only consciously; in the Unconscious he fears her" (94).

25. Freud adds, "as we see, both forms of the Oedipus complex . . . came to grief through the castration complex" (XX, 31).

26. The notion of the ego being overwhelmed (*Überwältigung*) goes back to some of Freud's earliest writings; see, for example, "The Neuro-Psychoses of Defense" (1894), III, 45–61; and Draft K of his January, 1896 letter to Fliess (*Origins*, 146–55).

27. "Clearly, [a danger situation] consists in the subject's estimation of his own strength compared to the magnitude of the danger and in his admission of

helplessness in the face of it—physical helplessness if the danger is real and psychical helplessness if it is instinctual. . . . Let us call a situation of helplessness of this kind that has been actually experienced a *traumatic situation*" (XX, 166; emphasis in original).

28. Somewhat less optimistically, as part of his analysis of the "table d'hôte" dream (*On Dreams*, V, 636–40) in which he mentions how uncomfortable he is to be reminded "of what [he] owe[s]" because his "debt seems to be growing too fast," Freud quotes the following lines from Goethe's *Wilhelm Meister*:

> Ihr führt ins Leben uns hinein,
> Ihr lasst den Armen schuldig werden.

Addressed in their original context to the Heavenly Powers, these lines appear to mean, "You lead us into life, / You make the poor creature guilty.'" But since *Armen* might also mean "poor" in a financial sense and *schuldig* might also mean "in debt," in the setting of Freud's dream the lines might make more sense as "you bring us into the world, you let the poor man fall into debt." (Freud quotes the lines twice in *On Dreams* [V, 637, 639] and then again in *Civilization and Its Discontents* [XXI, 133].) And as Freud goes further into the analysis he makes it clear that within the associations of the dream-thoughts the lines should be understood as being addressed to parents, though Freud, rather inexplicably, reverses the sense of burden suggested by the lines to place it on the parents rather than on the child who speaks: "Thus I was reminded of the *duties of parents to their children*" (V, 639; my emphasis). In applying the lines in the context of familial relations, Freud should have taken them to mean that, simply by the act of its having been brought into the world, a child is indebted to its parents and should be reminded of the gratitude it owes. As Freud concludes, his "own early life" is wrapped up in the dream as though his mother were saying to him, "there are children who would be only too pleased to have" what he has, the very existence for which he incurs the debt. Against this feeling of "being in debt" Freud also suggests that he is partly fantasizing through the dream that he might get something "without paying for it" (V, 638; original italics deleted), in other words without accruing a debt.

Chapter 3

1. Shakespeare is not merely repeating, but he does appear to be echoing three passages from *Julius Caesar*: 1.3.1–32, 43–78; 2.2.16–32. For example, Cassius mockingly refers to the omens preceding Caesar's death as "strange eruptions" (1.3.78); Horatio more seriously states that the Ghost "bodes some strange eruption to our state" (1.1.68).

2. Intriguingly, regarding the naming of children, in the *Interpretation of Dreams* Freud will note in passing that, for his own children at least, he "insisted on their names being chosen . . . in memory of people I have been fond of," that

is, in commemoration of others. Such names, Freud reflects, turn "the children into *revenants*," ghosts or, more literally, those who return (V, 421, 486).

3. The source of this notion was undoubtedly Plutarch's claim in the *Life of Brutus* that Caesar believed Brutus to be his son. But the possibility was widely enough credited to permit Shakespeare to give the following off-the-cuff remark to Suffolk in *2 Henry VI*: "Brutus' bastard hand / Stabb'd Julius Caesar" (4.1.136–37).

4. Viewing the carnage among his own troops at Philippi, Brutus cries out in words that strangely foreshadow the action of *Hamlet*: "O Julius Caesar, thou art mighty yet! / Thy spirit walks abroad, and turns our swords / Into our own proper entrails" (5.3.94–96).

5. Brutus's final lines suggest that Caesar's spirit can only find rest at the moment where the son, through a suicide that repeats the earlier killing, identifies himself most completely with his father: "Caesar, be still, / I kill'd not thee with half so good a will" (5.5.50–51). It is also worth noting that, while the stage direction refers to the apparition as the "Ghost of Caesar," the actual lines refer to it as Brutus's "evil spirit" (4.3.281), as though the ghost of his dead father were necessarily a part of himself.

6. In the *Interpretation of Dreams*, Freud imagines that through *Hamlet* Shakespeare expresses his own "bereavement" for the loss of both his father and his son (IV, 265–66).

7. "Psychoanalysis and Renaissance Culture," in *Literary Theory/Renaissance Texts*, ed. Patricia Parker and David Quint (Baltimore, MD, 1986), 210, 221.

8. In this apparently unconscious use of a later dream interpretation to censor an earlier dream interpretation, Freud is in a certain sense reenacting his understanding of Hamlet as a figure for the power of dreams to simultaneously reveal and conceal: "The Prince in the play, who had to disguise himself as a madman, was behaving just as dreams do in reality; so we can say of dreams what Hamlet says of himself, concealing the true circumstances under a cloak of wit and unintelligibility" (V, 444).

9. Saxo Grammaticus, *The History of the Danes, Books I–IX*, ed. Hilda Ellis Davidson, trans. Peter Fisher (Cambridge, 1996), 82–83.

10. *Will in the World: How Shakespeare Became Shakespeare* (New York, 2004), 311.

11. *Will in the World*, 315, 318; Watson, *The Rest is Silence: Death as Annihilation in the English Renaissance* (Berkeley, CA, 1994), ch. 2.

12. The passage from Thomas Lodge's *Wit's Misery and World's Madness* (1596) is quoted in *Narrative and Dramatic Sources of Shakespeare*, ed. Geoffrey Bullough, 8 vols. (New York, 1957–75), VII, 24. The play's disruption of the simple revenge story under the pressure of some psychological compulsion Shakespeare himself could not fully articulate is the foundation of T. S. Eliot's infamous claim that *Hamlet* is "most certainly an artistic failure" ("Hamlet and His Problems," in *Selected Essays* [New York, 1960], 123). For discussion of the general revenge-plot that Shakespeare's play swerves away from, see Michael Goldman, *Acting and Action in Shakespearean Tragedy* (Princeton, NJ, 1985), 17–45; for related discussion of the

play's complex relation to the revenge-tragedy tradition, see William Empson, *Essays on Shakespeare*, ed. David B. Pirie (Cambridge, 1986), 79–92.

13. *Will in the World*, 318.

14. For a fuller treatment of this issue, see Greenblatt's *Hamlet in Purgatory* (Princeton, NJ, 2002), especially ch. 5.

15. Although I do not have space to address Freud's Oedipal reading of *Hamlet*, I should observe that this reading could very well make sense in terms of Freud's 1896 dream in that the dream does clearly express repressed hostility toward the father. But Oedipalized hostility would only be fully meaningful in terms of repressed sexual love for the mother. Apart from my own deep reluctance to read *Hamlet* in this way, what an Oedipal reading fails to register is that hostility to the father can derive precisely from an original admiration, love, even idealization (though idealization might also be viewed, as Freud suggests, as a disavowal of a hostility that is perceived as forbidden). In her fine reading of the play, Janet Adelman shows how the son's over-idealization of the father functions as a central part of Shakespeare's story. But in focusing on how that over-idealization bespeaks an investment in masculine authority inseparable from an informing misogyny—a threat of annihilation posed by the mother to the male ego—Adelman does not consider that the over-idealization of his father might be a problem that Hamlet must deal with: *Suffocating Mothers: Fantasies of Maternal Origin in Shakespeare's Plays* (New York, 1992), 11–37.

16. For discussion of *Beyond the Pleasure Principle*'s concept of therapeutic mourning in the context of cognitive neurobiology, see Lisa J. Schnell, "Learning How to Tell," *Literature and Medicine* 23 (2004): 265–79.

17. As Freud notes, "forgetting impressions, scenes or experiences nearly always reduces itself to shutting them off." He adds that "in the many different forms of obsessional neurosis in particular, forgetting is mostly restricted to dissolving thought-connections, failing to draw the right conclusions and isolating memories" (XII, 148–49).

18. Therapeutically, the patient must learn to "put himself back into an earlier situation" but in such a way so as not "to confuse [it] with the present one." Freud later notes that what the "patient experiences . . . as something real and contemporary," the physician works on by "tracing it back to the past" (XII, 148, 152). We might also note that, for Freud, repetition itself is largely manifested in what he calls "acting out": "we may say that the patient does not *remember* anything of what has been forgotten [which is to say, repressed], but *acts* it out. He reproduces it not as a memory but as an action; he repeats it, without, of course, knowing that he is repeating it" (150).

19. Although Freud gives the phrase "*work through*" a specific technical meaning—the point at which resistance is overcome within the transference—its associations align it more broadly with the movement away from repression and repetition and toward conscious awareness and memory as remembering permits the patient to distinguish a past source of symptoms from the present experience of them. Working through entails "discover[ing] the repressed instinctual impulses

which are feeding the resistance" (XII, 155). For a description of this process, see Jean Laplanche, *Life and Death in Psychoanalysis*, trans. Jeffrey Mehlman (Baltimore, MD, 1976), 33–34.

20. Freud had discussed the core elements of the essay with Ernest Jones as early as January 1914; he presented a version of the piece at the Vienna Psycho-analytical Society in December 1914 (about the same time "Remembering, Repeating, and Working-Through" was published). By February 1915, Freud had a full working draft of "Mourning and Melancholia."

21. Freud adds: "one feels justified in maintaining the belief that a loss . . . has occurred, but [the physician] cannot see clearly what it is that has been lost, and it is all the more reasonable to suppose that the patient cannot consciously perceive what he has lost either" (XIV, 245).

22. As Freud adds, this inversion, often marked in a drive toward "self-punishment," is central to the patient's effort "to avoid the need to express . . . hostility [toward the lost love-object] . . . openly" (XIV, 251).

23. Thus Freud writes to Fliess on October 15, 1897:

> Only one idea of general value has occurred to me. I have found love of the mother and jealousy of the father in my own case too, and now believe it to be a general phenomenon of early childhood . . . If that is the case, the gripping power of *Oedipus Rex*, in spite of all the rational objections to the inexorable fate that the story presupposes, becomes intelligible . . . [T]he Greek myth seizes on the compulsion which everyone recognizes because he has felt traces of it in himself. Every member of the audience was once a budding Oedipus in phantasy, and this dream-fulfillment played out in reality causes everyone to recoil in horror. (*Origins*, 223–24)

Although Freud does not return explicitly here to the dream of his father's funeral, the association of his own or any son's hostility toward his father—three years later in the *Interpretation of Dreams* he will be more specific: "our first hatred and our first murderous wish is against our father" (IV, 262)—is linked directly to the "love of the mother." Anticipating one of the most famous claims he will make in the *Interpretation of Dreams*, in the 1897 letter he will make an explicit causal connection between sexual desire for the mother and murderous hatred for the father by reference to *Hamlet*:

> The idea has passed through my head that the same thing may lie at the root of *Hamlet*. I am not thinking of Shakespeare's conscious intentions, but supposing rather that he was impelled to write it as a real event because his own unconscious understood that of his hero. How can one explain the hysteric Hamlet's . . . hesitation to avenge his father by killing his uncle . . . ? How better than by the torment roused in him by the obscure memory that he himself had medi-

tated the same deed against his father *because* of his passion for his mother . . . ? (*Origins*, 224; my emphasis)

In short, seeing a relation between what happens in *Oedipus Rex* and what is repressed in Hamlet (and in *Hamlet*), Freud does not simply juxtapose love for the mother with hatred for the father but makes the former the cause of the later. We might note, finally, that between his letters of November 1896 and October 1897 Freud had already been observing the role sexual motives could play in a variety of otherwise inexplicable experiences and feelings: see, for example, *Origins*, 207–10.

24. Significantly, Freud also published "On Narcissism" in 1914. Noting that "narcissism was the concept whose development had precipitated Freud's self-revision," Harold Bloom suggests that Freud's key insight was that "narcissism, when severely wounded, transformed itself into aggressivity, both against the self and against others" ("Freud: Frontier Concepts, Jewishness, and Interpretation," in *Trauma: Explorations in Memory*, ed. Cathy Caruth [Baltimore, MD, 1995], 120).

25. A full consideration of this important issue is beyond the scope of this discussion. But a few citations are in order. In *Beyond the Pleasure Principle*, Freud hypothesizes that an "abstract idea of time" functions, indeed comes into existence, as a derivative "of the method of the working of the system *Pcpt.-Cs.* [*Perception-Consciousness*]" and that time so conceived "may perhaps constitute another way of providing a shield against stimuli" (XVIII, 28). Put in a different way, the evolutionary function of the human notion of time (of which memory is a key constitutive element) is precisely to protect the mind from being overwhelmed by stimuli, that is, from being traumatized by experience that cannot be temporally organized. What she calls Freud's "temporal definition of trauma" is thus, for Cathy Caruth, sufficient justification for her to define trauma as "a break in the mind's experience of time," or the failure of the mind to "plac[e] stimulation within an ordered experience of time" (*Unclaimed Experience: Trauma, Narrative, and History* [Baltimore, MD, 1996], 61). The temporal dissociation characteristic of traumatic recollection is to be distinguished from normal memory which integrates the potentially traumatic episode into a person's sense of time by organizing it in a particular form of language, namely narrative; for elaboration, see Bessel van der Kolk and Onno van der Hart, "The Intrusive Past: The Flexibility of Memory and the Engraving of Trauma," in Caruth, *Trauma*, 158–82.

26. In accounts of other incidents or dreams in which his ambivalent view of his father stands out, Freud often disguises his ambivalence toward his father by shifting it to other father figures. One such account in the *Interpretation of Dreams* is particularly noteworthy in that Freud's desire to get his father out of the way is masked in a series of other scenarios, including an episode from Shakespeare's *2 Henry IV* in which Prince Hal seems a little too eager to believe that his father, King Henry IV, is dead (V, 483–85).

27. If Hamlet must find a way to escape his father's shadow, it is worth noting that the first figure Shakespeare employs in the play to hint at this imperative points in the opposite direction: Hamlet's response to Claudius's query about

his excessive mourning is "I am too much in the sun" (1.2.67). The pun reveals what the play will then grapple with: in mourning (or more precisely melancholy), Hamlet is precisely too much in the *son*.

28. In "Mourning and Melancholia," Freud is interested in how melancholia often produces a "tendency to suicide." As we've noted, Freud explicitly mentions Hamlet as a prime instance of this melancholic temperament (XIV, 246). Even when, earlier in his career, Freud thought of Hamlet as a hysteric, he still saw Hamlet's drive to "bring . . . down his punishment on himself" as a repetition of King Hamlet's experience: "suffering the same fate as his father, being poisoned by the same rival" (*Origins*, 224).

29. *Rest is Silence*, 77–78. As Cavell observes, "the Ghost asks initially for revenge for his murder, a task the son evidently accepts as his to perform . . . But is this the son's business . . . ? Here the father asks the son to take the father's place, to make his life come out even for him, to set it right, so that he, the father, can rest in peace. It is a bequest of a beloved father that deprives the son of his identity" (*Disowning Knowledge in Seven Plays of Shakespeare* [Cambridge, 2003], 188).

30. It is interesting to note that, in his only occasionally coherent reading of the play, having first referred to Laertes as Hamlet's "double," Lacan appears to forget the symbolic valence of his own term when he later refers to the two as "warring *brothers*" ("Desire and the Interpretation of Desire in *Hamlet*," trans. James Hulbert, in *Literature and Psychoanalysis: The Question of Reading Otherwise*, ed. Shoshana Felman [Baltimore, MD, 1982], 31, 35).

31. It should be noted that the stage direction—"Hamlet leaps in after Leartes [sic]"—appears only in the First (or Bad) Quarto of 1603. Many modern editions (e.g., Riverside, Norton) include it even when basing their texts on either the Second Quarto or the Folio. Some editors have decided that dramaturgy and character development logically point to a different staging. Thus the most recent Arden edition, citing, among other things, the potential clumsiness of the staging, reassigns and so reverses the action: "[Laertes] *leaps out* and grapples with him." As will become apparent, it makes sense conceptually if not dramatically for Hamlet to jump into the grave precisely because he cannot yet separate himself from his dead father, which is the point of the scene.

32. *Will in the World*, 321. Greenblatt's cultural perspective on *Hamlet* might be said to borrow and then historicize the claims Lacan had earlier put forth about the play's concern with "insufficient mourning" ("Desire," 38–41).

33. We might note how Shakespeare goes out of his way to make other symbolic links between the deaths of King Hamlet and Ophelia. King Hamlet was murdered while sleeping in his orchard (1.5.35); Ophelia drowns after falling from the willow tree (4.7.166ff.). Ophelia's insanity and her death are associated with her picking of various flowers (4.5, 4.7), which she weaves into a crown (4.7.172) just before she dies; in what amounts to a totally gratuitous reference, we are told in the stage directions to the dumb-show that the king was lying "upon a bank of flowers" when he was murdered, an event marked in part by the murderer's theft of the crown (3.2).

34. *Rest is Silence*, 78.

35. Whether it is Hamlet in 1.2 "performing" mourning while acknowledging that the "show" may not accurately represent inward feelings, or the 3.2 play-within-the-play that only apparently repeats the preceding dumb-show, or Hamlet's attempt in 3.4 to distinguish the moral worth of two brothers (his father and his uncle) by simply looking at their pictures, *Hamlet* is constantly interrogating how one thing fails to be like what it appears to be like. In this context we might consider Freud's statement from *Totem and Taboo* as it offers perspective on Shakespeare's choice to rename his characters (King Hamlet/Prince Hamlet): "[C]hildren . . . consistently assume that if two things are called by similar-sounding names this must imply the existence of some deep-lying point of agreement between them" (XIII, 56).

36. Whatever its indebtedness to Freud's vocabulary, Greenblatt's claim that "Hamlet submits to an *uncanny* and yet actual link between himself and his dead father" (*Hamlet in Purgatory*, 217–18; my emphasis) owes more to the link Lacan makes between the Freudian uncanny and what he calls "depersonalization," an "experience . . . in the course of which the imaginary limits between subject and object change." Lacan adds that "an imbalance arises" in this experience, where the subject "cross[es] the limits originally assigned to it, and rejoins the image of the other subject" (22). For related discussion of the role of the uncanny in *Hamlet*, see Marjorie Garber, *Shakespeare's Ghost Writers: Literature as Uncanny Causality* (New York, 1987), ch. 6.

37. *Hamlet in Purgatory*, 207–08. Greenblatt grounds this assertion on the text of the Folio, which is the basis of the Norton edition, from which my own citation here comes. It should be noted that the slightly different version of the passage in the 1604 Quarto does in fact supply a subject for the sentence: "Haste me to know't, that *I* with wings as swift / As meditation, or the thoughts of love, / May sweep to my revenge" (quoted here from the Riverside edition; my emphasis).

38. In the interlineal comment in his published screenplay, Kenneth Branagh explicates this passage in a way that almost certainly matches our own intuitions, unexpected as these might be: Hamlet "has spoken with the heart-rending simplicity of a man who knows that he is going to die and probably very soon. He accepts the inevitability of it" (*Hamlet: Screenplay, Introduction, and Film Diary* [New York, 1996], 162).

39. Freud generalizes to say that his key "errors" or misrememberings "are derivatives of repressed thoughts connected with my dead father[,] . . . thoughts which would have contained unfriendly criticism of my father [and] dissatisfaction with my father's behavior" (VI, 219).

40. *Rest is Silence*, 79.

41. *Disowning Knowledge*, 186. For one of Freud's earliest musings on the relation between mourning and that ambivalence deriving from fear of the dead's continuing claim upon the living, see *Totem and Taboo*, XIII, 51–74. Reflecting at one point on the origin in the belief in and fear of demons and ghosts, Freud observes, "the fact that demons are always regarded as the spirits of those who have died *recently* shows better than anything the influence of mourning on the origin of

the belief in demons. Mourning has a quite specific psychical task to perform: its function is to detach the survivors' memories and hopes from the dead" (65). Freud adds in note: "In the course of psycho-analyses of neurotics who suffer (or who suffered in their childhood) from fear of ghosts, it is often possible to show without much difficulty that the ghosts are disguises for the patient's parents" (65n3). And to the extent ambivalence is at the heart of this relationship (at least filial ambivalence with respect to the deceased father), Freud's earlier explanation for the most commonly given reason for fear of the dead is instructive: "the dead . . . [seek to] drag the living in their train" (59).

42. As part of his analysis, Freud notes that he "had the dream only a few days after the unveiling of the memorial to [the late Ernst] Fleischl," a ceremony that had taken place on October 16, 1898 (V, 423). In what follows, I am particularly indebted to the account in Marthe Robert's *From Oedipus to Moses: Freud's Jewish Identity*, trans. Ralph Manheim (Garden City, NY, 1976). That said, while she offers a fine analysis of just how much the *Interpretation of Dreams* marked Freud's grappling with unresolved feelings for his father, throughout the study she interprets that struggle as Freud's lifelong effort to resolve his Oedipal conflict—at one point she refers to his personal "'Oedipean' triangle" (123)—without ever clarifying precisely what she means by that or even what Freud would have meant had he understood his filial position in those terms.

43. Given his own struggle with his feelings in the aftermath of his father's death, it is ironic that Freud will distinguish primitive from civilized times in saying that "it becomes obvious that there has been an extraordinary diminution in ambivalence [of the living toward the dead]. It is now quite easy to keep down the unconscious hostility . . . without any particular expenditure of psychical energy" (*Totem and Taboo*, XIII, 66).

44. Although Robert reads the entirety of the *Interpretation of Dreams* through the lens of Freud's ambivalent relation to his father, she more pointedly claims that "the whole 'non vixit' dream revolves around the father-phantom" (127). That said, Robert's reading relies so much on Freud's own labyrinthine account, one that does all it can *not* to acknowledge his father's presence, that, except for a couple noteworthy insights, she fails to document where and how Jacob Freud actually materializes in the dream.

45. On the process of screening generally, see V, 481, 482, 486.

46. The scene in question was from Schiller's play *Die Räuber*.

47. Addressing the question of the various "mistakes" that "slip]ped in" at various points in his dream-analyses, Freud observes that they should be understood as "substitute[s] for intentional falsification at some other point," that is, as unconscious markers of, even punishments for, his attempts to evade the truth elsewhere (*Interpretation of Dreams*, 3rd ed. [V, 456n2]). As we observed earlier, in elaborating on this point in the *Psychopathology of Everyday Life*, Freud confesses that, generally speaking, his key "errors" or misrememberings "are derivatives of repressed thoughts *connected with my dead father*" (VI, 219; my emphasis).

48. Robert, *From Oedipus to Moses*, 127–28.

49. "I had heard . . . that he was about to undergo an operation . . . The first reports I received after the operation were not reassuring and made me feel anxious. . . . The dream-thoughts now informed me that I feared for my friend's life. His only sister, whom I had never known, had, as I was aware, died in early youth after a brief illness" (V, 480–81). Later, Freud writes, "I was aware of how deeply he had mourned the sister he had so early lost" (486).

50. This is Freud's note in the original text: "It was this phantasy, forming part of the unconscious dream-thoughts, which so insistently demanded '*Non vivit*' instead of '*Non vixit*': 'You have come too late, he is no longer alive'" (V, 481n). We might say that it is Freud's own experience of coming late to his father's funeral that is the true revenant (what comes back) in the 1898 dream.

51. The "self-reproaches" Freud feels "for not going to *see*" Fliess (V, 481; my emphasis) also recollect the shop-notice in the 1896 dream, where closing one's eyes refers to the failure of doing one's duty toward the dead and thus a failure to mourn properly.

52. "Psychoanalysis and Renaissance Culture," 210, 217–18, 221.

53. *After Oedipus: Shakespeare in Psychoanalysis* (Ithaca, NY, 1993), 11.

54. One can see the explanatory role of the Oedipus complex taking shape as Freud moves from his letter to Fliess in 1896 to the draft-letter in May, 1897 and then to letter of October, 1897.

55. Although without explicit attention to sexual rivalry as the motive force of the son's antagonism toward the father, Paul Ricoeur's general view of the economy of desire governing the son's attitude is instructive: "First, there is the formation of the Oedipus complex as the obligatory landmark." But if the Oedipus complex is indeed a psychoanalytic landmark, as surely it is, in what sense is it obligatory? Obligatory for whom and in what form? Ricoeur is undoubtedly correct to add that "the Oedipus complex is in a certain sense the crucial question posed by psychoanalysis to its public." But the phrase "in a certain sense" hints at some uncertainty as to the precise nature of the question posed, and the concluding phrase "to its public" suggests that other formulations might have been considered or developed out of public view. More important, in going on to observe that the "initial constitution of [the son's] desire" moves toward "the phantasm of a father who would retain the privileges which the son must seize if he is to be himself," Ricoeur doesn't even mention the mother as part of, let alone as central to, the son's experience of desire ("Fatherhood: From Phantasm to Symbol," trans. Robert Sweeney, in *The Conflict of Interpretations: Essays on Hermeneutics*, ed. Don Ihde [Evanston, IL, 1974], 470). In what sense then is the Oedipal landmark truly expressive of the "critical question posed by psychoanalysis?"

56. *Disowning Knowledge*, 186–87; my emphasis.

57. "Psychoanalysis and Renaissance Culture," 216.

58. For broad discussion of this discursive transformation, see Timothy J. Reiss, *The Discourse of Modernism* (Ithaca, NY, 1982).

59. "Psychoanalysis and Renaissance Culture," 213, 220, 222.

60. *Love and its Place in Nature: A Philosophical Interpretation of Freudian Psychoanalysis* (New York, 1990), 4.

61. "Psychoanalysis and Renaissance Culture," 214.

Chapter 4

1. "Freud and the Sandman," in *Textual Strategies: Perspectives in Post-Structuralist Criticism*, ed. Josué V. Harari (Ithaca, NY, 1979), 319. Freud was at work on *Beyond the Pleasure Principle* while finishing up "The Uncanny" (XVII, 238).

2. "Freud and the Sandman," 318.

3. For a brief discussion of "the child's ambivalence toward his father" in relation to repetition compulsion, see Hertz, 303. The son's ambivalence toward his father in relation to Freud's understanding of the uncanny is a key issue in Sarah Kofman, *Freud and Fiction*, trans. Sarah Wykes (Boston, 1991), 121–62.

4. The *Standard Edition* has "Olympia" rather than "Olimpia." For the sake of consistency (and in conformity with Hoffmann's own spelling), I will use the latter throughout. The *Standard Edition* also has "Nathaniel" where Hoffmann has "Nathanael" (I will use the latter throughout). English citations from Jentsch are from "On the Psychology of the Uncanny," trans. Roy Sellars, *Angelaki* 2 (1996), 7–16; citations from the German original are from "Zur Psychologie des Unheimlichen" (Parts 1–2), *Psychiatrisch-Neurologische Wochenschrift* 22–23 (1906): 195–98, 203–05. As appropriate, subsequent page references will be provided in the text.

5. Even before he gets to his key disagreement with Jentsch, Freud associates the uncanny with "that which is obscure, inaccessible to knowledge" (XVII, 226).

6. At one point in the essay Freud states emphatically that the uncanny "can be traced without exception to something familiar that has been repressed" (XVII, 241).

7. German: *Der unheimliche Effekt . . . beruht zweifellos ebenfalls darauf, dass eine mehr oder weniger deutliche Vorstellung von dem Vorhandensein eines gewissen Associationzwanges (Mechanismus) im Menschen auftritt, die im Widerspruche mit der gewöhnlichen Anschauung von der psychischen Freiheit stehend an der Ueberzeugang der Beseelung des Individuums in voreiliger und ungeschickter Weise zu rütteln anfängt* ("Zur Psychologie des Unheimlichen," 205). In line with Jentsch's own phrasing, it makes more sense to take the phrase *voreiliger und ungeschickter Weise* as part of the description of how we experience a change in our normal way of thinking and not as a description of how that way of thinking (a conviction: *Ueberzeugang*) first formed (in a "hasty and careless" manner).

8. Looking ahead to Hoffmann's "The Sandman," we might observe that Freud's concept of being led back, so central to psychoanalysis generally, is imagined in the opening of the story: "You [the reader] will apprehend that this incident

must gain its significance from associations peculiar to myself [the protagonist, Nathanael], *reaching far back into my own life*" ("The Sandman," 86; my emphasis).

9. It is this paradox that leads Freud to cite Schelling's definition three times: the "'*Unheimlich*' is the name for everything that ought to have remained . . . secret and hidden but has come to light" (XVII, 224; also 225, 241).

10. For a synopsis of the plot of "The Sandman," see the Appendix to this chapter.

11. Stefani Engelstein aptly notes that Lothar, along with his sister, Clara, are characters without clear origin: they are orphans who, like this unidentified narrator, enter the story late and from places unknown (*Anxious Anatomy: The Conception of the Human Form in Literary and Naturalist Discourse* [Albany, NY, 2008], 164, 171); see Hoffmann, 99.

12. "Freud and the Sandman," 305.

13. Freud himself suggests that "Olimpia is, as it were, a dissociated complex of Nathanael's which confronts him as a person" (XVII, 232n1).

14. *Anxious Anatomy*, 145, 175.

15. Noting that "Nathanael . . . hardly seems human," Engelstein writes, for example, that "Nathanael and Olimpia are paired cyborgs linked through their transplanted and regenerated eyes" (163).

16. *Anxious Anatomy*, 175.

17. "The Uncanny Rendered Canny: Freud's Blind Spot in Reading Hoffmann's 'Sandman,'" in *Introducing Psychoanalytic Theory*, ed. Sander L. Gilman (New York, 1982), 223–24; my emphasis.

18. "Uncanny Rendered Canny," 227, 230. Kofman also understands the scene in Nathanael's father's study in terms of the Freudian primal scene (148–55). For the relevant passage in the story, see Hoffmann, 88–90.

19. Meltzer remarks, first, how, in his father's study, Nathanael is compelled to "*witness* . . . the primal scene"; later, as we have already noted, she claims that, in his final encounter with Olimpia, Nathanael is "only repeating the trauma of the conceptual primal scene which he *witnessed* from the closet"; and finally, she writes that in this encounter "Nathanael *witnesses* the Sandman *scène originaire* all over again, but he is now the spectator. Olimpia is substituted for him," a description she sums up with "a *scène originaire* is thus *witnessed* by the child" (225, 227, 230; my emphases).

20. See, for example, Meltzer, 235; and Kofman, 158.

21. As we noted in chapter 1, Cathy Caruth observes that in *Beyond the Pleasure Principle* Freud "moves from a speculation . . . that explains trauma as an interruption of consciousness . . . to an explanation of the origins of life as an 'awakening' . . . that precisely establishes the foundation of the [death] drive and of consciousness alike. This peculiar movement . . . traces a significant itinerary in Freud's thought from trauma as an exception, an accident that takes consciousness by surprise and thus disrupts it, to trauma as the very origin of consciousness and all life itself" (*Unclaimed Experience: Trauma, Narrative, and History* [Baltimore, MD, 1996], 104).

22. Anticipating the focus of part III, and of chapter 5 in particular, we might compare Hoffmann's description of Nathanael's (re)birth to the account of Adam's creation (Genesis 2:7) as elaborated by Milton in *Paradise Lost*. (This is the passage from which I draw the chapter's epigraph.) Adam is here recounting his memory of first coming to consciousness:

> For Man to tell how human life began
> Is hard: for who himself beginning knew?
> . . . *As new waked from soundest sleep*
> Soft on the flow'ry herb I found me laid
> In balmy sweat (*Paradise Lost*, 8.250–55; my emphasis)

Milton will again link Adam's creation—his condition of being animated—to awakening by contrasting it to a sleep that is indistinguishable from a return to inanimatedness:

> Pensive I sat me down. There *gentle sleep*
> First found me and with soft oppression seized
> My drowsèd sense, untroubled, though I thought
> I then was *passing to my former state*
> *Insensible*, and forthwith to dissolve. (8.287–91; my emphases)

Hoffmann's reference to the "warm, gentle breath" that "passed over [Nathanael's] face" thus causing him to awake "from a death-like sleep" might be alluding even more directly to Genesis 2:7: "the LORD God formed man from the dust of the earth. He blew into his nostrils the breath of life, and man became a living being."

23. German: . . . *denn die Begeisterung, in der man nur zu schaffen fähig sei, komme nicht aus dem eignen Innern* ("Der Sandmann," 21).

24. German: . . . *das Einwirken irgendeines außer uns selbst liegenden* ("Der Sandmann," 21).

25. See "Notes on Afterwardsness," in *Essays on Otherness*, ed. John Fletcher (New York, 1999), 260–65.

26. Laplanche, "Notes on Afterwardsness," 265; Caruth, *Unclaimed Experience*, 143n10; my emphases.

27. German: *was an diesen Wiederholungszwang mahnen kann* (XII, 251). Without explicit attention to repetition compulsion, Paul Ricoeur remarks in a related context that "the theme of anteriority pervades Freudianism" because "desire is in every respect prior . . . [T]his prior desire . . . pulls us backwards and insinuates the whole backward drift of affectivity on the level of familial relationships, fantasies and works of art, ethics and guilt, religion and the fear of punishment and the infantile wish for consolation." And to the extent the Freudian Unconscious is timeless, it is so because it is "rebellious to the temporalization which is linked to becoming-conscious" ("A Philosophical Interpretation of Freud," trans. Willis

Domingo, in Paul Ricoeur, *The Conflict of Interpretations: Essays in Hermeneutics*, ed. Don Ihde [Evanston, IL, 1974], 173).

28. Freud provides his own summary, XVII, 227–30.

29. Freud is absolutely correct in observing that "Hoffmann . . . leaves us in doubt whether what we are witnessing is the first delirium of the panic-stricken boy, or a succession of events which are to be regarded in the story as being real" (XVII, 229).

30. I would like to suggest that Hoffmann is calling attention here to what precisely is missing from the story and what especially troubles Nathanael because he cannot see it—or perhaps him. And what is missing is the Old Man (*Der Alte*) who, inexplicably, was present at Nathanael's creation. In short, it is his recognition of what he cannot see—can never see—that drives Nathanael to his final suicidal madness.

Part III Introduction

1. A full transcript of that episode appears in the book accompanying the series, *Genesis: A Living Conversation*, ed. Bill Moyers and Betty Sue Flowers (New York, 1996), 39–69; Professor Young's comments are cited on p. 50.

2. The poet, Stephen Mitchell, for example, takes this position: "There's something so beautiful and precious about early childhood, and part of a parent wants to make that last forever. That part grieves when a child grows up, reaches puberty, and becomes sexually aware. Emotionally, the story is meant to explain how it came about that we left the radiance of childhood, the clouds of glory, how it is that we are so close to God when we're born, and then somehow find ourselves living in a consciousness of separation and loss" (*Genesis: A Living Conversation*, 44).

3. *The Brothers Karamazov*, trans. Andrew R. MacAndrew (New York, 1981), 285.

4. Augustine had argued that death came about solely from an act of human will. But Julian saw death as part of the normal, prelapsarian dispensation. For a summary of this part of the debate, see Elaine Pagels, *Adam, Eve, and the Serpent* (New York, 1989), 142.

5. For a summary of Julian's position, see Pagels, 132–41.

6. While the accounts of creation (Genesis 2) and the Fall (Genesis 3) are different stories, we do well to remind ourselves that the J-narrative presents them as a continuous sequence.

7. *Ruin the Sacred Truths: Poetry and Belief from the Bible to the Present* (Cambridge, MA, 1989), 150.

8. This concern with how objects are made—even where objects might include human beings—might partly explain the Bible's interest in genealogies, more evidence that we have origins. These genealogies are linked to the Bible's privileging of memory and time over seeing and space, and they insist that authority resides in the present only to the extent it first existed in the past.

9. Both passages are from the Priestly narrative.

10. Genesis 6's story of "the sons of God" begetting the Nephilim hints that human divinity could be understood as residing in the capacity to sire children (obviously here more a male than a female capacity). If God is a father, then human fathers might be forgiven for thinking that they too are gods.

11. *The Book of J* (New York, 1990), 73; my emphasis.

12. Before moving from touching to seeing, we might remind ourselves that the first representation of this human-divine barrier is couched as the former, in Eve's otherwise unexplained addition in Genesis 3:3, "you shall not eat of it *or touch it*, lest you die." And an implicit prohibition on touching what God/the gods have forbidden to humankind then comes back in the Tower of Babel episode: "'They conceive this between them, and it leads up *until no boundary exists to what they will touch*.'" In *Totem and Taboo* (1913) Freud will write that "touching is the first step towards obtaining any sort of control over . . . a person or object" (XIII, 33–34). And if we read this statement in relation to the two stories in Genesis then we might imagine that what the gods forbid is the act of control or even possession by which humankind would claim a divine place for itself. Exodus 19 emphasizes seeing over touching, but it too appears to want to prevent people (here the Israelites) from crossing over to a place that does not and must not belong to them. In that sense, the Law begins with the people of Israel's renunciation of their desire to claim the place of god(s).

13. *A History of God: The 4000-Year Old Quest of Judaism, Christianity, and Islam* (New York, 1993), 9. We might compare this statement to a point Freud makes almost in passing in *Totem and Taboo*: "The notion of a man becoming a god . . . strikes us today as shockingly presumptuous; but . . . in classical antiquity, there was nothing revolting in it." Freud then quotes a passage from *The Golden Bough* in a footnote: "To us moderns, for whom the break which divides the human and the divine has deepened into an impassable gulf, such mimicry may appear impious, but it was otherwise with the ancients. To their thinking gods and men were akin, for many families traced their descent from a divinity" (XIII, 149 and 149n1; passage qtd. from J. G. Frazer, *The Golden Bough* [London, 1911], 177).

14. *The Art of Biblical Narrative* (New York, 1981), 154, 157.

15. This passage is most often viewed as belonging to the Priestly tradition, though perhaps originally deriving from the E or Elohist version and so first assimilated into scripture as part of the J-E epic. For efforts to resolve this debate, see Richard Elliot Friedman *Who Wrote the Bible?* (New York, 1987), 251, 258–59; and *The Bible with Sources Revealed* (New York, 2003), 153n.

16. Even to refer to these verses as the second commandment might be wrong. For various ways of establishing the particular *ten* commandments, see W. Gunther Plant's discussion in *The Torah: A Modern Commentary* (New York, 1981), 534–35.

17. The J-narrative's version of the Decalogue is quite different, though it does contain prohibitions both against the worship of other gods and against the making of graven images. The J-narrative's Decalogue comes after the story of the Golden Calf as though Yahweh decides on the necessity of the law after observing the Israelites' actual behavior rather than in anticipation of it.

18. In a general way, the commandment is a way of reminding the people of Israel of the fundamental incorporeality of their god (see, for example, Deuteronomy 4:15), just one of many reasons normative Judaism viewed Christianity as a heresy. In *Moses and Monotheism*, a text we shall consider in chapter 6, Freud linked the prohibition of images to Judaism's instinctual renunciation that "signified subordinating sense perception to an abstract idea; it was the triumph of spirituality over the senses" (144).

19. Alter, 32; Bloom, 148. Bloom adds that because, in the rabbinical tradition, "everything already is in the past, and nothing that matters can be utterly new," authority must "always reside in figures of the . . . past" (152, 147).

20. God's warning to the people not "to be drawn to" him, "to destroy boundaries" by "bursting through to see" (Exodus 19:21) is, we presume, a warning against gazing upon Yahweh himself. That strange image from the J-narrative (itself, I have suggested, echoing the Tower of Babel story) might be understood then as a very primitive version for which redacted Exodus 20:4–6 (perhaps from the much later P-narrative) then provides an elaboration or gloss. In other words, Exodus 19:21 warns the people against gazing on Yahweh himself, and this prohibition is subsequently extended to the making and worshipping of any "sculptured image, or likeness." Exodus 20:4 thus also effectively prohibits the mimicking of God's creative power, precisely the kind of power on display in the Golden Calf story: "[T]he people gathered against Aaron and said to him, "Come, *make us a god* '" (Exodus 32:1; my emphasis).

21. "Leviticus," in *Congregation: Contemporary Writers Read the Jewish Bible*, ed. David Rosenberg (New York, 1987), 29; subsequent page references will be cited in the text.

22. Wieseltier will go so far as to argue, in a way Emerson might have appreciated, that the very notion of the Fall within Jewish consciousness has almost nothing to do with sin in the later Christian sense and everything to do with a decline into temporality itself: "A fall need not connote sin, as in the Christian construction. It need only connote fate. But fate without sin: that is another way of describing *victimization by time*. Fate without sin is punishment by duration. You are not guilty, *you are merely late*" (30; my emphases).

23. Wieseltier particularly wants to distinguish scripture from later rabbinical commentary in the way the rabbis came to learn to read the former in such a way as to "honor . . . difference that cannot be overcome, a difference in kind between that world [God's world] and this world" (29). To the extent he sees rabbinical commentary as invested in the creation and enforcement of tradition as a specific form of compensation for lost immediacy, we might understand it precisely as part of the process by which Hebrew monotheistic discourse invents Alter's "absolute cleavage between man and God."

24. As an instance of what he generally terms Jewish "fatalism" ("a willingness to settle for something less than experience in a relationship with God"), Wieseltier remarks with some sense of pathos that "the impatient Jew . . . suffers his days in the deprivation of [divine] acknowledgement, or worse, in *its commemoration*" (27, 38; my emphasis). It is worth noting in this context that the Hebrew name for

Leviticus is *Vayikra*, "and he called," a concept glossed by rabbis to observe how God's voice is necessarily mediated: "The voice makes its way to Moses, and all of Israel does not hear it" (qtd. in Wieseltier, 37). Wieseltier adds: "Moses, of course, reported what he heard. It was precisely when the report of the voice did the work of the voice that tradition was born."

25. In *Paradise Lost*, the "'was' before the beginning" is a time before our world was even created, a time when human history merely existed as what Beelzebub calls "ancient and prophetic fame" (2.346).

Chapter 5

1. *On Free Choice of the Will*, trans. Anna S. Benjamin and L. H. Hackstaff (Indianapolis, IN, 1964), 145. Subsequent references to this text will be given by book, chapter, and section number(s).

2. *City of God*, ed. and trans. R. W. Dyson (Cambridge, 1998), XII.6; all references to *City of God* will be to this edition and cited by book and chapter.

3. For discussion of Milton's general indebtedness to Augustine on the matter of the angelic fall, see Peter A. Fiore, *Milton and Augustine: Patterns of Augustinian Thought in Paradise Lost* (University Park, PA, 1981), 12–22.

4. With regard to Milton specifically, William Kerrigan claims that *Paradise Lost* "interpreted psychoanalysis" (*The Sacred Complex: On the Psychogenesis of Paradise Lost* [Cambridge, MA, 1983], 162). Not going quite so far, Regina Schwartz argues that Milton was "deeply psychoanalytic before there was such a science," though she rightly observes that Milton himself subsumes his proto-psychoanalytic inquiry into his role as religious thinker (*Remembering and Repeating: On Milton's Theology and Poetics* [Chicago, 1993], xii). Subsequent references to Kerrigan's and Schwartz's studies will be cited in the text.

5. Schwartz, for example, analyzes Satan's problem as kind of traumatic neurosis (94–110).

6. *Disowning Knowledge in Seven Plays of Shakespeare* (Cambridge, 2003), 179.

7. The narrator will offer this diagnosis just a few lines later (5.659–65).

8. *Ruin the Sacred Truths: Poetry and Belief from the Bible to the Present* (Cambridge, MA, 1989), 104. Subsequent page references will be cited in the text.

9. For much fuller historical and/or theological assessments of Gnosticism, see Hans Jonas *The Gnostic Religion: The Message of the Alien God and the Beginnings of Christianity* (Boston, 1963); Elaine Pagels, *The Gnostic Gospels* (New York, 1979); Giovanni Filoramo, *A History of Gnosticism*, trans. Anthony Alcock (Oxford, 1990); and Bentley Layton, *The Gnostic Scriptures* (Garden City, NY, 1987).

10. The fullest account of what we might call the Gnostic dream is provided in Harold Bloom's *Omens of Millennium: The Gnosis of Angels, Dreams, and Resurrection* (New York, 1996). Milton, not surprisingly, views that dream in negative terms; in *De Doctrina Christiana* he will argue that Adam and Eve were "sac-

rilegious and deceitful, cunningly *aspiring to divinity* although thoroughly unworthy of it" (VI, 384; my emphasis).

11. *The Alternative Trinity: Gnostic Heresy in Marlowe, Milton, and Blake* (Oxford, 1998), 83. Subsequent page references will be cited in the text. In the end, however, Nuttall's account, especially in regard to *Paradise Lost*, is so broad as to render the notion of "Gnostic heresy" a bit misleading. Not only is he not particularly interested in what precisely constitutes *gnosis* as a secret or mystical redemptive knowledge, but, with respect to *Paradise Lost*, he effectively equates Milton's position with a series of broader heresies that have no immediate connection to historical Gnosticism.

12. As Bloom has particularly shown, Gnostic myth was generally obsessed with proclaiming some reversal in the priority of creation, a reversal in which what would normally "come after" precisely because created by what came before (the self-existent god) could be reimagined as having temporal and/or ontological precedence: see *Omens of Millennium*, especially 35–53, 85–93, and 145–72. Following Bloom's thought, Kerrigan has noted the "distinctive intensity" Milton brings to the valuing of "earliness"; "Milton designs the poem so as to catch up his readers in an excited search for priority" by taking "his plot further back into the recesses of extrabiblical history" (157–58).

13. Although I take their arguments in a different direction, what follows is indebted in various ways to the work of Kerrigan, Schwartz, and John Guillory (*Poetic Authority: Spenser, Milton, and Literary History* [New York, 1983], especially ch. 5; page references to Guillory's study will be cited in the text).

14. Citing a number of biblical source-texts in support, Milton makes exactly this point in *De Doctrina Christiana*, VI, 206.

15. While celebrating "of all Creation first, . . . Divine Similitude" in their Book 3 hymn of praise, the unfallen angels will observe that the "Heav'n of Heavens and all the Powers therein" were "created" by the "Begotten Son" (3.383–84, 390–91). But despite coming earlier in the poem's narrative, in terms of the poem's temporal ordering this recognition comes after the events that lead to the rebellion and expulsion of the rebel angels.

16. We might compare Adam's first thoughts to Augustine's statement in his *Confessions*: "I do acknowledge you, Lord of heaven and earth, and I praise you for my first beginnings, *although I can not remember them*" (*Confessions*, trans. R. S. Pine-Coffin [Baltimore, MD, 1961], 26; my emphasis). Tellingly, in *Paradise Lost* Adam earlier refers to what happened prior to his existence as what "was done / Before . . . memorie" (7.65–66).

17. Although he is simply following traditional Christian theology on this point, Milton seems to want to give special stress to the notion of angelic belatedness by emphasizing the fact that all of creation is doubly belated: God isn't even its immediate creator; that distinction belongs to God's only begotten Son, who is himself brought into existence—begotten if not created—and so "later" than God. Generally speaking, Milton sees the Son as the firstborn offspring of God.

18. Guillory points out that, to the extent Satan and his cohort's longing not to have been created leads to their fall, the fantasy that they have effectively fathered themselves functions as a kind of parody of Gnostic self-realization: "The already fallen angels no longer know the time when they were not, as now, *fallen*. . . . Lucifer becomes Satan, and in the gap between these two identities is the origin Satan seeks. He does indeed create himself as Satan, self-authored, self-begotten" (119).

19. From Charles Leslie's preface to his *History of Sin and Heresy*; reprinted in *Milton: The Critical Heritage*, ed. John T. Shawcross, 2 vols. (London, 1970–72), I, 117–18.

20. As Milton concludes in *De Doctrina Christiana*, "For a supreme God is self-existent, but a God who is not self-existent, who did not beget but was begotten, is not a first cause but an effect, and is therefore not a supreme God" (VI, 263–64).

21. Although Wieseltier is actually referring to the God-time prior to the creation of earth as recounted in Genesis 1, for Milton and indeed for many Gnostics, the " 'was' before the beginning" actually goes back even further (Wieseltier, "Leviticus," in *Congregation: Contemporary Writers Read the Jewish Bible*, ed. David Rosenberg [New York, 1987], 31). Of course, stories of a war in heaven prior to the creation of humankind would necessarily demand some imagining of that earlier "was."

22. In *De Doctrina Christiana*, Milton observes that "in scripture there are two senses in which the Father is said to have begotten the Son: one literal, with reference to production; the other metaphorical, with reference to exaltation" (VI, 205).

23. What we might call Milton's deliberate confusion over just what the Son's begetting means in the context of God's proclamation of Book 5 is traceable in particular to Psalm 2:7,

> Let me tell of the decree:
> the LORD said to me,
> "You are My son,
> I have fathered you this day."

The basic image of the Psalm, undoubtedly a celebration of Davidic kingship, is of a divine son (king/messiah) ruling over other nations. But while the proclamation of the king-messiah's special filial relationship to the Lord—"You are My son"— seems to be part of a ritual of royal investiture (we might compare the language of 2 Samuel 7 or Psalm 89), the final phrase, "I have fathered you this day" (more commonly translated as "This day I have begotten you") might be interpreted as distinguishing the (begetting-)enthronement from the (begetting-)fathering, as though they were separate acts.

24. In its unwillingness or inability to narrate the true beginning, the poem itself experiences Satan's own dilemma (and Adam's and Uriel's): it only *knows of* an earlier time ("with report") without actually knowing it (seeing it, remembering it).

25. We might recall in this context how the reference to the mysterious "Old Man" (*der Alte*) in the account of Nathanael's construction in "The Sandman" similarly suggested an aspect of the origin that was inaccessible or even, more radically, had to be formerly acknowledged as inaccessible, mysteriously and inexplicably out-of-bounds.

26. That Milton wants us to see Gabriel's portrayal of Satan's past actions *as* a misinterpretation is borne out by the fact that Milton offers us Gabriel's perspective only after (and very much at odds with) Satan's own confession as to his actual motives. The fact that Milton puts both of these in Book 4 only serves to highlight the contrast.

27. *Thus Spoke Zarathustra*, trans. Adrian del Caro (Cambridge, 2006), 110–11. We might recall Satan's heroic self-fashioning from the opening of *Paradise Lost*:

> What though the field be lost?
> All is not lost; the unconquerable Will,
> And *study of revenge*, immortal hate,
> And courage never to submit or yield:
> And what is else not to be overcome? (1.105–09; my emphasis)

28. Freud himself was not oblivious to Milton's significance to his own thought. In a 1907 response to the Viennese publisher Hugo Heller, for example, he had written: "You ask me to name 'ten good books' for you, and refrain from adding to this any word of explanation. . . . You did not say: 'the ten most magnificent works (of world literature)' . . . Nor did you say the 'ten most significant books' . . . You did not even ask for 'favorite books,' among which I should not have forgotten Milton's *Paradise Lost*" ("Contribution to a Questionnaire on Reading," *Standard Edition*, IX, 245). And in an August, 1882 letter to his then fiancée, Martha Bernays, Freud had explicitly mentioned only *Paradise Lost* as among "the works of the men who were my real teachers" (qtd. in Ernest Jones, *The Life and Work of Sigmund Freud*, 3 vols. [New York, 1953–57], I, 179).

Chapter 6

1. *Moses and Monotheism* makes several direct references to *Totem and Taboo*, e.g. 65, 68, 71, 102–08, 167–69, 171–72.

2. We shall examine Freud's analysis in more detail subsequently. For now we might just note Freud's summary of his own long considerations on the topic: "After these considerations I have no qualms in saying that men have always known . . . that once upon a time they had a primeval father and killed him" (*Moses and Monotheism*, 129). The killing of the primeval father subsequently fuels a guilt that, under the force of repression (and so disguising a continuing hostility), will return in the highly distorted form of a collective neurosis. This return of the

repressed in what Freud calls "mass psychology" then creates a range of religious beliefs and practices that mark the "father deity" as a "restoration of the [slain] primeval father" (106, 109).

3. Marthe Robert has convincingly argued that it was the self-analysis initiated by the death of Jacob Freud that was the true foundation of psychoanalysis as both a content of ideas and a method of interpretation: see *From Oedipus to Moses: Freud's Jewish Identity*, trans. Ralph Manheim (Garden City, NY, 1976), 63–64, and 120–22. Robert's addition that as early as 1896 Freud's ambivalence toward his father was bound up with "the contradictory nature of his Jewish sentiment" (133) is not so well grounded, although, as we shall see, that "sentiment" will get drawn into later works, especially *Moses and Monotheism*.

4. This is the central contention of Robert's study which argues that Freud's ambivalence toward his father was fueled by an Oedipal struggle as traditionally conceived, where "the infant's desire for the parent of the opposite sex" is balanced, even caused by, "hatred of the other parent seen as a rival to be eliminated" (133). For related discussion, see Marianne Krüll, *Freud and his Father*, trans. Arnold J. Pomerans (New York, 1986); Dennis B. Klein, *Jewish Origins of the Psychoanalytic Movement* (New York, 1981); and Emanuel Rice, *Freud and Moses: The Long Journey Home* (Albany, NY, 1990). Freud's feelings for his father as caught up in the complex relationship between psychoanalysis and Jewish identity is at the heart of Yosef Hayim Yerushalmi's consistently insightful *Freud's Moses: Judaism Terminable and Interminable* (New Haven, CT, 1991).

5. Both in his own description and in his borrowings from others, Freud keeps returning to this scorn, elsewhere describing it as "wrath," "indignation," "anger," "contempt."

6. Freud ventures that Michelangelo's depiction of what he takes to be a very particular episode from the life of Moses has the paradoxical effect of rendering Moses "in his wrath forever" (XIII, 221).

7. In the analysis proper, Freud claims that Michelangelo's Moses starts up to "annihilate" those against whom his anger has been kindled (XIII, 225).

8. Exodus 32:19 ("As soon as Moses . . . saw the calf and the dancing, he became enraged; and he hurled the tablets from his hands and shattered them at the foot of the mountain") becomes the following in Freud's version of Michelangelo's artistic intention:

> [T]he resting Moses is startled by the clamor of the people and the spectacle of the Golden Calf. . . . Now wrath and indignation lay hold of him . . . What we see before us is not the inception of a violent action but the remains of a movement that has already taken place. In his first transport of fury, Moses desired to act, to spring up and take vengeance and forget the Tables [of the Law]; but he has overcome the temptation, and he will now remain seated and still, in his frozen wrath and in his pain mingled with contempt. Nor will he throw the Tables so that they will break on the stones, for it is on the especial

account that he has controlled his anger; it was to preserve them that he kept his passion in check. In giving way to his rage and indignation, he had to neglect the Tables, and the hand which upheld them was withdrawn. They began to slide down and were in danger of being broken. This brought him to himself. He remembered his mission and for its sake renounced an indulgence of his feelings. . . . [I]n this attitude Michelangelo has portrayed him[.] (XIII, 224–30)

9. While Freud notes that "such deviations from the scriptural text . . . were by no means unusual or disallowed to artists" even in more overtly religious times (XIII, 232), his very recognition of that fact suggests his awareness of the right of readers of the bible not to be limited by the authority of tradition. More to the point, although his work on *Moses and Monotheism* is still some twenty years away, Freud here seems to imagine Michelangelo's "deviation from the scriptural text" as precisely the kind of bold act—"an act of blasphemy" (230)—that he too might perform.

10. The preface was first published in German in 1934 (*Gesammelte Shriften*, 12 vols. [Vienna, 1922–34], XII.385), perhaps not so coincidentally the same year in which Freud completed a draft of *Moses and Monotheism* (September, 1934). We might even imagine that the 1930 preface to the translation of *Totem and Taboo* into "the language of holy writ" prompted Freud to revisit the book's argument in the more specific context of the origins on Hebrew monotheism. The Hebrew translation of *Totem and Taboo* was not actually published until 1939 (Jerusalem: Kirjeith Zefer), the same year in which the full text of *Moses and Monotheism* was published.

11. Freud was not the only Jewish son whose ambivalence toward his father was caught up in and expressed through Judaism. In a 1921 critique of contemporary German-Jewish literature, Kafka had drawn as one of the key lessons of psychoanalysis "the observation that the father complex from which more than one Jew draws his spiritual nourishment relates not to the innocent father but to *the father's Judaism*. What most of those who began to write in German wanted was to break with Judaism, . . . but their hind legs were bogged down *in their fathers' Judaism*, and their front legs could find no ground" (*Briefe, 1902–1924* [New York, 1958], 337; my emphases). Although there is no reason to believe that Freud would have been particularly sensitive to this idea, it is worth bearing in mind that the God of the Hebrew Bible is often less a father figure himself than the deity "of the fathers," a particularly common phrasing in the prophetic writings (but see also Genesis 26:23, 28:13, 31:5, 32:10, 46:1–3, 48:15–16, and Exodus 3:6). (Surprisingly, the reference to God as "father" appears rather infrequently in the Hebrew Bible.) We might note in this context Paul Ricoeur's (re)reading of Freud's figure of the Oedipal father through the lens of Hegel's *Phenomenology of Spirit*. Remarking that the "recognition of fatherhood is shifted to the Penates" (ancestral or household gods), Ricoeur glosses the Penates as "the dead father raised to a representation; it is when he is dead, when he is absent, that he passes into the symbol of fatherhood." Ricoeur concludes that this movement from the literal

if now dead father to the father as symbol (what is of *the fathers*) "raises fatherhood above the contingency of individuals . . . [T]he death of the [literal] father is thus blended into the representation of the bond of fatherhood which dominates the sequence of the generations" ("Fatherhood: From Phantasm to Symbol," trans. Robert Sweeney, in *The Conflict of Interpretations: Essays on Hermeneutics*, ed. Don Ihde [Evanston, IL, 1974], 480, 492).

12. Although she comes at the issue from the perspective of what she sees as Freud's final *postmodern* commitments, Regina Schwartz has similarly traced how *Moses and Monotheism* grapples with the problematic nature of the origin: see "Freud's God," in *Post-Secular Philosophy: Between Philosophy and Theology*, ed. Philip Bond (New York, 1998), especially 282–83, 293.

13. Six years later, Freud would still be making this claim: "the miraculous thing . . . [that] makes the Jew" is nevertheless "inaccessible to analysis" (*Letters*, 428).

14. We might put this in exactly the opposite way: Freud cannot find words to express his own Jewishness (it remains inaccessible to him) because he is not as estranged as he believes. For the very metonymy he employs (Judaism as the "religion of his fathers") tells us that he is inescapably lodged within that very identity.

15. Freud was not the first to suggest this possibility. For broad discussion of related views that predate *Moses and Monotheism*, see Paolo Rossi, *The Dark Abyss of Time: The History of the Earth and the History of Nations from Hooke to Vico*, trans. Lydia G. Cochrane (Chicago, 1984), ch. 17 ("The Egyptian Culture of Moses").

16. For Freud's various descriptions, see 13, 17–18, 31–32, 74.

17. As an example of the confusion (or irrelevance) regarding Moses's ethnic identity, Freud borrows from Eduard Meyer's *Die Israeliten und ihre Nachbarstämme* (1906) the notion that there was a second Moses, a priest of Midian, who was instrumental in bringing the volcano-god, Yahweh, to the Israelites: *Moses and Monotheism*, 38ff. That said, while Freud himself appears to have believed that he had stumbled across a major secret in Moses's Egyptian origins, most of his account of the post-Exodus/pre-Conquest period would make as much (or as little) sense even if Moses had been an Israelite. Even the single most shocking detail of Freud's speculation—that Moses had been murdered by the rebellious Israelites at the oasis of Meribah-Kadesh—could just as easily have happened had Moses been exactly as the biblical account depicts him. Freud borrows the claim of the murder of Moses and other important ideas from a 1922 work by Ernst Sellin: see *Moses and Monotheism*, 42–43 and *passim*. But, as Freud himself recognizes, Sellin never suggests that Moses was not an Israelite.

18. In reference to this stage in their history, it would be more accurate to call the biblical people Israelites rather than Jews. From this point on, I will follow Freud's own usage and refer to the pre-Conquest people as the Jews. But the fact that Freud himself does not make the distinction even as he fully grasps its historical basis is telling: he wants to insist, in short, on a very real transhistorical or perhaps ahistorical connection between those who left Egypt with Moses and Freud's own Jewish contemporaries.

19. *Letters of Sigmund Freud and Arnold Zweig*, ed. Ernst L. Freud, trans. Elaine Robson-Scott and William Robson-Scott (New York, 1970), 98. At the close of part II of *Moses and Monotheism*, Freud will write that his "sole purpose" was "to fit the figure of an Egyptian Moses into the framework of Jewish history" (64). But the addition two years later of part III (more than twice the length of parts I and II combined) suggests that this was not his sole purpose.

20. Borrowing or directly quoting from Otto Rank's 1909 *Myth of the Birth of the Hero*, Freud writes, for example: "*the hero is the son of parents* of the highest station"; "*his conception* is impeded by difficulties . . . *his parents practice intercourse* in secret because of prohibitions or other external obstacles"; "*during his mother's pregnancy* or earlier an oracle or a dream *warns the father of the child's birth*" (7–8; my emphases). Freud offers this summary: "The inner source of the [exposure] myth is the so-called 'family romance' of the child, in which the son reacts to the change of his inner relationship to his parents" (9).

21. It is worth noting in this context that even as Freud cites the Oedipus story as one of many instances of the exposure myth, the conventions of the myth Freud focuses on have nothing to do with the son's relationship to the mother and everything to do with the father, especially the son's hostile relationship toward his father (9–10). Later in the text, in referring to the "longing for the father that lives in each of us from his childhood days" (140), he makes no mention of a sexual longing for the mother.

22. Freud again quotes much of this material from Rank's *Myth of the Birth of the Hero*.

23. Freud unwittingly captures the duality of Moses's identity when, in generalizing about the role of the father in both individual and mass psychology (with particular relevance to his understanding of the origin of religion), he observes almost casually that "it is the longing for the father that lives in each of us from childhood days, for *the same father whom the hero of legend boasts of having overcome*" (140; my emphasis). In short, Moses is for Freud at once the great father for whom the son longs and, as represented in the exposure myth, the son-hero who, as an adult, will overcome the father.

24. At the very beginning of *Moses and Monotheism*, Freud endorses the traditional history at least in broadest terms: "[T]he great majority of historians have expressed the opinion that Moses did live and that the exodus from Egypt, led by him, did in fact take place. . . . [T]he later history of Israel could not be understood if this were not admitted" (4).

25. We might consider the particular case of the Levites. As Freud interprets their pre-Exodus identity, the Levites were not originally a Jewish tribe at all but rather Egyptian followers of Moses (44–45). Just prior to that, in reference to a "tribe returning from Egypt" to Canaan, he also says that the "people of Israel" proper did not come into existence until that group combined with other tribal groups living south of Palestine, though he does imagine the two groups as culturally/ethnically related in terms of a shared Canaanite ancestry (44). In short, Freud

doesn't think that the Jewish people as we retrospectively understand them truly existed until after the Exodus.

26. What Freud consistently depicts as the "essence" of Jewish identity across time derives from what Moses imposed: the intellectual, spiritual, and moral rigor of a religion based in abstraction and various commitments to instinctual renunciation. Among the elements of Jewish monotheism Freud most admires, especially in contrast to Egyptian and other forms of pagan-polytheism but also in contrast to a later Christianity, are its surrender of the hope of an afterlife and its refusal of magical rites by which what Freud in *Totem and Taboo* calls "the omnipotence of thoughts" substitutes fantasy for reality.

27. For other descriptions of this process, see 3, 18, 29, 36, 136, 158; for other images of Moses as founder, see 16, 18, 31, 32, 35, 42.

28. *Letters of Sigmund Freud and Arnold Zweig*, 91.

29. Freud returns to the concept of chosenness over and over again: 32–34, 51n1, 55, 74, 79, 134–35, 142–44, 147, 158.

30. It is worth noting in this context the title Freud gives to part III of *Moses and Monotheism*: "Moses, *His People* [*Sein Volk*], and Monotheistic Religion" (66; my emphasis).

31. Yerushalmi, *Freud's Moses*, 29.

32. In regard to religious experience generally, Freud had argued in the *Psychopathology of Everyday Life* (1901) that "a large part of the mythological view of the world, which extends a long way into the most modern religions, *is nothing but psychology projected into the external world.*" He would add that "the obscure recognition . . . of psychical forces and relations in the unconscious is mirrored—it is difficult to express it in other terms, and here the analogy with paranoia must come to our aid—in the construction of *supernatural reality*, which is destined to be changed back once more by science into the *psychology of the unconscious*" (VI, 258).

33. See also 18, 21–26, and 61–62 for Freud's understanding of the original Aton religion.

34. While Moses, Freud surmises, "forced [the people] to adopt a new religion" (18), he also imagines that Moses's own version of the Aton-religion "was still more uncompromising than that of his master," Ikhnaton. For "he had no need to retain any connection with the religion of the sun-god since the school of On would have had no importance for his alien people" (57).

35. For Freud's full account, see 42–49. Freud writes later: "Moses met with the same fate as Ikhnaton, the fate that awaits all enlightened despots. . . . But while the tame Egyptians waited until fate had removed the sacred person of their Pharaoh, the savage Semites took their destiny into their own hands and did away with the tyrant" (57–58).

36. So Freud argues, "the religion of Moses did not achieve it effects immediately, but in a strangely indirect manner. . . . It took a long time, many centuries, to do so." Indeed, after the "Jewish people shook off the religion of Moses," the Mosaic tradition existed only as "a sort of memory," but it "survived, obscured and distorted" (159). Earlier, he had generalized to say that "recent events [may]

produce impressions or experiences which are so much like the repressed material that they have the power to awaken it. Thus the recent material gets strengthened by the latent energy of the repressed, and the repressed material produces its effect behind the recent material and with its help" (121). He then applied this model to Jewish tradition following the murder of Moses (129).

37. Freud clearly thinks that such repressed memories had been passed down as the phylogenetic heritage of all human beings: see, for example, *Moses and Monotheism*, 101–02. For related comments, see *Three Essays on the Theory of Sexuality*, VII, 131.

38. Freud writes of "religious phenomena" in general that they "are to be understood only on a model of the neurotic symptoms of the individual . . . as a return of long-forgotten happenings in the primeval history of the human family . . . [T]hey owe their obsessive character to that very origin" (71). In taking the origins of Jewish monotheism as his particular test-case, he will add that for it to have become a tradition with a fully compulsive character it "must first have suffered the fate of repression, that state of being unconscious, before it could produce such mighty effects on its return, and force the masses under its spell" (130).

39. That said, even to the extent Moses returns as the Father-God, the true archetype remains the "primeval father" (115). As Freud summarizes this process within Jewish history, "the great deed and misdeed of primeval times, the murder of the father, was brought home to the Jews, for fate decreed that they should repeat it on the person of Moses, an eminent father substitute" (113).

40. For a simple summary statement, see 167.

41. Freud acknowledges that he "argue[s] as if there were no question that there exists an inheritance of memory—traces of what our forefathers experienced, quite independently of direct communication and of the influence of education." But he then "admit[s] . . . that [he] cannot picture biological development proceeding without taking this factor ["acquired qualities being transmitted to descendants"] into account" (127–28).

42. For Freud's earlier reliance on Lamarckism, see "Overview of the Transference Neuroses" (1915), published in *A Phylogenetic Fantasy: Overview of the Transference Neuroses*, ed. Ilse Grubitch-Simitis, trans. Axel Hoffer and Peter T. Hoffer (Cambridge, MA, 1987), 5–20; and *Outline of Psycho-Analysis*, XXIII, 167, 190n1, 200–02, 207. For discussion, see Frank J. Sulloway, *Freud, Biologist of the Mind: Beyond the Psychoanalytic Legend* (New York, 1979); Ilse Grubitch-Simitis, "Metapsychology and Metabiology: On Sigmund Freud's Draft Overview of the Transference Neuroses," in *A Phylogenetic Fantasy*, 75–107; and Henry Edelheit, "On the Biology of Language: Darwinian/Lamarckian Homology in Human Inheritance (with some thoughts about the Lamarckism of Freud)," in *Psychoanalysis and Language* (Psychiatry and the Humanities, v. 3) (New Haven, CT, 1978), 45–74. Freud makes many direct references to Lamarck, for example in letters to Sándor Ferenczi on January 6, and December, 22, 1916, and January 28, March 2, May 29, and December 27, 1917. Ferenczi himself is still referring to the joint work on Lamarck as late at May 18, 1918.

43. In "Overview of the Transference Neuroses," for example, Freud writes that "one can justifiably claim that the inherited dispositions [of the human psyche] are residues of the acquisition of our ancestors," in other words a "phylogenetic disposition." "In this sense," Freud concludes, "neurosis is . . . a cultural acquisition" (*Phylogenentic Fantasy*, 10, 19).

44. *Freud's Moses*, 31; my emphases. Yerushalmi had earlier cited Freud's half-question from a 1932 letter in which he pondered "what heritage from this land [Israel] we have taken over into our blood and nerves" (*Letters of Sigmund Freud and Arnold Zweig*, 40).

45. *Freud's Moses*, 10; my emphasis.

46. *Unclaimed Experience: Trauma, Narrative, and History* (Baltimore, MD, 1996), 17; my emphasis. Subsequent page references will be cited in the text.

47. On this point, Ruth Leys is particularly scathing in her observation that Caruth turns what for Freud is a "crime" (*Moses and Monotheism*, 109)—parricide/murder—into an experience of loss, even victimhood. Imagining the "murder of Moses" as "traumatic separation," Caruth argues that "separation from the father figure in the murder is . . . an endlessly incomprehensible violence that is suffered, repeatedly, . . . as the traumatic repetition of the violent separation" (69). As Leys puts it, Caruth imagines the murderers as "victims and survivors of a completely unexpected, unintended, exogenous accident" (*Trauma: A Genealogy* [Chicago, 2000], 279–80). But what Leys misses, partly because Caruth herself is so unclear on this point, is that Caruth does not locate the trauma in the violent act itself. Rather, as we shall explore in more detail, she views the trauma as residing in the experience of chosenness.

48. Caruth later writes that "trauma, as a historical experience of a survival exceeding the grasp of the one who survives, engages a notion of history exceeding individual bounds" (66). We might remind ourselves here that Freud himself admitted that there was something foundationally inaccessible in the essence of Judaism.

49. Although Caruth is here applying her revised understanding of trauma specifically in the context of Jewish history, elsewhere she presents a general theory of trauma in similar terms: trauma, that is, defined by or as a fundamental "inaccessibility," a "resistance to full . . . understanding," inseparable from the "impossibility of knowing that first constituted it," what is experienced as a "temporal delay" because of an "inherent belatedness," the experience of "hav[ing] been *chosen* by it [the trauma], *before* the possibility of mastering it with knowledge" (Introduction to *Trauma: Explorations in Memory*, ed. Cathy Caruth [Baltimore, MD, 1995], 10–11).

50. So Freud describes the impulse behind the murder of Moses: "those who felt themselves kept in tutelage, or *who felt dispossessed*, revolted, and threw off the burden of a religion that had been forced on them" (58; my emphasis).

51. To clarify, although I agree with Caruth's contention that there is always an "inherent belatedness" in the "history of a trauma" (*Trauma*, 11)—indeed, a trauma may necessarily be an experience of belatedness—I distinguish my views from hers here precisely because Caruth yet imagines, as Freud himself does, that

there is an actual experience at the origin that is subsequently, even immediately, forgotten. In "Remembering, Repeating, and Working-Through," Freud writes that "in these processes, it particularly happens that something is 'remembered' which could never have been 'forgotten' because it was never at any time noticed" (XII, 149). Though focused on the psychical process of dissociation rather than that of repression, Caruth similarly refers to the "inherent forgetting" through which a person first experiences a trauma (*Unclaimed Experience*, 17). In other words, a person was literally present for that moment (that scene, incident, encounter), but in being traumatized psychically lost sight of it (set it in a parallel stream of consciousness from which conscious memories could not be retrieved). But in the terms I have argued throughout this study, Freud's phrase "could never have been 'forgotten' because . . . never at any time noticed" could refer to a literal missing of an event that subsequently (re)emerges under new circumstances as an experience of belatedness: the uncanny recollection through a having not been there of what was never experienced in the first place. In revising Freud's efforts to grapple with the traumatic origins he associates with Jewish tradition, my argument is that the trauma resides in the burden of being originated in the act of another ("from outside, from a great stranger" [63]), a burden that becomes the foundational crisis of Jewish consciousness itself. This moment is experienced as traumatic precisely because what is absent at the scene of the origin is one's own choice to exist.

52. In a 1926 letter to the Vienna lodge of the B'nai B'rith, Freud would write: "That you are Jews could only be welcome to me, for I was myself a Jew, and it has always appeared to me not only undignified, but outright foolish to deny it. What tied me to Jewry was . . . not the faith, not even the national pride, for I was always an unbeliever, have been brought up without religion . . . But there remained enough to make the attraction of Judaism and the Jews irresistible, many dark emotional powers all the stronger the less they could be expressed in words, as well as the clear consciousness of an inner identity, the familiarity of the same psychological structure" (*Letters*, 366–67).

53. *Freud's Moses*, 7.

54. *From Oedipus to Moses*, 98, 160, 166.

55. It is instructive that the Oedipal explanation is more an assumption on Robert's part than a conclusion drawn from any detailed analysis. In writing, for example, that his first mention of the Oedipus complex in 1897 marked an idea "toward which [Freud] had long been groping" (92), she suggests that his pairing of incest–parricide offered the definitive psychical foundation for the filial ambivalence he had felt after his father's death a year earlier. In other words, she appears to be arguing that the 1896 dream on the night after Jacob Freud's funeral simply awaited its proper Oedipal interpretation.

56. *From Oedipus to Moses*, 146, 165.

57. Schwartz similarly observes how the very ambivalence Freud locates in the figure of his Egyptian Moses functions both within the broader father-son conflict at the heart of the psychoanalytic project and as a sort of allegory of Freud's act

of filial impiety against the authority of the biblical text itself ("Freud's God," 295, 299–301).

58. We might remind ourselves that Amenhotep IV had changed the name given him through his paternal lineage to become Ikhnaton.

59. It is hard not to recall here Freud's reflection in the *Psychopathology of Everyday Life* on his childhood fantasies regarding Hannibal "of how different things would have been if I had been born the son not of my father" (VI, 219–20). In that reference to Hannibal Freud himself is recollecting an incident in which his father's restrained response to an anti-Semitic taunt had led the young Freud to an awareness not just of the social consequences of Jewish identity generally but also of his own critical feelings towards the "unheroic conduct" of his father (*Interpretation of Dreams*, IV, 197).

60. Just as important, Freud could, when pressed, imagine that valiant streak as still available in the present. For example, when asked by the father of Little Hans if the worsening climate of anti-Semitism might reasonably prompt him to raise his son as a Christian, Freud responded: "If you do not let your son grow up as a Jew, you will deprive him of those sources of energy which cannot be replaced by anything else. He will have to struggle as a Jew, and you ought to develop in him all the energy that he will need for that struggle" (Max Graf, "Reminiscences of Professor Sigmund Freud," *Psychoanalytic Quarterly* 11 [1942]: 473).

61. If as Yerushalmi suggests, Freud saw the Jewish retention of a "pure monotheism" as a "stubborn" clinging "to the Father" in contrast to the Christian uprising marked by its "deifying [of] the Son" (*Freud's Moses*, 50), that stubbornness, while an act of perpetual submission on one level, yet had its compensations. The experience of having been chosen by Moses would be transformed, via the distorted return of the repressed, into "the proud feeling" among the Jews "of being God's chosen people," a status that, in Freud's view, produced a "self-confidence," even a feeling of superiority, that enabled them to survive through their long history of adversity (*Moses and Monotheism*, 147). The collective feeling, passed down through the ages, of thus being in "the secret possession of a precious gift" (chosenness as closeness to God) also explained for Freud why despite that history the people were yet "animated by a special trust in life," a "kind of optimism" that "religious people would call . . . trust in God" (134).

62. Although Freud himself would not have given much attention to the historical realities underlying biblical political theory, it is worth noting in the context of this collective act of choosing Michael Walzer's observations regarding the "covenant of law" made between Moses and the Jewish people at Sinai. This covenant, as opposed to the covenant of flesh made between God and Abraham's descendants (a covenant based more on kinship and ethnic separatism) "is open to anyone prepared *to accept its burden*; hence it isn't entirely implausible to say that there is no chosen people, *only a people who choose*" (*In God's Shadow: Politics in the Hebrew Bible* [New Haven, CT, 2012], 3; my emphases). We might contrast Walzer's position to that of Emmanuel Levinas who argues that "the teaching that

is Tora[h] . . . cannot come to the human person through the effect of a choice: what has to be received in order to make free choice possible cannot have been chosen, except *après-coup* ["after the event," though, significantly, this is also the French term for Freud's concept of "Nachträglichkeit" or deferred action]." For, as Levinas will later conclude, "to hear the voice [of the father-god] is *ipso facto* to accept the obligation with regard to him who speaks" (*Quatre lectures talmudiques* [Paris, 1968]; qtd. in Jean-François Lyotard, "Jewish Oedipus," trans. Susan Hanson, *Genre* 10 [1977], 403–04). To the extent Freud himself would have taken Levinas's position it would have been because the Jewish son could only ever *respond to* the father-god, for the son was not present—was never present—to have spoken first. Working off Levinas's claim that it is the "very egoism of the Self" to "pos[e] as its own origin" ("Humanisme et anarchie" [1968]), Lyotard himself will argue that in Jewish thought "the son's possession of the voice" ("the Father who has spoken") must be recognized as "older than his liberty," for the son's very "liberty [is] the sin, the crime, of the impossible repossession." The Jewish son, then, can claim his liberty—a self-possession that is limited because divided—only in a belated recognition that he is always in some sense possessed in and by the Other/the Father who comes before. In that sense, as Lyotard puts it, that son "knows himself dispossessed of origin" ("Jewish Oedipus," 402–03).

Epilogue

1. In reality, the benches in the Etruscan grave had been made of stone, but in the dream they become "wooden benches" as though to emphasize that the house in the dream symbolizes a coffin. This detail appears to be linked to the "two wooden boards" next to which the Alpine guide sets down the decrepit Freud.

2. This idea seems to be part of what is conveyed in the dream's closing image of the "two children sleeping" who now replace the "two wooden boards" that Freud had thought to use to cross over to the wooden house. As part of the subsequent analysis, Freud writes: "the thought that I should have to leave it to my children to reach the goal of my difficult journey forced its way through to representation at the end of the dream" (V, 478).

3. The two dreams are linked together by the journey-motif, the cab of the "dissection/wooden house" dream now replaced by the carriage of the "train to Marburg" dream. In the latter, the haughty husband-and-wife travelers of the dream-thoughts become a much more agreeable "English brother and sister" whom Freud associates with a visible "row of books" and a pleasant conversation about writers. Freud recalls that in the dream, "referring to a particular work," he said to the pair, in English, " 'It is from . . .', but corrected myself: 'It is by . . .' 'Yes,' the man commented to his sister, 'he said that right' " (IV, 456). Not only does Freud receive confirmation of his views about a published work from a true gentleman (and an English one at that), but the correction ("from" becomes "by") suggests

that the issue at stake is who the writer is rather than from where the writer comes. In other words, the exchange suggests that Freud wants to be recognized as the producer of works that might merit even international approbation.

4. As Freud comments, in transforming a coffin or grave into a house, "the dream-work achieved a masterpiece in its representation of this most unwished-for of all thoughts by a wish-fulfillment." "The replacement," he adds, "transformed the gloomiest of expectations into one that was highly desirable" (V, 454–55). In short, he should not have woken up in a mental fright especially since the dream also contained what should have been a pleasing thought: a father's pride in the success of his children.

5. Against this more radical possibility, we might simply opt for the more obvious one that, to the extent the "dissection/wooden house" dream depicts Freud himself in the guise of a feeble old man, his main concern is that he will not create a sufficient monument to achieve the immortality he longs for, regardless of what this might mean in terms of Jacob Freud. If that is the case, Freud might here be anticipating the portrait he will offer of King Lear in his 1913 "Theme of the Three Caskets." Although there is no direct connection to *King Lear*, in the image of Freud himself the "dissection/wooden house" dream similarly features a feeble man who grapples with the necessity of dying. And as in Shakespeare's revision of the primitive myth, Freud discovers in his own dream's "replacement" of a coffin/grave by the small wooden house the same sort of reversal, a substitution of the "most unwished-for . . . by a wish-fulfillment," a transformation of "the gloomiest of expectations into one that [is] highly desirable" (V, 454–55).

6. It is telling in this context that in *Moses and Monotheism* Freud appears to understand modern Judaism as the result of a cultural evolution that began after the Roman destruction of the Second Temple: "Immediately after the destruction of the Temple in Jerusalem by Titus, Rabbi Jochanan ben Sakkai asked for permission to open at Jabneh the first school for the study of the Torah. From now on, it was the Holy Book, and the study of it, that kept the scattered people together . . . through two thousand years" (147).

7. In his unpublished "Overview of the Transference Neuroses" (1915), Freud writes that "the [son's] triumph over the father must have been planned and fantasized *through countless generations*" (in *A Phylogenetic Fantasy: Overview of the Transference Neuroses*, ed. Ilse Grubitch-Simitis, trans. Axel Hoffer and Peter T. Hoffer [Cambridge, MA, 1987], 20; my emphasis).

8. Freud comments that although "the impressions . . . experienced at an early age and forgot later . . . are called traumata[,] . . . it may be an open question whether the aetiology of the neuroses should in general be regarded as a traumatic one" (*Moses and Monotheism*, 91). Freud presents the case of the primal scene (effectively a summary of the case of the Wolf Man) soon after (98–101), and at that stage explicitly connects the emergence of a traumatic neurosis to the Oedipus complex. It is worth noting in this context that the full development of the complex in the case of the Wolf Man did not occur until "after his father's death" (100). We might consider, then, whether the experience of mourning might

be just as or even more important to the son's traumatic experience as the release of barely contained incestuous feelings for the mother. Freud observes that, minimally, a trauma must be understood as formed through "an unusual reaction to experiences and demands." But precisely what those demands are, even if, as he adds, "the genesis of the neurosis *always* goes back to the very early impressions in childhood" (91; my emphasis), remains an open question.

    9. *Freud's Moses: Judaism Terminable and Interminable* (New Haven, CT, 1991), 2.

Works Cited

Adelman, Janet. *Suffocating Mothers: Fantasies of Maternal Origin in Shakespeare's Plays*. New York: Routledge, 1992.
Agamben, Giorgo. *Remnants of Auschwitz: The Witness and the Archive*. Trans. Daniel Heller-Roazen. New York: Zone Books, 1999.
Alter, Robert. *The Art of Biblical Narrative*. New York: Basic Books, 1981.
Armstrong, Karen. *A History of God: The 4000-Year Old Quest of Judaism, Christianity, and Islam*. New York: Ballantine Books, 1993.
Augustine. *Confessions*. Trans. R. S. Pine-Coffin. Baltimore, MD: Penguin Books, 1961.
———. *On Free Choice of the Will*. Trans. Anna S. Benjamin and L. H. Hackstaff. Indianapolis, IN: Bobbs-Merrill Publishing, 1964.
———. *City of God*. Ed. and trans. R. W. Dyson. Cambridge: Cambridge University Press, 1998.
Bellamy, Elizabeth J. "From Ficino to Freud: Egyptian/Greek/Jew in Cultural History." In *Repossessions: Psychoanalysis and the Phantasms of Early Modern Culture*. Ed. Timothy Murray and Alan K. Smith. Minneapolis, MN: University of Minnesota Press, 1998. 23–46.
Bloom, Harold. *Ruin the Sacred Truths: Poetry and Belief from the Bible to the Present*. Cambridge, MA: Harvard University Press, 1989.
———. "Freud: Frontier Concepts, Jewishness, and Interpretation." In *Trauma: Explorations in Memory*. Ed. Cathy Caruth. Baltimore, MD: Johns Hopkins University Press, 1995. 113–27.
———. *Omens of Millennium: The Gnosis of Angels, Dreams, and Resurrection*. New York: Riverhead Books, 1996.
Blum, Harold. "On the Concept and Consequences of the Primal Scene." *Psychoanalytic Quarterly* 48 (1979): 27–47.
Branagh, Kenneth. *Hamlet: Screenplay, Introduction, and Film Diary*. New York: Norton, 1996.
Bullough, Geoffrey. Ed. *Narrative and Dramatic Sources of Shakespeare*. 8 vols. New York: Columbia University Press, 1957–75.
Cameron, Sharon. "Representing Grief: Emerson's 'Experience.'" *Representations* 15 (1986): 15–41.

Caruth, Cathy. Ed. *Trauma: Explorations in Memory.* Baltimore, MD: Johns Hopkins University Press, 1995.

———. *Unclaimed Experience: Trauma, Narrative, and History.* Baltimore, MD: Johns Hopkins University Press, 1996.

Cavell, Stanley. *Disowning Knowledge in Seven Plays of Shakespeare.* Cambridge: Cambridge University Press, 2003.

———. *This New Yet Unapproachable America: Lectures after Emerson after Wittgenstein.* Albuquerque, NM: Living Batch Press, 1989.

Derrida, Jacques. "The Animal That Therefore I Am (More to Follow)." Trans. David Wills. *Critical Inquiry* 28 (2002): 369–418.

Edelheit, Henry. "Mythopoesis and the Primal Scene." *Psychoanalytic Study of Society* 5 (1972): 212–33.

———. "On the Biology of Language: Darwinian/Lamarckian Homology in Human Inheritance (with some thoughts about the Lamarckism of Freud)." In *Psychoanalysis and Language* (Psychiatry and the Humanities, v. 3). New Haven, CT: Yale University Press, 1978. 45–74.

Eliot, T. S. *Selected Essays.* New York: Harcourt, Brace & World, 1960.

Emerson, Ralph Waldo. *Selections from Ralph Waldo Emerson.* Ed. Stephen E. Whicher. Boston: Houghton Mifflin, 1957.

Empson, William. *Essays on Shakespeare.* Ed. David B. Pirie. Cambridge: Cambridge University Press, 1986.

Engelstein, Stefani. *Anxious Anatomy: The Conception of the Human Form in Literary and Naturalist Discourse.* Albany: State University of New York Press, 2008.

Felman, Shoshana. "To Open a Question." In *Literature and Psychoanalysis: The Question of Reading Otherwise.* Ed. Shoshana Felman. Baltimore, MD: Johns Hopkins University Press, 1982. 5–10.

Filoramo, Giovanni. *A History of Gnosticism.* Trans. Anthony Alcock. Oxford: Basil Blackwell, 1990.

Fiore, Peter A. *Milton and Augustine: Patterns of Augustinian Thought in Paradise Lost.* University Park, PA: Pennsylvania State University Press, 1981.

Frazer, J. G. *The Golden Bough: A Study in Magic and Religion.* 3rd ed. 12 vols. London: Macmillan, 1906–15.

Freud, Sigmund. *Standard Edition of the Complete Psychological Works of Sigmund Freud.* Ed. and trans. James Strachey, et al. 24 vols. London: Hogarth Press, 1953–74.

———. *The Origins of Psycho-Analysis: Letters to Wilhelm Fliess, Drafts and Notes, 1887–1902.* Ed. Marie Bonaparte, Anna Freud, and Ernst Kris. Trans. Eric Mosbacher and James Strachey. New York: Basic Books, 1954.

———. *Moses and Monotheism.* Trans. Katherine Jones. New York: Vintage, 1954.

———. "Theme of the Three Caskets." Trans. C. J. M. Hubback. In *The Collected Papers.* Ed. Joan Riviere, 5 vols. New York: Basic Books, 1959. IV, 244–56.

———. *Letters of Sigmund Freud.* Ed. Ernst L. Freud. Trans. Tania and James Stern. New York: Basic Books, 1960.

———. *Gesammelte Werke*. 18 vols. Ed. Marie Bonaparte, Anna Freud, et al. Frankfurt am Main: S. Fischer, 1968–78.

———. "Overview of the Transference Neuroses." In *A Phylogenetic Fantasy: Overview of the Transference Neuroses*. Ed. Ilse Grubitch-Simitis. Trans. Axel Hoffer and Peter T. Hoffer. Cambridge, MA: Harvard University Press, 1987. 5–20.

Freud, Sigmund, and Arnold Zweig. *The Letters of Sigmund Freud and Arnold Zweig*. Ed. Ernst L. Freud. Trans. Elaine and William Robson-Scott. New York: Harcourt, Brace & World, 1970.

Friedman, Richard Elliot. *Who Wrote the Bible?* New York: HarperOne, 1987.

———. *The Bible with Sources Revealed*. New York: HarperOne, 2003.

Garber, Marjorie. *Shakespeare's Ghost Writers: Literature as Uncanny Causality*. New York: Methuen, 1987.

Goldman, Michael. *Acting and Action in Shakespearean Tragedy*. Princeton, NJ: Princeton University Press, 1985.

Graf, Max. "Reminiscences of Professor Sigmund Freud." *Psychoanalytic Quarterly* 11 (1942): 465–76.

Greenblatt, Stephen. "Psychoanalysis and Renaissance Culture." In *Literary Theory/ Renaissance Texts*. Ed. Patricia Parker and David Quint. Baltimore, MD: Johns Hopkins University Press, 1986. 210–24.

———. *Will in the World: How Shakespeare Became Shakespeare*. New York: Norton, 2004.

———. *Hamlet in Purgatory*. Princeton, NJ: Princeton University Press, 2002.

Guillory, John. *Poetic Authority: Spenser, Milton, and Literary History*. New York: Columbia University Press, 1983.

Hertz, Neil. "Freud and the Sandman." In *Textual Strategies: Perspectives in Post-Structuralist Criticism*. Ed. Josué V. Harari. Ithaca, NY: Cornell University Press, 1979. 296–321.

Hoffmann, E. T. A. "The Sandman." In *The Golden Pot and Other Stories*. Trans. Ritchie Robertson. New York: Oxford University Press, 1992. 85–18.

———. "Der Sandmann." In *Poetische Werke*, 12 vols. Ed. Walter Wallerstein. Berlin: Walter de Gruyter, 1957. III, 3–44.

Jentsch, Ernst. "On the Psychology of the Uncanny" (1906). Trans. Roy Sellars. *Angelaki* 2 (1996): 7–16.

———. "Zur Psychologie des Unheimlichen" (Parts 1–2). *Psychiatrisch-Neurologische Wochenschrift* (1906). 22–23: 195–98, 203–05.

Jonas, Hans. *The Gnostic Religion: The Message of the Alien God and the Beginnings of Christianity*. Boston: Beacon Press, 1963.

Jones, Ernest. *The Life and Work of Sigmund Freud*. 3 vols. New York: Basic Books, 1953–57.

Justin Martyr. *First Apology*. In *Ante-Nicene Fathers*. 10 vols. Ed. Alexander Roberts and James Donaldson. Buffalo, NY: Christian Publishing, 1885–87. I, 163–87.

Kafka, Franz. *Briefe, 1902–1924*. New York: Schocken Books, 1958.
Kearney, Richard. *On Stories*. London: Routledge, 2002.
Kerrigan, William. *The Sacred Complex: On the Psychogenesis of Paradise Lost*. Cambridge, MA: Harvard University Press, 1983.
Klein, Dennis B. *Jewish Origins of the Psychoanalytic Movement*. New York: Praeger, 1981.
Kofman, Sarah. *Freud and Fiction*. Trans. Sarah Wykes. Boston: Northeastern University Press, 1991.
Krüll, Marianne. *Freud and his Father*. Trans. Arnold J. Pomerans. New York: Norton, 1986.
Lacan, Jacques. *The Language of the Self: The Function of Language in Psychoanalysis*. Trans. Anthony Wilden. New York: Delta Books, 1968.
———. "Desire and the Interpretation of Desire in *Hamlet*." Trans. James Hulbert. In *Literature and Psychoanalysis: The Question of Reading Otherwise*. Ed. Shoshana Felman. Baltimore, MD: Johns Hopkins University Press, 1982. 11–52.
———. *The Seminar of Jacques Lacan, Book III: The Psychoses (1955–56)*. Ed. Jacques-Alain Miller. Trans. Russell Grigg. New York: Norton, 1993.
Langer, Lawrence. *Holocaust Testimonies: The Ruins of Memory*. New Haven, CT: Yale University Press, 1991.
Laplanche, Jean. *Life and Death in Psychoanalysis*. Trans. Jeffrey Mehlman. Baltimore, MD: Johns Hopkins University Press, 1976.
———. *Essays on Otherness*. Ed. John Fletcher. New York: Routledge, 1999.
Laplanche, Jean, and Jean-Bertrand Pontalis. *The Language of Psycho-analysis*. Trans. Donald Nicholson-Smith. New York: Norton, 1974.
Layton, Bentley. *The Gnostic Scriptures*. Garden City, NY: Doubleday, 1987.
Lear, Jonathan. *Love and its Place in Nature: A Philosophical Interpretation of Freudian Psychoanalysis*. New York: Farrar, Strauss, & Giroux, 1990.
Leys, Ruth. *Trauma: A Genealogy*. Chicago: University of Chicago Press, 2000.
Lukacher, Ned. *Primal Scenes: Literature, Philosophy, Psychoanalysis*. Ithaca, NY: Cornell University Press, 1986.
Lupton, Julia Reinhard, and Kenneth Reinhard. *After Oedipus: Shakespeare in Psychoanalysis*. Ithaca, NY: Cornell University Press, 1993.
Lyotard, Jean-François. "Jewish Oedipus." Trans. Susan Hanson. *Genre* 10 (1977): 395–411.
McMillin, T. S. *Our Preposterous Use of Literature: Emerson and the Nature of Reading*. Urbana, IL: University of Illinois Press, 2000.
Meltzer, Françoise. "The Uncanny Rendered Canny: Freud's Blind Spot in Reading Hoffmann's 'Sandman.'" In *Introducing Psychoanalytic Theory*. Ed. Sander L. Gilman. New York: Brunner/Mazel, 1982. 218–39.
Milton, John. *Complete Prose Works*. Ed. Don M. Wolfe, et al. 8 vols. New Haven, CT: Yale University Press, 1953–82.
———. *The Riverside Milton*. Ed. Roy Flannagan. Boston: Houghton Mifflin, 1998.

Moyers, Bill, and Betty Sue Flowers. Ed. *Genesis: A Living Conversation*. New York: Doubleday, 1996.
Nägele, Rainer. *Reading after Freud*. New York: Columbia University Press, 1987.
Nietzsche, Friedrich. *The Birth of Tragedy and the Genealogy of Morals*. Trans. Francis Golffing. Garden City, NY: Doubleday Anchor Books, 1956.
———. *Thus Spoke Zarathustra*. Trans. Adrian del Caro. Cambridge: Cambridge University Press, 2006.
Nuttall, A. D. *The Alternative Trinity: Gnostic Heresy in Marlowe, Milton, and Blake*. Oxford: Oxford University Press, 1998.
Obholzer, Karin. *The Wolf-Man: Conversations with Freud's Patient—Sixty Years Later*. Trans. Michael Shaw. New York: Continuum, 1982.
Packer, B. L. *Emerson's Fall*. New York: Continuum, 1982.
Pagels, Elaine. *The Gnostic Gospels*. New York: Random House, 1979.
———. *Adam, Eve, and the Serpent*. New York: Vintage, 1989.
Plant, W. Gunther. *The Torah: A Modern Commentary*. New York: Union of American Hebrew Congregations, 1981.
Poirier, Richard. *The Renewal of Literature: Emersonian Reflections*. New Haven, CT: Yale University Press, 1988.
Rank, Otto. *The Trauma of Birth*. Trans. James E. Lieberman. New York: Robert Brunner, 1952.
Reiss, Timothy J. *The Discourse of Modernism*. Ithaca, NY: Cornell University Press, 1982.
Rice, Emanuel. *Freud and Moses: The Long Journey Home*. Albany: State University of New York Press, 1990.
Ricoeur, Paul. *The Conflict of Interpretations: Essays in Hermeneutics*. Ed. Don Ihde. Evanston, IL: Northwestern University Press, 1974.
Robert, Marthe. *From Oedipus to Moses: Freud's Jewish Identity*. Trans. Ralph Manheim. Garden City, NY: Anchor Books, 1976.
Rosenberg, David. *The Book of J*. New York: Vintage, 1990.
Rossi, Paolo. *The Dark Abyss of Time: The History of the Earth and the History of Nations from Hooke to Vico*. Trans. Lydia G. Cochrane. Chicago: University of Chicago Press, 1984.
Santner, Eric. *On the Psychotheology of Everyday Life: Reflections on Freud and Rosenzweig*. Chicago: University of Chicago Press, 2001.
Saxo Grammaticus. *The History of the Danes, Books I–IX*. Ed. Hilda Ellis Davidson. Trans. Peter Fisher. Cambridge: D. S. Brewer, 1996.
Schnell, Lisa J. "Learning How to Tell." *Literature and Medicine* 23 (2004): 265–79.
Schwartz, Regina M. *Remembering and Repeating: On Milton's Theology and Poetics*. Chicago: University of Chicago Press, 1993.
———. "Freud's God." In *Post-Secular Philosophy: Between Philosophy and Theology*. Ed. Philip Bond. New York: Routledge, 1998. 281–304.
Sellin, Ernst. *Mose und seine Bedeutung für die israelitisch-jüdische Religionsgeschichte*. Leipzig: A. Deichert, 1922.

Shakespeare, William. *The Riverside Shakespeare*, 2nd ed. Ed. G. Blakemore Evans, et al. Boston: Houghton Mifflin, 1996.
———. *The Norton Shakespeare*. Ed. Stephen Greenblatt, et al. New York: Norton. 1997.
———. *Hamlet*. Ed. Ann Thompson and Neil Taylor. London: Arden Shakespeare, 2006.
Shawcross, John. Ed. *Milton: The Critical Heritage*. 2 vols. London: Routledge, 1970–72.
Sulloway, Frank J. *Freud, Biologist of the Mind: Beyond the Psychoanalytic Legend*. New York: Basic Books, 1979.
Tanakh: A New Translation of the Holy Scriptures According to the Traditional Hebrew Text. New York: The Jewish Publication Society, 1985.
Van der Kolk, Bessel, and Onno van der Hart. "The Intrusive Past: The Flexibility of Memory and the Engraving of Trauma." In *Trauma: Explorations in Memory*. Ed. Cathy Caruth. Baltimore, MD: Johns Hopkins University Press, 1995. 158–82.
Walzer, Michael. *In God's Shadow: Politics in the Hebrew Bible*. New Haven, CT: Yale University Press, 2012.
Watson, Robert. *The Rest is Silence: Death as Annihilation in the English Renaissance*. Berkeley, CA: University of California Press, 1994.
Wieseltier, Leon. "Leviticus." In *Congregation: Contemporary Writers Read the Jewish Bible*. Ed. David Rosenberg. New York: Harcourt Brace Jovanovich, 1987. 27–38.
Yerushalmi, Yosef Hayim. *Freud's Moses: Judaism Terminable and Interminable*. New Haven, CT: Yale University Press, 1991.
Young, Kay, and Jeffrey L. Saver. "The Neurology of Narrative." *SubStance* 30 (2001): 72–84.

Permissions

Cover art

René Magritte, "La reproduction interdite" (1937)
Museum Boijmans Van Beuningen, Rotterdam, The Netherlands
© 2016 C. Herscovici/Artists Rights Society (ARS), New York
Photo Credit: Banque d'Images, ADAGP/Art Resource, NY

Text is reprinted from the following sources with permission as noted:

Material in chapter 1

"Coming Too Late: Freud, Belatedness, and Existential Trauma" was originally published in *SubStance* 41.2 (2012): 119–38. © 2012 by the Board of Regents of the University of Wisconsin System. Reproduced courtesy of the University of Wisconsin Press.

Material in chapter 3

"Tardy Sons: Hamlet, Freud, and Filial Ambivalence" was originally published in *Comparative Literature*, vol. 65: pp. 220–41. © 2013, University of Oregon. All rights reserved. Republished by permission of the copyright holder, and the present publisher, Duke University Press. www.dukeupress.edu.

Material in chapter 4

"'After the Event': Freud's Uncanny and the Anxiety of Origins" was originally published in *Psychoanalytic Quarterly* 84 (2015): 975–1006.

Material in chapter 5

"Cringing before the Lord: Milton's Satan, Samuel Johnson, and the Anxiety of Worship" was originally published in *The Sacred and Profane in English Renaissance Literature*, ed. Mary A. Papazian, pp. 321–44. © 2008, University of Delaware Press.

Index

Adelman, Janet, 255*n*1, 263*n*15
afterwardsness, 3, 6–7, 9, 17–18, 26, 33, 39, 48, 143–44, 147, 163, 166, 173, 180, 185, 191, 216, 224–25, 228–29, 240, 245*n*2
Agamben, Giorgio, 25–26, 155, 250*n*1
Alter, Robert, 158–58, 161–62, 165, 274*n*14, 275*n*19
Amenhotep IV (Ikhnaton), 213–14, 217–18, 241, 284*n*35, 288*n*58
anxiety, 40, 52, 57–63, 66–69, 71, 257*n*11, *n*13, *n*14, 257–58*n*15, 258–59*n*17, 259*n*19, 260*n*22
Armstrong, Karen, 157–58, 274*n*13
Aton-religion (Egyptian monotheism), 212, 214, 217–18, 284*n*33, *n*34
(St.) Augustine, 153, 167, 173, 192–93, 273*n*4
 City of God, 170–72, 185, 276*n*2
 Confessions, 277*n*16
 On Free Choice of the Will, 169–70, 172–73, 276*n*1
belatedness, 2, 4–9, 11, 14–19, 26, 28, 33–34, 38–41, 48, 50–52, 54–55, 70, 73–74, 109–10, 113, 116–19, 121, 126–27, 129, 133–36, 143–47, 151, 154–56, 163–66, 172–73, 184–85, 189, 191, 193–95, 201, 212–13, 216, 221–23, 226, 228–30, 240, 242–43, 248*n*20, 251*n*4, 256*n*4, *n*5, 277*n*17, 286*n*47, 287*n*51, 289*n*62
Bellamy Elizabeth, 17, 250*n*36
Bernays, Martha, 279*n*28
Bible
 2 Samuel, 159, 278*n*23
 Deuteronomy, 155, 167, 275*n*18
 Ecclesiasticus, 170, 172
 Exodus, 18, 155, 157, 159–66, 204–06, 209, 213, 218, 274*n*12, *n*16, 275*n*20, 280*n*8, 281*n*11
 Genesis, 18, 147, 152–58, 162, 205, 226, 272*n*22, 273*n*6, 274*n*10, *n*12, 278*n*21, 281*n*11
 Isaiah, 149
 John, 23, 158–59, 166–67, 241–42
 Job, 159
 Leviticus, 159, 162–63, 276*n*24
 Matthew, 99, 196
 Numbers, 218
 Psalms, 159, 176, 188, 278*n*23
 E-narrative, 274*n*15
 J-narrative, 152–57, 209, 273*n*6, 274*n*17, 275*n*20
 P-narrative, 156, 159, 274*n*9, *n*15, 275*n*20

Bloom, Harold, 35, 155, 161, 165, 178, 180, 185–89, 193–94, 265*n*24, 273*n*7, 275*n*19, 276*n*8, *n*10, 277*n*12

Blum, Harold, 246n10
Branagh, Kenneth, 267n38
Brücke, Ernst, 103–05, 108–12, 203–04, 231, 234–35, 237–38

Cameron, Sharon, 246n7
Caruth, Cathy, 28, 34, 37–41, 44–49, 51–52, 143, 221–24, 251n1, 252–53n5, 253n6, n7, n9, n10, 254n12, n13, n16, 265n25, 271n21, 272n26, 286n46, n47, n48, n49, n51, 287n51
castration / castration anxiety, 9, 28, 52, 54–56, 59, 62–64, 66–70, 73, 117–18, 123, 131, 138, 201, 248n21, 251n4, 256n9, 259n19, 260n25
Cavell, Stanley, 94, 101–02, 115, 117, 173, 193, 245n5, 266n29, 267n41, 269n56, 276n6

death drive, 28, 32, 37, 46–48, 65, 72, 137–39, 143, 253n10, 254n13, n16, 271n20, n21
deferred action (see also *Nachträglichkeit*), 10–11, 13–14, 17–18, 34, 37–40, 120, 127, 133–34, 246–47n14, 250n37, 252n4, 253n7, 289n62
Derrida, Jacques, 1, 6–8, 13, 19, 121, 135, 246n8
Descartes, René, 3, 245n3
disavowal, 249n29
dissociation, 34–38, 221, 224–25, 251n2, 252n3, n4, 287n51
Dostoevsky, Fyodor, 152, 273n3

Edelheit, Henry, 246n10, 285n42
Eliot, T. S., 262n12
Emerson, Ralph Waldo, 1, 4–8, 13, 15, 17, 33–34, 48, 50–51, 73, 118, 155, 173, 228, 240, 245n4, 246n9

Empson, William, 263n12
Engelstein, Stefani, 132, 271n11, n14, n15, n16
Enuma Elish, 157
exposure-myth (myth of birth of hero), 209–11, 225, 228–29, 283n20, n21, n23

Felman, Shoshana, 18–20, 250n39, n40
Ferenczi, Sándor, 285n42
fetish, 256n4
filial ambivalence, 16–17, 19, 52, 69, 71, 73–74, 81, 88–89, 98, 101, 104, 106–07, 109, 111–13, 115, 117, 121, 166–67, 172, 180, 194–95, 197, 200–01, 208, 210–11, 218–19, 225–26, 229, 237–39, 241–43, 256n5, 263n15, 264n22, 265n26, 268n41, 270n3, 283n21, 287n55, 287–88n57
Filoramo, Giovanni, 276n9
Fiore, Peter A., 276n3
Fleischl von Marxow, Ernst, 103–04, 106, 108, 268n42
Fliess, Wilhelm, 16–17, 81, 84, 88–89, 103–04, 107–11, 115, 135, 197, 239, 260n26, 264n23, 269n49, n51
Frazer, J. G., 274n13
Freud, Anna, 251n4
Freud, Ernst, 226
Freud, Jacob, 16, 73, 80, 88, 100–01, 103–04, 107, 109, 111, 113, 196–97, 200, 203, 206–08, 212, 226–27, 235–43, 251n4, 268n44, 280n3, 287n55, 290n5
Freud, John, 104–05, 107, 112–13
Freud, Sigmund
"Analysis of a Phobia in a Five-Year-Old Boy," 257n13
Beyond the Pleasure Principle, 18, 28, 32–33, 35, 40, 46–50, 53,

55, 70, 72–73, 86–87, 117, 120, 137–39, 144, 200, 241, 253*n*10, 253–54*n*11, 254*n*12, *n*14, *n*16, 263*n*16, 265*n*25, 271*n*21
Civilization and Its Discontents, 261*n*28
"Contributions to a Questionnaire on Reading," 279*n*28
"Contributions to the Psychology of Love," 70–71, 194, 257*n*13
"Disturbance of Memory on the Acropolis," 236
Ego and the Id, 70, 260*n*20, *n*22
"Fragment of an Analysis of a Case of Hysteria," 58
"From the History of an Infantile Neurosis," 9, 11, 16, 59, 119–20, 137, 200, 246*n*10, *n*11, *n*12, 246–47*n*14, 247*n*15, *n*16, *n*17, *n*18, *n*19, 248*n*21, *n*23, *n*24, *n*25, *n*26, *n*28, 249*n*29, *n*30
Inhibitions, Symptoms and Anxiety, 18, 24, 27–28, 30, 33, 55, 57–64, 68–70, 200, 233, 249*n*29, 256*n*7, 257*n*14, 257–58*n*15, 258*n*16, 258–59*n*17, 259*n*19, 260*n*23, *n*25, 261–62*n*27
Interpretation of Dreams, 16, 41–46, 48, 58, 67, 73, 77, 80, 82–83, 88–89, 100–01, 103–13, 196–97, 200–01, 227, 235, 242, 246*n*10, 249*n*33, 260*n*21, 261–62*n*2, 262*n*6, *n*8, 264*n*23, 265*n*26, 268*n*42, *n*44, *n*45, *n*47, 269*n*49, *n*50, *n*51, 288*n*59
  "burning child" dream, 41–46, 48, 253*n*10
  "non vixit" dream, 103–13, 202–04, 235, 268*n*44, 269*n*50, *n*51
  "train to Marburg" dream, 234, 289–90*n*3
  "dissection/wooden house" dream, 231–38, 289*n*1, *n*2, *n*3, 290*n*4, *n*5

Introductory Lectures, 257*n*13
Moses and Monotheism, 3, 16, 18, 20, 40, 113–14, 152, 197, 199–201, 206–30, 240–43, 253*n*9, *n*10, 275*n*18, 279*n*1, 279–80*n*2, 280*n*3, 281*n*9, *n*10, 282*n*12, *n*16, *n*17, *n*18, 283*n*19, *n*20, *n*23, *n*24, 283–84*n*25, 284*n*26, *n*27, *n*29, *n*30, *n*34, *n*35, 284–85*n*36, 285*n*37, *n*38, *n*39, *n*40, *n*41, 286*n*47, *n*50, 288*n*61, 290*n*6, *n*7
"Moses of Michelangelo," 201–06, 208, 228–29, 280*n*5, *n*6, 280–81*n*8, 281*n*9
"Mourning and Melancholia," 87–91, 98, 111, 115, 200, 264*n*20, *n*21, *n*22, 266*n*28
"Neuro-Psychoses of Defense," 260*n*26
On Dreams, 261*n*28
"On Narcissism," 265*n*24
Outline of Psycho-Analysis, 249*n*29, 285*n*42
"Overview of the Transference Neuroses," 285*n*42, 290*n*7
Project for a Scientific Psychology, 253*n*8
Psychopathology of Everyday Life, 100–01, 267*n*39, 268*n*47, 284*n*32, 288*n*59
"Remembering, Repeating, and Working-Through," 34, 87–88, 90, 111, 200, 263*n*17, *n*18, 264*n*20, 287*n*51
"Theme of the Three Caskets," 28–33, 50, 53–55, 65, 68, 70, 169, 200, 251*n*3, *n*4, *n*5, *n*6, 260*n*22, 290*n*5
Totem and Taboo, 24, 151, 200, 207–08, 212, 216–18, 220, 233, 267*n*35, 267–68*n*41, 268*n*43, 274*n*12, *n*13, 279*n*1, 284*n*26
  Preface to the Hebrew edition, 201, 206–08, 226, 243, 281*n*10

Freud, Sigmund *(continued)*
  Three Essays on the Theory of Sexuality, 257*n*13, 285*n*37
  "The Uncanny," 18, 20, 73, 114, 117, 120, 122–24, 126–28, 131–32, 135, 137–40, 200, 270*n*4, *n*5, *n*6, 273*n*28, *n*29
Freud, Sigmund, and Josef Breuer, 15
Friedman, Richard Elliot, 274*n*15

Garber, Marjorie, 251*n*4, 267*n*36
Gnostic / Gnosticism, 159, 178–80, 182, 185, 187, 193–96, 241–42, 276*n*9, *n*10, 278*n*18, *n*21
Goethe, Johann Wolfgang, 261*n*28
Goldman, Michael, 262*n*12
Graf, Max, 288*n*60
Greenblatt, Stephen, 80–81, 85–86, 91, 94, 96, 101, 114, 116–17, 262*n*7, *n*10, *n*11, 263*n*14, 266*n*32, 267*n*36, *n*37, 269*n*52, *n*57, 270*n*59, *n*61
Grubitch-Simitis, Ilse, 285*n*42
Guillory, John, 192, 277*n*13, 278*n*18

Haggard, H. Rider, 232–33, 235, 237
Heine, Heinrich, 199
Hertz, Neil, 120–21, 130, 137, 270*n*1, *n*2, *n*3, 271*n*12, *n*13
Hoffmann, E. T. A.
  "Die Automate," 132
  "The Sandman," 18–19, 73, 117–18, 121–23, 129–36, 138–39, 142–45, 147–48, 172, 239, 241, 270–71*n*8, 271*n*11, *n*18, 272*n*23, *n*24, 273*n*28, *n*29, *n*30, 279*n*25

isolation, 249*n*29

Janet, Pierre, 253*n*6
Jentsch, Ernst, 73, 117–18, 121–30, 132–33, 137–43, 145, 147, 193, 270*n*4, *n*7, 272*n*23

Jonas, Hans, 276*n*9
Jones, Ernest, 61–62, 257*n*13, 257–58*n*15, 259*n*17, *n*18, 264*n*20
Josephus, 209
Julian of Eclanum, 153, 273*n*4, *n*5
Justin Martyr, 21, 50–51, 255*n*21

Kafka, Franz, 281*n*11
Kearney, Richard, 252*n*3
Kerrigan, William, 8–10, 14, 182, 246*n*13, 247*n*16, 248*n*22, *n*23, 276*n*4, 277*n*12, *n*13
Kierkegaard, Søren, 199
Klein, Dennis B., 280*n*4
Kofman, Sarah, 137, 270*n*3, 271*n*18, *n*20
Krüll, Marianne, 280*n*4

Lacan, Jacques, 15–16, 45–46, 245*n*3, 250*n*35, *n*37, 255*n*1, 256*n*4, 266*n*30, *n*32, 267*n*36
Lamarck, Jean-Baptiste, 220, 285*n*42
Lamarckism, 220, 223, 285*n*41, *n*42
Langer, Lawrence, 253*n*6
Laplanche, Jean, 50, 143–44, 245*n*2, 252*n*4, 253–54*n*11, 255*n*17, *n*19, 264*n*19, 272*n*25, *n*26
Laplanche, Jean, and Jean-Bertrand Pontalis, 9–10, 14, 247*n*19, 250*n*37, 252*n*4, 253*n*7
latency, 34, 40, 50, 221–25
Layton, Bentley, 276*n*9
Lear, Jonathan, 116, 270*n*60
Leslie, Charles, 187, 278*n*19
Levinas, Emmanuel, 288–89*n*62
Leys, Ruth, 286*n*47
Little Hans, 62, 68–69, 288*n*60
Lodge, Thomas, 85, 262*n*12
Lukacher, Ned, 11–14, 248*n*27, *n*28, 249*n*31, 250*n*34
Lupton, Julia Reinhard, and Kenneth Reinhard, 53–54, 68, 114, 255*n*1, *n*2, *n*3, 255–56*n*4, 269*n*53

Index   305

Lyotard, Jean-François, 289*n*62

Magritte, René, 1–4, 10, 15, 245*n*1
McMillin, T. S., 246*n*6
Meltzer, Françoise, 133–34, 136–37, 271*n*17, *n*18, *n*19, *n*20
memory, 15, 60–61, 78–80, 85–87, 90–93, 98, 100–02, 109, 224, 248*n*25, 249*n*29, 252*n*4, 253*n*6, 258–59*n*17, 263*n*18, 263–64*n*19, 265*n*25
   narrative memory, 36, 252*n*3, 265*n*25
   traumatic memory, 36–39, 252*n*3
Meyer, Eduard, 282*n*17
Milton, John
   De Doctrina Christiana, 151, 155, 169, 173, 188, 276–77*n*10, 277*n*14, 278*n*20, *n*22
   Paradise Lost, 18–19, 25, 52, 119, 145–47, 152, 166–67, 169, 171–97, 215, 225, 241, 243, 272*n*22, 276*n*25, 276*n*7, 277*n*11, *n*15, *n*16, *n*17, 278*n*24, 279*n*26, *n*27, *n*28
Mitchell, Stephen, 273*n*2
Moses, 113, 157, 160, 163, 203, 205–06, 208–19, 221, 223–30, 239, 241–42, 276*n*24, 280*n*6, 282*n*17, 283*n*19, 284*n*27, *n*34, 287–88*n*57, 288*n*62
mourning, 73, 80–81, 85–93, 100–02, 107–08, 110–12, 114–17, 246*n*7, *n*9, 254*n*11, 266*n*27, 267–68*n*41, 290–91*n*8
Moyers, Bill, 152

Nachträglichkeit (*see also* deferred action), 9, 17, 37, 39, 54, 120, 245*n*2, 248*n*20, 289*n*62
Nägele, Rainer, 247–48*n*20, 248*n*24, 250*n*38
narcissism, 193

Nietzsche, Friedrich, 11, 27, 57, 65, 67, 193–95, 250*n*2, 279*n*27
Nuttall, A. D., 179–80, 194–95, 277*n*11

Obholzer, Karin, 249*n*29
Oedipus complex, 9–10, 16–17, 19, 28, 32, 54–55, 58–59, 62–64, 68–69, 72, 74, 89, 91, 114–15, 120–21, 200–02, 227, 239–40, 242, 247*n*15, *n*18, 248*n*23, 255*n*3, 257*n*13, 259*n*18, 260*n*25, 263*n*15, 264–65*n*23, 268*n*42, 269*n*54, *n*55, 287*n*55, 290–91*n*7
Oedipus Rex, 17, 264–65*n*23
origins (crisis of), 1, 3–4, 6, 8, 10–18, 26–28, 32–33, 49–51, 53–55, 58, 68, 70, 72, 74, 115–17, 121, 125, 129–30, 133–36, 138–39, 145–47, 159, 166–67, 172, 180, 184–85, 189, 194–97, 208, 212–13, 224–29, 240–43, 282*n*12, 287*n*51, 289*n*62

Packer, B. L., 245*n*5
Pagels, Elaine, 273*n*4, *n*5, 276*n*9
Paneth, Josef, 104, 106, 108–09, 112, 203–04
Plant, W. Gunther, 274*n*16
Plutarch, 262*n*3
Poirier, Richard, 245*n*5
primal scene
   as existential problem, 1, 9–16, 19, 26, 28, 33, 50, 70, 73, 136, 144–47, 173, 195, 240, 249*n*31, 250*n*34
   Freudian concept, 7–8, 10–14, 16–17, 59, 119, 134–35, 137, 240, 246*n*10, 246–47*n*14, 247*n*17, *n*18, *n*19, 247–48*n*20, 248*n*23, *n*25, *n*26, *n*28, 249*n*29, *n*32, 249–50*n*33, 250*n*38, 271*n*18, *n*19, 290*n*8

Rank, Otto
  Myth of the Birth of the Hero, 229, 283n20, n22
  Trauma of Birth, 18, 28, 52, 55–69, 72–73, 256n6, n8, 256–57n11, 257n12, n13, 257–58n15, 258n17, 259n18, 260n22, n24
reaction-formation, 30, 33
Reiss, Timothy J., 269n58
repetition compulsion, 36–40, 49, 57, 65, 86–87, 90, 93, 120, 144, 240, 252–53n5, 253n7, 263n18, 263–64n19, 270n3, 272n27, 286n47
repression, 34–37, 58–59, 66, 69, 86–89, 93, 98, 118, 123, 126, 128, 201, 219, 221, 224, 240, 249n29, 251–52n2, 263n18, 263–64n19, 270n6, 279–80n2, 285n36, n37, n38, 287n51
  return of the repressed, 118, 120, 123, 126, 128, 219–20, 222, 240, 279–80n2, 285n36, n38, 288n61
repudiation, 249n29
Rice, Emmanuel, 280n4
Ricoeur, Paul, 75, 245n3, 250n37, 255n18, 255n3, 269n55, 272–73n27, 281–82n11
Robert, Marthe, 104, 106, 227, 268n42, n44, 269n48, 280n3, n4, 287n54, n55, n56
Rosenberg, David, 157, 274n11
Rossi, Paolo, 282n15

Santer, Eric, 51–52, 255n20, n22
Sartre, Jean-Paul, 21, 27–28, 52, 72, 167
Saxo Grammaticus, 84–85, 95, 262n9
Schelling, Friedrich, 271n9
Schiller, Friedrich 234, 268n46
Schnell, Lisa J., 263n16
Schopenhauer, Arthur, 24, 233

Schwartz, Regina, 276n4, n5, 277n13, 282n12, 287–88n57
Sellin, Ernst, 210, 212, 225, 282n17
Shakespeare, William
  2 Henry IV, 105, 108–09, 265n26
  2 Henry VI, 53, 262n3
  As You Like It, 149
  Coriolanus, 231
  Hamlet, 18–19, 52, 73, 77–81, 84–87, 91–102, 107, 109, 113–18, 136, 193, 196, 202–04, 232, 235, 238–39, 241–43, 262n6, n8, 264–65n23, 265–66n27, 266n28, n31, n33, 267n35
  King Lear, 23, 28–30, 32–33, 255n2, 290n5
  Julius Caesar, 78, 80, 105–07, 261n1, 262n4, n5
  Merchant of Venice, 28–29, 251n3
  Richard III, 80
sibling rivalry (in *Paradise Lost*), 176, 195
Smith, Adam, 234
splitting of the ego, 249n29
Sulloway, Frank, 285n42

temporality, 2–3, 5–6, 14, 39–40, 51–52, 53, 143, 163, 250n34, n37, 253n6, 265n25, 272n27, 275n22
trauma, 8, 10, 14–16, 18, 33–41, 45–52, 54–58, 61–62, 65–67, 70, 73, 87, 100, 117, 138, 143, 172, 185, 195, 217, 221–25, 240–41, 252n3, n4, n5, 253n10, 253–54n11, 254n16, 256n7, n9, 257n14, 261–62n27, 265n25, 271n21, 276n5, 286n47, n48, n49, 287n51, 290–91n7

uncanny (as existential problem), 15, 73, 117–18, 121–30, 132–33, 135–47, 172, 180, 185, 193,

226, 228, 240–42, 270n3, 271n9, 287n51

Van der Kolk, Bessel, and Onno van der Hart, 35–37, 251n1, 251–52n2, 252n3, n4, 253n6, n7, 265n25

Walzer, Michael, 288n62
Watson, Robert, 85, 94–96, 101, 262n11, 266n29, 267n34, n40
Wieseltier, Leon, 162–66, 187, 275n21, n22, n23, 275–76n24, 278n21
wish-fulfillment, 42–45

Wolf Man, 11, 16, 59, 63, 68–69, 119, 137, 246n10, n11, n14, 247n15, n17, n18, n19, 248n24, n26, n28, 249n29, n30, 290n8
working-through, 87, 91, 263–64n19

Yerushalmi, Yosef Hayim, 216–17, 220–21, 223–24, 227, 242, 280n4, 284n31, 286n44, n45, 287n53, 288n61, 291n9
Young, Kay, and Jeffrey L. Saver, 252n3
Young, Robyn Darling, 152

Zweig, Arnold, 215

www.ingramcontent.com/pod-product-compliance
Ingram Content Group UK Ltd.
Pitfield, Milton Keynes, MK11 3LW, UK
UKHW041924140426
5217IPUK00014B/308